The Integrated Behavioral Health Continuum

Theory and Practice

The Integrated Behavioral Health Continuum

Theory and Practice

Edited by

Laurel J. Kiser, Ph.D., M.B.A.
Paul M. Lefkovitz, Ph.D.
Lawrence L. Kennedy, M.D.

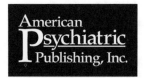

Washington, DC
London, England

Copyright © 2001 American Psychiatric Publishing, Inc.
ALL RIGHTS RESERVED

Manufactured in the United States of America on acid-free paper
04 03 02 01   4 3 2 1
First Edition

American Psychiatric Publishing, Inc.
1400 K Street, N.W.
Washington, DC 20005
www.appi.org

Library of Congress Cataloging-in-Publication Data
The integrated behavioral health continuum : theory and practice / edited by Laurel J. Kiser, Paul M. Lefkovitz, Lawrence L. Kennedy.
    p. ; cm.
  Includes bibliographical references and index.
  ISBN 0-88048-945-6 (alk. paper)
    1. Mental health services. 2. Continuum of care. I. Kiser, Laurel J., 1955- II. Lefkovitz, Paul M. III. Kennedy, Lawrence L., 1925-
  [DNLM: 1. Mental Health Services--organization & administration. 2. Continuity of Patient Care--organization & administration. 3. Delivery of Health Care, Integrated--organization & administration. WM 30I59507 2001]
  RA790. .I525 2001
  362.2--dc21

                                                             2001022958

British Library Cataloguing in Publication Data
A CIP record is available from the British Library.

Contents

Contributors

Melissa E. Abraham, M.S.
Research Fellow, Mental Health Services and Policy Program, Institute of Health Services Research and Policy Studies, Northwestern University, Chicago, Illinois

Joan Betzold, M.Ed., A.B.Q.A.U.R.P., A.B.R.M.
President, Professional Services Consultants, Inc., Bel Air, Maryland

Allen S. Daniels, Ed.D.
Professor, Department of Clinical Psychiatry, University of Cincinnati College of Medicine; and Chief Executive Officer, Alliance Behavioral Care, Cincinnati, Ohio

Susan L. Ettner, Ph.D.
Associate Professor, Department of Medicine, Division of General Internal Medicine and Health Services Research, University of California–Los Angeles, Los Angeles, California

Joanne Forbes, R.N., M.S.
Director of Program Development, South Beach Psychiatric Center, Staten Island, New York

Trevor Hadley, Ph.D.
Professor, Department of Psychiatry, Center for Mental Health Policy and Services Research, University of Pennsylvania, Philadelphia, Pennsylvania

Eunice Hartman, R.N., M.S., C.S., C.N.A.A.
President and Chief Executive Officer, Hartman and Associates, Inc., Boston, Massachusetts

Michael A. Hoge, Ph.D.
Associate Professor of Psychology (in Psychiatry) and Director, Managed Behavioral Health Care, Yale University School of Medicine, New Haven, Connecticut

Edna Kamis-Gould, Ph.D.
Clinical Associate Professor, Department of Psychiatry, Center for Mental Health Policy and Services Research, University of Pennsylvania, Philadelphia, Pennsylvania

Lawrence L. Kennedy, M.D.
Former Director, Partial Hospitalization Services, Menninger Memorial Hospital, Topeka; private practice, Topeka; and Training and Supervising Analyst, Greater Kansas City Psychoanalytic Institute, Leewood, Kansas

Laurel J. Kiser, Ph.D., M.B.A.
Associate Professor of Psychiatry, Center for Mental Health Services Research, University of Maryland School of Medicine, Baltimore, Maryland

Edward L. Knight, Ph.D.
Consultant, ValueOptions, Colorado Springs, Colorado

Paul M. Lefkovitz, Ph.D.
Executive Director, St. Vincent Stress Centers, St. Vincent Hospital; and Clinical Associate Professor of Psychology (Psychiatry), Indiana University School of Medicine, Indianapolis, Indiana

John S. Lyons, Ph.D.
Director, Mental Health Services and Policy Program, Institute of Health Services Research and Policy Studies, Northwestern University, Chicago, Illinois

Margaret Moran, R.N., M.H.S.A.
Principal, Moran and Associates, Wilmington, Massachusetts

David E. Ness, M.D.
Medical Director, Psychiatry Service, Mercy Hospital of Pittsburgh, Pittsburgh, Pennsylvania

Ike Powell
Director of Training, Mental Health Empowerment Project, Albany, New York

Andres J. Pumariega, M.D.
Professor and Director, Child and Adolescent Psychiatry, James H. Quillen College of Medicine, East Tennessee State University, Johnson City, Tennessee

David F. Raney, M.D.
GCS Group, Inc., Pittsburgh, Pennsylvania

Mark S. Salzer, Ph.D.
Assistant Professor, Department of Psychiatry, Center for Mental Health Policy and Services Research, University of Pennsylvania, Philadelphia, Pennsylvania

Karl W. Stukenberg, Ph.D.
Assistant Professor, Xavier University, Cincinnati, Ohio

Mark Tidgewell, C.P.A.
President, Tidgewell Associates, Columbia, Maryland

Anthony M. Trachta, M.S.W.
Principal, Atrium Management Team Consultants, Boston, Massachusetts

Preface

The years surrounding the start of the new millennium may very well be thought of as the era of the health care continuum. Attention to the importance and role of the continuum of care abounds in journals, conferences, and private dialogues. The health care industry has embraced the continuum as a vehicle for enhanced quality, efficiency of operation, and responsiveness to community and industry needs.

In the same way the richness of impressionistic art grew out of the overly restrictive and defined art forms that preceded it, contemporary views of the continuum of care provide a palette of possibilities that explodes with creative energy, placing new definitions on the boundaries of health care delivery. In behavioral health, the continuum renders obsolete its dichotomous heritage of inpatient and outpatient care, a system that, for years, failed to mirror the range and complexity of human experience and clinical needs.

A continuum, by its very nature, is infinite; between every two points on a continuum a third can be found. Levels of care, such as inpatient services, partial hospitalization, and outpatient treatment, define the conventionally accepted points on the continuum. These levels of care constitute the structure of a continuum. Yet structural elements can essentially stand alone without relating to one another in any meaningful way. In fact, that is an apt description of many behavioral health service providers.

It is also possible to call forth various processes to establish meaningful linkage among these discrete structural elements. Those processes are collectively known as *service delivery integration*. The result of service delivery integration is an organized system of care that is rooted in a common vision and defined by processes intended to promote continuity of care, coordination of efforts, efficiencies of operation, and seamless patient movement through a range of services.

The integrative processes described herein serve to bind the structural elements of the continuum together into an orderly, collective whole. These forces can make powerful contributions to quality, patient satisfaction, staff morale, and cost effectiveness. When service delivery is properly integrated, the whole truly becomes greater than the sum of its parts.

This book differs from those that address the development of integrated delivery systems. Those works tend to concentrate on the macrostructure of alignments between hospitals, physicians, and other entities that are drawn together to achieve certain financial or strategic objectives. Although those issues will not be ignored, this volume will be more operationally focused.

The health care marketplace will increasingly require the kind of operational efficiencies, coordinated efforts, and heightened quality that can be brought about through a carefully engineered strategy of integration. These strategies will be particularly valuable to those who not only deliver direct services but also manage the integrated financing and delivery of quality care. The pervasive and powerful market pressures toward collaboration, vertical integration, alliances, and other forms of partnership in health care delivery make the content of this book relevant. The concepts described herein are as applicable to multiorganizational alliances as they are to single entities.

This book can be used by those wishing to harness operational forces in establishing an effective integrated behavioral health continuum. It can serve as an introduction to the conceptualization and operationalization of integrated service delivery. It can also be used by those already familiar with system-oriented thinking who seek input in specific content areas. Whether the need is strategic or "nuts-and-bolts" in nature, this volume may be used to derive perspectives and information related to service delivery integration.

In summary, the delivery of behavioral health care is at a crucial juncture where impediments to efficiency and quality must be addressed carefully. Coordination must be maximized and focused around the varied and changing needs of those served. The integrated behavioral health continuum offers one vehicle for achieving these vital objectives. It is hoped this volume represents a modest contribution to that cause.

Laurel J. Kiser, Ph.D., M.B.A.
Paul M. Lefkovitz, Ph.D.
Lawrence L. Kennedy, M.D.

1

Toward Integration

Laurel J. Kiser, Ph.D., M.B.A.

Evolution will be what we want it to be. If we can envision it, we can achieve it.

Jonas Salk

Those who survived the 1990s will define the future of behavioral health care. Health care reform is placing tremendous pressure on mental health and substance abuse professionals and providers to alter their practice styles. Both the pace of change and the amount of change required are extensive. Many clinicians, clinical administrators, and others are responding to this pressure, not because they are convinced that all the changes will result in better quality of care for their patients, but because they are afraid that if they do not make modifications their practice or program will not survive.

We begin this book on integrated behavioral health service delivery by exploring this revolution or reform process. We start by addressing the critical questions: What is driving the change? Where are we going? What are we going to become?

WHAT IS DRIVING THE CHANGE?

As in all other areas of health care, change in the delivery of behavioral health care is driven by a combination of factors (Devers et al. 1994; Tonges 1998).

Economic Pressures and Models

Health care costs rose by 16.8% yearly from 1988 through 1991 and by 11%–12% yearly from 1992 to 1994 (Crane 1995; Hay Study Group 1998). Sky-

1

rocketing costs provided the impetus for multiple cost-containment strategies that slowed this growth to only 0.7% yearly from 1994 through 1997 (Hay Study Group 1998) and to less than 0.5% during 1998.

Behavioral health care will feel and has already felt the brunt of these cost-containment efforts (Hay Study Group 1998; McDaniel et al. 1995). Two cost trends highlight this statement:

- In the 1990s the benefit costs of behavioral health care decreased 670% more than the costs of general health care.
- Over that same period, behavioral health fell from 6.2% to 3.1% of the total health care benefit.

Given the rapidly changing economic landscape in behavioral health care understanding, cost-containment strategies and their related effects on the delivery of mental health and substance abuse treatment are critical. Two cost-containment strategies appear particularly consequential: managed care and prospective payment systems. Both strategies, as illustrated in the next sections, support movement toward the development of integrated delivery systems.

Managed Care

Employers and other purchasers of health care view managed care as a powerful mechanism to slow or control health care costs and as such either mandate that employees participate in managed care plans or offer them incentives to do so. The rapid growth of managed care has placed enormous pressures for change on medical and behavioral health providers (Middlebrook 1996). How does managed care achieve cost savings? The managed care industry uses three basic tools: 1) change in the use of expensive services, 2) change in access to services, and 3) change in the flow of dollars through the system.

First, managed care has significantly affected our medical care delivery system by severely restricting the use of hospital-based care. This restriction is creating fundamental change in medical care by shifting care delivery from a hospital-driven to a managed care–driven system. Behavioral health care has seen the most dramatic decreases in inpatient use: Mutual of Omaha reported drops of as much as 68.8% between 1991 and 1996 (Hay Study Group 1998). The threat to hospital systems created by this downward trend in use is causing many to form partnerships and alliances with other care providers (Oss and Moghul 1997; Schreter 1998; Teisberg et al. 1994; Tonges 1998). Additionally, development and systematic use of an integrated continuum of services allow patients to receive adequate intensity of treatment without inappropriate dependence on hospital-based care.

Second, the use of "gatekeepers" to control access to specialty care is another cost-containment strategy used extensively by managed care. Through use of gatekeeper models, managed care has affected relationships among physician specialists and thus altered traditional referral mechanisms (Pincus et al. 1998). For behavioral health care, the gatekeepers are often primary care physicians who make the initial referral for behavioral health care services. Often managed care builds in incentives that reward these primary care physicians for limiting their use of specialty services. The introduction of strict precertification and utilization review criteria is another gatekeeping mechanism used by managed care. In many instances, these external evaluations create significant barriers to access to and use of mental health and substance abuse services (see Chapter 5).

Managed care also affects access to care and use of services through contract negotiations. Patients enrolled with managed care organizations are typically referred for treatment based on contractual relationships rather than established referral relationships (Schreter 1998). Managed care companies show a clear preference toward negotiating a single contract with a network of providers (Moskowitz 1997). This preference is clearly linked to administrative efficiency and the ability to leverage discounts for volume guarantees. Thus, to remain viable in highly penetrated managed care markets, providers must be competitive in terms of ease and efficiency of access, variety of services offered, and ability to serve large numbers of clients (Manderscheid 1996).

Third, managed care has changed the flow of money through the system. Traditionally, providers have contracted directly with purchasers of health care. Managed care essentially becomes a middleman—an intermediary between the purchaser and the provider of care. Not only does it control the flow of dollars to providers, it also retains a percentage of the money (for administration, operations, profit) that previously went to providers. The provider community, with fewer dollars available for the provision of care, must choose either to provide fewer services or to devise more cost-efficient service delivery mechanisms. Through centralization and standardization of administrative and clinical processes, integrated service delivery models attempt to do more with less.

Shared Risk

Shared risk is another method for pressuring systems to control or reduce medical costs and prepayment systems with shared risk change care delivery models. Fiscal incentives that drive care delivery are inherent in all payment systems. Under traditional fee-for-service payment models, the needs of individual patients are prioritized, whereas under prospective payment systems, the needs of populations are elevated in priority (Bennett 1996). Thus, under traditional fee-for-service payment models, overuse is an inherent potential, whereas prospective reimbursement systems such as global case rates and cap-itation models create fiscal incentives that support underuse or rapid move-ment of patients from more expensive, intensive levels of care to least expensive levels of care. Bennett (1996) framed this incentive as the need for "parsimony in planning a course of treatment. The main reason for this par-simony is the need to keep something in reserve for the next patient who has not yet arrived. Parsimony, which may be understood as a form of rationing, places responsibility on the therapist to allocate justly and as needed rather than arbitrarily" (p. 967). (See Chapters 12 and 13.)

This focus on population-based care has multiple effects. Effective and effi-cient processes that support parsimony in treatment planning and delivery without jeopardizing quality or outcome develop in response to the pressure to contain costs (Moskowitz 1997; Shortell et al. 1994). These processes tend to minimize the importance of the one-to-one relationship between therapist and patient, creating more collaboration and teamwork. They also tend to balance the role of prevention, recovery, and rehabilitation with the curative aspects of care. Thus, an integrated service delivery approach is well suited for population-based payment systems.

Policy

With the death of sweeping national health reform came an explosion of health care changes driven by federal beneficiaries and state and local politics. Most current policy initiatives stem from concerns about the costs of health care (Clark 1996) and move consumers from fee-for-service plans to managed care arrangements. Although these reforms help control costs, they fall short of reaching the broader goals envisioned by leaders of the national reform, including universal coverage and portable insurance that would guarantee long-term, uninterrupted coverage to all.

Although the success of managed care in regard to cost containment is unquestionable, the side effects of its cost-cutting strategies are becoming more evident and creating additional policy initiatives. Consumer and pro-vider advocacy initiatives are attempting to balance quality of care with bottom-line fiscal administration.

Consumer Rights Movement

Consumerism is partly responsible for the changes taking place in the health care industry. Patients are demanding to be treated with a new respect as con-sumers of a costly service. Their slogan, "Not about us without us," sums up this sentiment. Consumers are demanding increasing levels of partnership with their health care providers, including access to information necessary for educated decision making.

Consumerism has also increased pressure on the health care delivery system to become more user friendly. Ease of access, convenience (both geographic and time of day/week), choice of provider, and so on are competitive issues in the current marketplace. Guarantees are being demanded, including access to providers of choice, to emergency care, and to new and innovative technologies such as advanced therapies and pharmaceuticals (Coile 1998).

Interest in patient satisfaction with services is another outgrowth of consumerism. Customer satisfaction is one of the major areas of monitoring on health care report cards, and providers and facilities are being graded on how satisfied their customers are with the care they receive. Preliminary evaluations of integrated systems of care suggest increased consumer satisfaction is a major benefit (see Chapter 14).

Application of Business Principles

As for-profit medicine and cost cutting were introduced to our health care system, managers and management strategies from business and industry greatly influenced the delivery of care. Health care in the United States has undergone an industrialization or corporatization (Cummings 1995; McDaniel et al. 1995; Tonges 1998). We took our science and superimposed business principles on it. In the process of industrialization, we moved from an independent practitioner model with caring professionals to an industry focused on standardization and efficiency. Consolidation, downsizing or rightsizing, quality improvement, and customer-oriented care are outgrowths of this movement.

According to McDaniel et al. (1995), "The current corporate revolution is transforming health care from a cottage industry of small group practices to a big business dominated by highly competitive regional and national corporations" (p. 283). One result of this process has been consolidation. Mergers and acquisitions within the behavioral health care industry have occurred at an astonishing rate and with amazing variety in the types of organizations joining forces. Consolidation within the industry has involved horizontal, vertical, and backward integration, creating a dramatically changed behavioral health care landscape (Oss and Moghul 1997). The blurring of distinctions between private and public mental health systems of care is one of the major effects of consolidation, creating multiple opportunities and challenges for collaboration and integration of services.

Along with consolidation comes a necessary restructuring of management and business practices. A primary objective in many consolidations is increased operational efficiencies and economies of scale. Thus, behavioral health care has been introduced to the concept of downsizing or rightsizing.

> Despite the serious dangers of institutional "downsizing" as a means to increase short-term profitability and its potentially negative effects on employee morale and patient care, the restructuring and reorganizing of human service delivery within hospitals may powerfully change the organizational culture by prominently emphasizing the importance of building interdependencies and accountability among various types of professionals. (Francoeur et al. 1997, p. 8)

Two other aspects of health care have been significantly affected by the adoption of business principles. Introduction of total quality management principles borrowed from manufacturing has changed the way we both implement and study new care delivery processes. Customer-centered approaches to service provision also affect current practice patterns and styles (McDaniel et al. 1995; Tonges 1998).

Advances in Science and Technology

Advances in science and technology have substantially altered the delivery of behavioral health care during the 1980s and 1990s. Specifically, advances in pharmacotherapy and information technology made important contributions to improving the outcomes of behavioral health care.

Advances in the pharmacotherapy of serious mental illness as well as of the mild to moderate range of disorders continue at a rapid pace. Improvements in many classes of psychotropic medications, including increased drug specificity and decreased side effects, reduce the need to place patients in restrictive treatment settings when initiating and titrating medications. Increased effectiveness of medications for controlling psychotic and mood disturbances means that fewer patients experience acute crises that require the intensity of hospitalization, and those who do can be stabilized more quickly, thus reducing lengths of stay (Clark 1996). Additionally, the antidepressant drug class termed *selective serotonin reuptake inhibitors* has had a major impact on prescribing practices of both behavioral and general medical practitioners (Pincus et al. 1998).

Computer and electronic technologies have revolutionized the information services industry. The explosion in technology results in greater access to information, in availability of enormous amounts of information, and in rapid changes in substantive knowledge. In addition to demands for effective management of all of this information, advances in electronic communications have facilitated quick, even real-time, exchanges of information. As in many other industries, advances in the information services industry affect the delivery of behavioral health care (Franklin and Schwab 1995).

The effects of this information explosion on behavioral health care involve the ability to collect and analyze large patient data sets that improve our knowledge of the disease process, of the burden of mental health and sub-stance abuse, and of treatment approaches that effect positive change. The ability to capture and manipulate large amounts of data increases our ability to track population-based indices of disease and to understand prevalence, risk, and treatment effectiveness at the population level versus the individual level. Integrated care takes advantage of this expanded capacity. Additionally, advanced electronic technologies stimulate interest in the concept of tele-health, with mental health ranking toward the top in its use (Stamm 1998). Diverse applications range from real-time transfer of clinical patient data for remote consultation to on-line testing and monitoring to technology-mediated face-to-face contact (Brown 1998; Stamm 1998). Telehealth has important implications for access to services and information, especially in rural settings.

Ethical Issues

Fraud and abuse of the health care system have been estimated to account for up to 25% of the costs associated with Medicaid (Crane 1995). This statistic alone points to a major problem in the delivery of health care. During the 1980s the behavioral health care industry was plagued by overuse of expensive services, particularly inpatient care. Investigations into the practices used by some to fill inpatient beds led to complaints of arbitrary links between treat-ment received and treatment needed, at best, and to unethical and illegal behavior on the part of providers, at worst (Bennett 1996; Weithorn 1988). These allegations and practice violations led to cries for change in the system. During the 1990s, under managed care, delivery of behavioral health care ser-vices was characterized by sharp restrictions in use of services, raising con-cerns of underuse.

Without strong empirical evidence of treatment effectiveness, such wide variations in the use of services raise concerns about provider ethics. Ethical issues in the practice of behavioral health care create demands for accountabil-ity. Consumers, employers, payors, and other stakeholders are demanding increased accountability for services provided. They are looking for overall improvements in the health and well-being of the population. They are look-ing for value in terms of positive outcomes for dollars spent (General Accounting Office 1994). They are looking for treatments based on scientific data of effectiveness. Reliance on decision-assistance tools, medical necessity criteria, treatment protocols, and best practice standards to provide more objective guidelines for when and how mental health treatments are adminis-tered is a response to the need for accountability (see Chapters 6, 7, 8, and 15 for more information).

WHERE ARE WE GOING?

Evolution of Health Care

> Chaos. In nature it is the cauldron of creativity. Few metaphors so aptly describe health care....Stable structures, predictable programs, the most solid organizations—all are caught in the throes of unprecedented turbulence, "rightsizing," reconfiguration, and redesign.
>
> **Carlson 1996, p. 10**

In response to the pressures described earlier, the delivery of health care in the United States is changing rapidly. Table 1–1 presents an overview of this changing industry. The three foci outlined in the table—individual program, episode of care, and management of health—represent conceptualizations of the way health care services were or will be delivered. Movement from one focus to the next occurs through a series of paradigm shifts that alter the way we view health care and thus deliver services.

INDIVIDUAL PROGRAM FOCUS

Historically, delivery of health care focused on the program level. Limited responsibility and accountability, heavy competition, hospital dominance, and high cost characterized delivery of care. This focus of health care is most noted for fragmentation. "Our healthcare system is organized around treatment of different body parts" (McDaniel et al. 1995, p. 285). The biggest split in our health care system has been between the body and the mind, giving rise to the fragmentation between treatment of physical illnesses and mental illnesses. Lack of parity in benefits, continued stigmatization of mental illness, and the existence of freestanding psychiatric hospitals result from this way of thinking.

Within behavioral health care, fragmentation is a way of life. It translates into a dichotomous system of care. Patients with mental illnesses are typically treated either in a hospital-based inpatient service or in a clinic or office setting using traditional outpatient models. Some intermediate treatment modalities, such as partial hospitalization and intensive outpatient programs, have been defined and standardized in response to this dichotomy. As intermediate levels of care and the treatment modalities that fall within them become more mature and familiar, use of a service continuum to treat an episode of illness becomes more acceptable (Kiser et al. 1999). (See Chapter 8.)

However, despite growth in a continuum of services, the design of mental health insurance benefits defines fragmentation for behavioral health care.

TABLE 1–1. Evolution of behavioral health care

	Individual program focus	Episode of care focus	Management of health focus
Focus	Defining, developing, and standardizing programs and modalities of care	Developing processes of care and practice guidelines	Understanding prevention and managing population health
Goals	Program-specific treatment goals	Episode of care goals developed at initial assessment	Long-term goals for managing health and illness Management of illness averts need for emergency care
Responsibility	Provider responsible for care only during admission to program	Provider responsible for care only during current episode	Provider responsible for care over entire course of illness or lifetime
Service function	Specific program of care with notion of "aftercare"	Use of continuum until "no further intervention is necessary"	Prevention and wellness
System	Independent providers Freestanding programs	Integrated behavioral health systems Carve-outs	Holistic health care delivery networks with connections to workplace, community, and social services
Cost	Escalating costs with lack of coordination	Cost efficiency Economies of scale	Medical and social cost offset
Resources	Benefit dollars support inpatient and outpatient	Percentage of medical dollars allocated for behavioral health care	Management of health care resources, both expenditures and costs
Accountability	Program evaluation	Outcomes measurement Provider profiles	System performance scorecard Outcomes management

Source. Data from Shortell et al. 1996 and Seelig and Pecora 1995.

For the most part, mental health benefit plans specify limits for inpatient and outpatient care. Typically, there is little or no coordination of these benefits. Often, there is little flexibility in benefits for treatments that fall outside the inpatient or outpatient description but provide essential care for a patient during the course of an illness.

Flowing from this fragmented model of service delivery, treatment of an illness is broken down into discrete segments based on the specific program used. Fragmentation results in duplication of services, such as the separate, often extensive, assessments repeated each time a patient moves from one program to another. Fragmentation results in poor coordination of services, such as limited discharge planning between an inpatient admission and outpatient treatment, even within the same facility (Tonges 1998). This lack of coordination between intensive, restrictive treatment settings and return to the community is the point at which treatment fails (Francoeur et al. 1997).

EPISODE OF CARE FOCUS

Within this evolutionary schema, the episode of care focus represents a midpoint, requiring a shift to more holistic approaches for providing care. The episode of care focus maintains the split between the mind and the body while concentrating on putting the behavioral health care industry house in order. The paradigm shifts necessary to achieve an episode of care focus require resolution of the fragmentation faced during the individual program focus.

This is a period of innovation and rapid change, characterized by intense pressure to form or join large provider networks and to change traditional practice patterns. Focused on providing care for an episode of illness across a variety of treatment modalities, these newly formed networks are working to provide comprehensive service systems and improve the coordination of care across the system.

Promulgation of disease management is a manifestation of the shifting emphasis. Disease management focuses on understanding and altering the natural course of diseases. Disease management programs empower consumers to learn how to control an illness and to minimize the effects of an illness on their lifestyles. These programs encourage providers to assume responsibility for multiple stages of illness care from prevention through cure (see Chapter 7).

Within the episode of care focus, the pressure to maintain separate service delivery and funding streams for physical health care and behavioral health care continues. Thus we see the popularity of carve-outs and behavioral health organizations (managed care organizations that deal only with behavioral health care) and the ongoing debate over cost offset.

MANAGEMENT OF HEALTH FOCUS

The long-term goal—the pot of gold at the end of the rainbow—is a focus on management of health. This focus requires the greatest shifts in thinking along with significant changes in financing and structuring of health care delivery. Movement to the management of health focus necessitates mending the split between the mind and body and providing holistic health and wellness services. In this era, wellness providers will have a "shared perspective of seeing patients as biological entities, psychological beings, and social systems participants" (Strozier and Walsh 1998, p. 27).

A major shift required for a management of health focus moves the system from caring for individuals to caring for populations. Population-based care is not a new concept; the Community Mental Health Act of 1963 provided a good example of this model. Community mental health centers were given responsibility for publicly funded mental health care provided to consumers within specific geographic boundaries (see Chapter 5).

A focus on illness and disease has dominated health care, so along with the shift to a population focus, a shift from managing disease to improving health is required. As opposed to the emphasis on illness and problems, strength and wellness are stressed. "The concern here is that the majority of health care resources are being spent in treating illnesses once they occur. Many argue that significant savings could be achieved by increased emphasis on preventive measures such as routine physical examinations, immunizations, prenatal care, and so forth" (Crane 1995, p. 117).

Finally, the health care industry, including behavioral health care, must shift to a focus on managing resources for population health. This is a multifaceted endeavor that requires achieving a balance between support of wellness and prevention initiatives with curative processes. To achieve this balance, learning systems will become increasingly competent at matching treatment with patient needs using the most efficient means possible, thus freeing dollars for prevention and education.

However, the art, science, and technology of health care have not reached that point yet. Structural elements and policy issues hamper movement toward a management of health focus. Several examples illustrate the difficulties. First, the major funding streams for health, behavioral health, and social services are still separate and not easily coordinated, creating problems in designing and paying for holistic health care programs. Second, employment and thus insurance contracts are still short term (usually 1 year). This short-term focus raises fiscal uncertainties for payors about who will benefit from health care strategies designed to improve general health and to prevent illnesses. Therefore, prevention and wellness initiatives, a conceptual mainstay of this period, are theoretically attractive but difficult to fund.

WHAT WILL WE BECOME?

In direct response to the pressures outlined in this chapter, health care delivery is changing rapidly. Because of the scope and complexity of the changes needed, reengineering of the delivery system is taking place (Bologna et al. 1998). "Most health care executives are no longer in denial. They know that radical reform—integration of healthcare's fragmented delivery and financing systems—is necessary" (Ummel 1997, p. 73). Thus, health care providers and organizations preparing for the future are creating new delivery systems in response to the demands for *one-stop shopping* (i.e., full continuum of services, single contracting agency, wide geographic access); *low cost* (i.e., shared infrastructure—low administrative overhead—and efficient care guided by protocols), and *risk assumption* (i.e., capitation, aligned incentives, cash flow).

Creating Systems of Care

In this section I examine the various ways organizations are proceeding with restructuring. Specifically, I will try to separate 1) delivery systems created through consolidations, 2) those created to address funding models such as capitation, 3) those created as provider networks, and 4) those created based on a model of clinical service delivery. The first three probably achieve structural integration through organizational alignment, whereas the goal of the fourth is functional integration requiring "a much more fundamental change in clinical practices and processes throughout the organization" (Dixon 1998, p. 38).

Consolidation

Consolidation, as mentioned earlier, is occurring rapidly in behavioral health care. In many instances, consolidation results in the necessary joining of several organizations that offer multiple, discrete, and often competing services. The newly consolidated organization then announces that it provides a full array of integrated services. Decisions about the service system offered under the newly formed organization are often made during the contractual phase of the consolidation or early in the operationalization phase. Such decisions often are based on business plans and financial data without much thought to clinical process issues such as theoretical or philosophical compatibility, barriers to patient movement within the system, and competitive or overlapping admission and discharge criteria.

Financial Models

Some organizations develop clinical delivery systems designed to address the incentives inherent in different financial models. For example, organizations accepting at-risk arrangements under capitation agreements quickly develop service systems that use the least expensive services for the fewest number of days or visits possible. Meeting the challenges of capitation requires increasing levels of efficiency from a system of care, with rapid movement of patients to less intensive levels of care or out of the system of care. Thus behavioral health care provider organizations considering accepting at-risk arrangements often implement or contract for new services, such as intensive outpatient programs or case management, to achieve these objectives. They put together a continuum of services and/or structure mechanisms to manage service use without necessarily tying all the pieces together into a coherent service system.

Provider Networks

Many systems of care are created today by managed care companies. Network managers must "contract with an array of resources to support the needs of an identified patient population" (Sederer and Bennett 1997, p. 33). These systems of care involve a variety of independent providers agreeing to participate in a contracted network. Current accreditation standards stipulate various ways in which coordination of care is to be facilitated by network providers and by the managed care company. However, these networks experience difficulty achieving functional integration.

Model-Driven

Another model for the reengineering of behavioral health care stems from clinical models of system integration. In such systems care delivery is based on a definition of integrated service delivery and a set of principles of care that drive development and operationalization of processes of care at every level—structural and clinical.

This book presents one such model of integrated service delivery based on the following definition and principles of care:

Definition of *Integrated Service Delivery*

An organization or network of organizations that provides or arranges to provide a coordinated service system based on a continuum of care to a defined population and is willing to be held clinically and fiscally accountable for the outcomes and the health status of the population served (Shortell et al. 1994).

Principles of Care

- Integrated delivery systems are designed with a longitudinal focus on disease management and health promotion at both the individual and the community level.
- Access to care at all levels of intensity is maximized through efficiencies of clinical process and effective management of resources.

- An emphasis on creating healthy environments permeates all levels of service delivery and treatment domains.
- Partnerships are cultivated between organizations, including payors, to support development of effective systems of care.
- Clinical decision making about the course of care resides primarily and fundamentally within the partnership between the client and the clinician.
- A wide variety of services at various levels of intensity, including behavioral health and other support services, operate in a coordinated fashion.
- Care delivery is integrated within community settings, such as primary care clinics, work, or school, to ensure consistency and continuity and to cause the least disruption in the client's daily routine.
- Multidisciplinary teams, sharing a coherent treatment philosophy and speaking and understanding a common language, plan and implement an individualized set of treatment recommendations.

Building on this definition and the principles of care, the authors of this book present a coherent strategy for service system reengineering. In the initial chapters we offer a conceptual foundation for service delivery integration and the barriers that impede its fulfillment. In these chapters we also provide the structural foundation for building integrated systems of care, allowing the reader to experience different models for developing the basic infrastructures necessary to support integrated systems.

In Chapters 5 through 9 we take the reader through the clinical processes and mechanisms fundamental to caring for patients within a seamless continuum of services. We go beyond a review of the levels of care, detailing the decisions, processes, and practices necessary to match patient care needs smoothly and efficiently with available services. Of particular importance are the chapters that analyze and discuss the changes inherent in therapeutic and milieu processes as a patient moves from one level of care to another. This group of chapters mixes theory and technique to provide the reader with a comprehensive understanding of quality patient care within an integrated delivery system.

In Chapters 10 through 13 we provide an overview of the administrative and management structures central to the delivery of behavioral health care within an integrated system. Specific chapters are dedicated to the critical components of staffing, documentation, and financial matters. Behavioral health care solutions and challenges are highlighted.

In the last four chapters we provide an overview of our current understanding of integrated service delivery based on research and quality of care efforts, and we explore how integrated behavioral health delivery systems relate to various other systems, spotlighting the individual consumer and other segments such as social/welfare, criminal justice, and education. In these chapters we provide a vision for how behavioral health care can sensitively address the needs of each individual within the broader medical and sociocultural context. In the epilogue we discuss the future of behavioral health care as it progresses along its evolutionary path.

ORGANIZATIONAL CHANGE

Organizational change is a process that begins with the realization that change is necessary and ends with an evaluation of the final product. Where is your organization in the health care evolution process?

REFERENCES

Bennett MJ: Is psychotherapy ever medically necessary? Psychiatr Serv 47:966–970, 1996

Bologna NC, Barlow DH, Hollon SD, et al: Behavioral health treatment redesign in managed care settings. Clinical Psychology: Science and Practice 5:94–114, 1998

Brown FW: Rural telepsychiatry. Psychiatr Serv 49:963–964, 1998

Carlson LK: Chaos and the emerging order in health care. Surgical Services Management 2:10–13, 1996

Clark, R: Searching for cost-effective mental health care. Harv Rev Psychiatry 4:45–48, 1996

Coile J: Access to the Future. Keynote address at the 1998 annual conference of the Association for Ambulatory Behavioral Health Care, Washington, DC, August, 1998

Crane DR: Health care reform in the United States: implications for training and practice in marriage and family therapy. J Marital Fam Ther 21:115–125, 1995

Cummings N: The next ten years: what can we expect? Inside AABH, Newsletter of the Association for Ambulatory Behavioral Health Care. 19:1–14, 1995

Devers KJ, Shortell SM, Gillies RR, et al: Implementing organized delivery systems: an integration scorecard. Health Care Manage Rev 19:7–20, 1994

Dixon K: The roles of the behavioral health professional in integrated systems. Behav Healthc Tomorrow 7:35–39, 1998

Francoeur RB, Copley CK, Miller PJ: The challenge to meet the mental health and biopsychosocial needs of the poor: expanded roles for hospital social workers in a changing health care environment. Soc Work Health Care 26:1–13, 1997

Franklin C, Schwab AJ: Information clearinghouses and resource centers: an emerging practice trend. Journal of Applied Social Sciences 19:17–24, 1995

General Accounting Office: Health Care Reform: "Report Cards" Are Useful but Significant Issues Need to Be Addressed. Report to the Chairman, Committee on Labor and Human Resources, U.S. Senate. Washington, DC, General Accounting Office, 1994

Hay Study Group: The Hay Study Group on Health Care Plan Design and Cost Trends 1997–98. Washington, DC, National Association of Psychiatric Health Systems, 1998

Kiser LJ, Lefkovitz PM, Kennedy LL, et al: The Continuum of Behavioral Health Care Services. Washington, DC, Association for Ambulatory Behavioral Health Care, 1999

Manderscheid R: Improving the Quality of Managed Care: What Providers Can Do. Keynote address at the annual conference of the Association for Ambulatory Behavioral Health Care. Minneapolis, MN, August, 1996

McDaniel SH, Campbell TL, Seaburn DB: Principles for collaboration between health and mental health providers in primary care. Family Systems Medicine 13:283–298, 1995

Middlebrook MR: Some answers to the big questions in health care. Mod Healthc 26:80, 1996

Moskowitz D: The urge to merge: providers and insurers find creative ways to integrate, in Behavioral Managed Care Sourcebook. New York, Faulkner and Gray, 1997, pp 80–83

Oss ME, Moghul A: The managed behavioral health care industry: overview and future prospects, in Behavioral Managed Care Sourcebook, New York, Faulkner and Gray, 1997, pp 3–29

Pincus HA, Tanielian TL, Marcus SC, et al: Prescribing trends in psychotropic medications: primary care, psychiatry, and other medical specialties. JAMA 279:526–531, 1998

Schreter RK: Reorganizing departments of psychiatry, hospitals, and medical centers for the 21st century. Psychiatr Serv 41:1429–1433, 1998

Sederer LI, Bennett MJ: Managed mental health in the United States: a status report, in Behavioral Managed Care Sourcebook. New York, Faulkner and Gray, 1997, pp 30–39

Seelig WR, Pecora P: The changing world of services to children and families, in Quality Improvement and Evaluation in Child and Family Services: Managing Into the Next Century. Edited by Davis SM, Pecora PJ, Seeling WR, et al. Washington, DC, Child Welfare League of America, 1995

Shortell SM, Gillies RR, Anderson DA: The new world of manage care: creating organized delivery systems. Health Aff 13:46–64, 1994

Stamm BH: Clinical applications of telehealth in mental health care. Professional Psychology: Research and Practice 29:536–542, 1998

Strozier M, Walsh M: Developmental models for integrating medical and mental health care. Families, Systems and Health 16:27–40, 1998

Teisberg EO, Porter ME, Brown GB: Making competition in health care work. Harv Bus Rev July/August:131–141, 1994

Tonges MC: Clinical integration in organized delivery systems: responding to new challenges in health care, in Clinical Integration: Strategies and Practices for Organized Delivery Systems. Edited by Tongues MC. San Francisco, CA, Jossey-Bass, 1998, pp 3–17

Ummel SL: Pursuing the elusive IDN. Health Care Forum Journal May/June:73–76, 1997

Weithorn LA: Mental hospitalization of troublesome youth: an analysis of skyrocketing admission rates. Stanford Law Rev 40:773–838, 1988

2

A Model of Service Delivery Integration

Paul M. Lefkovitz, Ph.D.

As a concept, service delivery integration is paradoxical; it is obvious yet subtle, simple yet complex, attainable yet elusive. In any health care organization the need to coordinate efforts is obvious, yet disorganization is commonplace. Cooperation is a simple courtesy taught in childhood, yet factions within organizations compete with one another. Well-intentioned efforts to address these issues begin with attainable objectives clearly in sight, yet all too often they end in failure.

A clear vision for service delivery integration is essential in resolving these paradoxes. At best, the concept of service delivery integration is moving from infancy into a stage of youthful exuberance. It is a novel but ambiguous idea that brings forth a fresh and idealistic view of the world as a place where cooperation and synergy can be the norm. Exuberance extends the concept into many realms, always with energy and enthusiasm, but often without direction or boundaries.

Such is the current status of integrated service delivery as a scientific construct and as a conceptualized paradigm of care. Several models have been advanced; however, a common language for integration has not yet evolved. Some speak of the "integrated delivery system" (Shortell et al. 1994); others refer to the "coordinated service system" (Evashwick 1996), the "continuum of care" (Kiser et al. 1993), the "organized delivery system" (Shortell et al. 1993), the "Galatea Model" (Hamm 1993), "service lines" (Scott 1996), "product lines" (Bowers 1990), and the "integrated continuum" (Lefkovitz 1995). These terms connote very different concepts on the basis of their focus, scope, and intent. Often, when professionals discuss integrated care, the conflicting underlying constructs impede communication. The resultant Tower of Babel poses an interesting irony, because the very notion of integration is to seek alignment and understanding among individuals.

In this chapter I attempt to offer a more unified vision for integrated service delivery in behavioral health. I also present a conceptual model for consideration, drawing on the excellent work of others in the field. To do so I must turn to the broader health care literature because of the paucity of published material in the behavioral health realm.

A model for integrated service delivery rightly begins with the concept of *integration* itself. Integration is in some ways a mind-set, a way of thinking about things. Integration suggests bringing parts together into a whole. The possibilities inherent in the concept are best reflected in the maxim "the whole is greater than the sum of its parts." This is the *raison d'être* for service delivery integration. When parts are integrated, their respective potentials are amplified, releasing the power of a whole new range of possibilities.

In systems of care, therefore, potency can emanate from the collective strength of the integrated components. Isolation is an attenuating factor, creating vulnerability much like that faced by the straggler in an antelope herd. In a care delivery system components exist in myriad forms, including the functional, programmatic, financial, political, personnel, and physical environment. Integration can involve any or all of these aspects. Any component of organization life, properly integrated with others, enhances the power of the whole.

The current model is therefore based on the relationship between organizational components and what is referred to as *integrative mechanisms* (Conrad and Dowling 1990). Organizational components represent building blocks of activity within health care settings. In and of themselves, they tend to be static and unrelated to one another. For example, access to services is an organizational component inherent in all health care systems. The broad integrative possibilities emerge only when access is viewed as a centralized and coordinated process. Another component is the physical environment. It can be viewed simply as an artifact of bricks and mortar that serves the needs of a particular program. Conversely, its relationship to the community or its functional interaction with varied clinical operations can bring this organizational component to life.

Therefore I offer the following definition of *service delivery integration*: a planned and coordinated approach toward the alignment of key organizational components and processes so as to optimize the collective efficiency and effectiveness of the health care system. This definition addresses the alignment of organizational components and the role that integrative mechanisms can play in harnessing the dynamics among them. As such, this generic definition would appear to apply equally as well to a small agency with limited services as it would to a large multihospital/multiagency collaboration. The principles, dimensions, and components of service delivery integration are ubiquitous, although the settings in which they are applied will differ in scope, magnitude, and complexity.

The current model recognizes two primary organizational domains: functional/administrative and clinical. These are largely drawn from the extensive and seminal work of Stephen Shortell and his colleagues (Shortell et al. 1996).

There are three components within the functional/administrative domain and eight in the clinical domain. These components are reviewed in the sections that follow. Also, the integrating mechanisms that reside within each component are addressed and explored. Table 2–1 presents an overall road map of this conceptualization.

Functional/Administrative Dimensions

The functional/administrative dimensions relate to the organization's infrastructure. They represent the essential building blocks of the system of care, including 1) organizational structure, 2) finance management, and 3) information management.

Organizational Structure

Organizational structure defines the formal relationships and boundaries among an entity's components and provides the basic foundation for service delivery integration. Integrating mechanisms can be called on to affect the structure of the organization, whether the setting is a large multihospital system or a modest single agency.

Organizational alignment is the principal integrative mechanism to facilitate service delivery integration. The degree to which organizational components are aligned with one another determines the potential for this integration. According to Shortell et al. (1993), "A final major barrier to system integration is a lack of alignment or match between various components or dimensions of a system's strategy, particularly in regard to its orientation toward the market versus its administrative or managerial control of the strategy" (p. 460).

The most obvious vehicles for achieving organizational alignment are mergers, partnerships, strategic alliances, and joint ventures among organizations seeking to achieve mutual business, economic, or strategic objectives. However, although the resultant entity may bring about aspects of structural alignment, the arrangement may or may not actually achieve the aim of full organizational alignment. Also, within single organizations, the concept of organizational alignment may not even be recognized as a vehicle for service delivery integration. Organizational alignment is defined by a number of characteristics, as reflected in Table 2–2.

TABLE 2–1. Dimensions of service delivery integration

	Component	Integrating mechanisms
Functional/administrative dimensions	Organizational structure	Organizational alignment (e.g., mergers, partnerships, joint ventures, strategic alliances, physician–hospital organizations)
		Leadership and vision
	Finance management	Financial alignment
		Uniform financial management processes
		Alignment of provider incentives
	Information management	Centralized information management platform and processes
		Full integration of registration, master patient index, billing, finance, reporting and decision-support functions
Clinical dimensions	Continuum of care	Comprehensive range of coordinated, complementary services
	Access	Centralized patient access to all system components 24 hours per day
	Program boundaries	Flexible program boundaries that allow for permeability of resources
	Patient flow	Coordination of care across all service components
		Shared clinical protocols or pathways
		Case management
		Systemwide milieu
	Personnel resources	Uniform policies that emphasize cross-training and flexible deployment
		Redefining the team
	Facility resources	Space design that promotes patient flow, efficiency, and sharing of resources
	Programming resources	Continuum-based programming that extends across levels of care
	Clinical information	Continuous medical record
		Clinical electronic medical record

TABLE 2–2.	Characteristics of organizational alignment
Common vision	Overarching expression of vision that offers strategic direction, establishes priorities and boundaries for the organization's activities, and provides support for service delivery integration
Shared mission and values	Agreed-on expression and understanding of why the organization should exist, the values that make it distinct from others, and how those values shape the work of the organization
Communication channels	Establishment of processes to disseminate information quickly and uniformly throughout all parts of the system
Decision-making structures	Uniform, clear set of processes for the application of authority throughout the system, typically reflected in the organizational table

A common unifying vision is a vital ingredient of organizational alignment. The teleological drivers underlying organizational behavior are very powerful. Lethargy, ambiguity, and stasis will prevail if vision is absent. However, it is not sufficient for a common vision to merely exist; it must emanate from and be supported by the very top. In organizations in which multiple representations of vision exist, fragmentation and conflict are likely. Frequent changes in vision contribute to a lack of commitment and to frustration. Occasionally, vision will be in conflict with established values, which can beget an ambivalent organization. These potential difficulties are summarized in Table 2–3.

Shared mission and values merit careful attention in the creation of systems of care. These dimensions are generally recognized as crucial factors in affiliations between religious and secular entities, for-profit and not-for-profit organizations, and academic and nonacademic institutions. However, in other types of environments, these factors are often overlooked. The need for a shared sense of mission and values is vital in all organizations that seek service delivery integration. Shared purpose provides a link, a commonality among all parts of the system that serves to nurture cohesion, galvanize commitment in the face of hardship, and guide decision making.

Communication flow is also an important component of organizational alignment. In ancient times successful civilizations such as the Roman and the Inca understood the unifying role of communication by building networks of roads throughout their realms. Communication is even more important today, with the growing complexities of information in all its forms. Organizational alignment is facilitated by processes and systems that transfer information efficiently and effectively. An increasingly rich array of technologies assist in this task, including audio and video conferencing, faxes, e-mail, and voice

TABLE 2–3.   Pitfalls of organizational vision

Pitfall		Organizational impacts
Lack of a clear vision	→	Lethargy
		Ambiguity
		Stasis
		Lack of direction
Vision not actively supported by senior leadership	→	Initiatives without follow-through
		Lack of awareness of vision within organization
Multiple representations of vision within organization	→	Fragmentation
		Conflict
		Disharmony
		Competition
Frequent changes in vision	→	Lack of commitment
		Confusion
		Frustration
Clash between vision and values	→	False starts
		Ambivalence

mail. Whatever the means, communication represents a key component of organizational alignment.

Decision-making structures, by definition, must serve the well-being of the overall system. Organizational alignment brings all system components under the purview of a central decision-making structure to achieve that end. That does not mean all decisions are centralized. Decision making should, in fact, be delegated to the most appropriate level within the organization. However, organizational alignment implies that reserved powers of the organization are retained to ensure that conflicting interests among the ranks do not undermine the overall vision. To support service delivery integration, such centralization of authority is necessary. Often integration requires giving up local control over certain processes in the interests of the "greater good." Without centralized decision making, such compromise becomes difficult to achieve. The system's decision-making structure is typically reflected in its organizational table.

Finance Management

All organizations must manage their financial resources in a way that supports their continued viability. How those finances are managed determines the opportunities for integration within the organization. Integrative mechanisms exist in many forms. Uniform financial and accounting processes serve to establish a level playing field among all parts of the system. In multihospital systems, this may be a considerable challenge.

Provider incentives within those systems should also be aligned. For example, in a highly capitated environment, fee-for-service reimbursement to physicians represents an inherent conflict. It is necessary to alter reimbursement formulas to bring the provider's incentives in line with those of the organization. This may be achieved through a subcapitated arrangement or other risk-sharing model.

Similarly, financial alignment calls for mechanisms that minimize competition among components or programs within the system. For example, in the system with which I am affiliated, the program ("cost center") was traditionally the primary unit of financial accountability. Since reorganizing around population-focused service lines (adults, youth, chemical dependency, and geriatric), accountability has been shifted to the service line level. As a result, levels of care (e.g., inpatient, partial hospitalization) no longer compete with one another for patients and the financial resources they bring. Success entails all of them working together effectively to meet the targets they establish as a service line. As a group they can decide that a "loss" in one area is acceptable if they can compensate elsewhere.

Information Management

Managing information has become increasingly complex in today's taxing environment. Technology has not kept pace with the need for information systems that provide a coherent and uniform platform for understanding the organization's operations. "Best of breed" thinking continues to dominate the information management market, leading to the acquisition of multiple systems that are only partially interfaced and fragmented in the overall picture they provide. This challenge is particularly daunting when several organizations, supported by different systems, attempt to establish a composite picture of their combined operations.

The integrative mechanisms for information management would be the presence of a centralized information system and supporting processes. The system should have full integration of relevant functions, including scheduling, registration, precertification management, master patient index, billing, accounts receivable, financial reporting, and decision support.

CLINICAL DIMENSIONS

Clinical dimensions provide the "meat" on the framework of the organization's infrastructure. They define the work carried out and the methods by which it takes place. The clinical dimensions include 1) levels of care, 2) access, 3) program boundaries, 4) patient flow, 5) personnel resources, 6) facility resources, 7) programming resources, and 8) clinical information.

Levels of Care

Central to the notion of an organized system of care is a range of services. Coordinated and complementary levels of care represent a potent integrative mechanism that affects the structure of service delivery. As we move along in our journey from the bifurcated inpatient–outpatient system that has historically dominated behavioral health, the richness and diversity of the continuum of care continues to grow.

It is not uncommon, in many of today's markets, for providers to be expected to provide (or arrange for) at least four levels of care for a given population: inpatient care, partial hospitalization, intensive outpatient programming, and outpatient services. In the most comprehensive systems, a variety of other beneficial levels of care are also offered, such as home-based care, residential facilities, halfway houses, assertive case management, outpatient detoxification, and 23-hour observation.

These therapeutic alternatives help ensure that "patients are treated at the right point in the continuum of care—that point at which the greatest value is added" (Shortell 1994, p. 1). It may be difficult for any one provider, particularly in small communities, to be able to offer a sufficient range of services. In such instances it may be necessary to pursue agreements among providers within the community.

A rich and diverse array of services provide the necessary foundation for highly individualized and tailored care. More in-depth discussions about the avenues for enhancing the continuum of services appear in Chapters 8 and 9.

Access to the System

Access to services is controlled by multiple sources. Third-party payors, employers, regulatory bodies, and providers all influence access. Control points will generally be aligned with the locus of financial responsibility and accountability. In traditional indemnity markets, the employer and third-party payors will exert primary influence. Where providers carry financial risk for a given population, they will generally be the drivers of control over access to services.

Access is a key component of service delivery integration. The primary integrative mechanism is the concept of a centralized "intake" process that provides access to the system 24 hours/day, 7 days/week. This may exist in the form of one-stop shopping, with a centralized number and a specialized, dedicated team. It may also be operationalized as a single set of procedures carried out uniformly at various locations throughout the system.

In an integrated system it is important for initial patient placement to be driven by the patient's presenting problems as opposed to economic or political factors. That will result in the most appropriate use of the available levels of care. This aim may best be achieved by placing the access function outside the treatment continuum. In some systems the access function is tied to one of the teams, for example, inpatient or outpatient. However, it is better to avoid such ties if possible, because placement decisions can be influenced by clinical, political, and financial biases that exist within each level of care. Various models for understanding and operationalizing access are provided in detail in Chapter 5.

Program Boundaries

One of the hallmarks of continuum evolution is the movement away from focusing on boundaries that serve to separate organizational components. Instead, it is more helpful to emphasize mechanisms that can serve to enhance flow and integration among program elements. Although proper boundaries are very important in helping to ensure appropriate matching of patient need with service intensity, they should also be permeable enough to meet a variety of clinical and financial needs.

In an integrated continuum the system is service driven rather than program driven. The needs of patients function as the driver rather than the needs of the program, department, or discipline. Turf-oriented thinking is avoided and is viewed as a dynamic that creates conflict and dissension.

A term that has diagnostic value in suggesting the presence of rigid program boundaries and the presence of turf-oriented thinking is *dumping* (e.g., an inappropriate referral). If impassioned discussions about dumping exist within a system, they indicate the presence of organizational components that are overprotective of their boundaries. In an integrated system the concept of dumping has little meaning because all components proactively work together on behalf of efficient and effective patient care.

Program boundaries also have a great deal of impact on staff identification. In an integrated environment staff members identify primarily with the overall mission of the organization, or perhaps the target patient population, as opposed to their own program, unit, or discipline.

My system provides an example of how program boundaries can change when the continuum becomes integrated. For many years the system was organized around levels of care, as in most other psychiatric hospitals. Also, as in most other hospitals, certain tensions and competition could be observed between the various levels of care. This problem became particularly evident when a new residential program was established for those with chemical dependency. Not long after, the organization was completely redesigned around service lines, including one for chemical dependency services. Leaders of the various levels of care within the chemical dependency continuum then began to meet together as an empowered team to bring about efficient and effective patient movement through the continuum. One could literally see the old and established boundaries dissolving over a period of weeks.

A situation arose that served as testimony to the changes that had taken place. The inpatient detoxification unit wanted to refer a patient to the residential program but found that no beds would be available for 2 or 3 days. This created a bind for the patient, who was ready to leave the hospital; the managed care company, which was pressing for release; and the unit staff, who were feeling the pressure from both sides.

The inpatient manager and residential coordinator collaborated and soon arrived at a plan that offered a possible resolution to the problem. They proposed housing the patient on the inpatient unit until a bed was available in the residential program. The facility would charge the managed care company the agreed-on rate for the residential program. They explored the proposal with the patient, the attending physician, the managed care company, and the Patient Finance Department. All parties were agreeable, and the plan worked to everyone's satisfaction.

This scenario serves to illustrate the vital impact of removing rigid program boundaries. It also celebrates the dedication and creativity of those who worked together on behalf of the patient's best interests. In all likelihood that solution would have been impossible 6 months earlier. Concerns over who the patient "belonged to," who was responsible for solving the problem, who got "credit" for the patient, and the like may have bogged down the discussion. Because of the redesign, it was recognized that the patient "belonged" to both the inpatient manager and the residential coordinator, and their alignment made it possible for a creative solution to emerge.

Patient Flow

In behavioral health settings, many patients are exposed to multiple levels of care. Although levels of intensity certainly exist in other domains of health care, behavioral health has evolved a particularly rich array of programs and services. Yet the behavioral health industry has largely ignored the patient's need for coordinated and seamless movement among those programs and services.

In traditional behavioral health systems, transfers into a program are treated as entirely new episodes of care. Patients feel as though they are starting over, even if they have been extensively treated elsewhere within the same building. Frequently the transfer process is fraught with ambiguity, a sense of disorganization, or even open tension. For a patient population that already feels helpless and out of control, such frustrations adversely affect patient care outcomes.

Seamless patient movement represents an important ideal in any integrated system of care. It is pursued by identifying and removing any "bumps" that might interfere with the patient's journey through the system. Such bumps include any aspect of care that may be experienced by the patient as disruptive, unclear, repetitive, inconvenient, conflictual, or uncomfortable, particularly at juncture points. Ideally, junctures in levels of care should not be noticeable to the patient. The patient should experience the movement among programs as subtle shifts in intensity and focus. Seamlessness translates into a feeling of continuity.

Coordination of care represents a primary integrative mechanism for bringing about seamless patient movement. Unlike many of the concepts of recent origin described in this chapter, coordination of care was established many years ago when it was included as a requirement under the Community Mental Health Centers Act of 1963. *Coordination of care* refers to a centralized set of procedures for treatment planning and implementation that aligns activities across settings, providers, and programs.

There are many models and approaches available for facilitating coordination and continuity of care. Some are based on the establishment of guidelines that unify the activities of various providers along the continuum. Patient care pathways, shared clinical protocols, and Caremaps serve as good examples. Other models, such as integrated treatment team meetings, emphasize the communications and planning process among care providers.

Formalized case management represents another integrative mechanism for aligning patient care processes. *Case management* is "a flexible and dynamic approach to managing the care of individual patients and patient populations. Case management is a continuum and episode-focused strategy to manage both clinical and cost outcomes" (Bower 1998, p. 179). Specialized professionals may carry out case management or those functions may be incorporated into the providers' role. This topic is explored in detail in Chapter 7.

Repetitive activities for patients or staff, such as the completion and signing of forms, should also be avoided. When programs operate independently, many redundant processes emerge. However, integrative thinking produces refinements that result in less work for both patients and staff. For example, many systems are not aware that it is not necessary to create a new medical record every time a patient transfers from one program to another. Assessments, instruments, and forms need only be updated. Appropriate reference to information that appears elsewhere in the record is acceptable, as long as it is noted that the information has been reviewed, is complete, and is accurate. Further discussion about medical records that support seamless patient movement appears in Chapter 11.

Mutual support and respect among the various organizational components also enhance coordination of care and seamless patient movement. In some systems of care, outright conflict among programs can result in devaluation and sabotage. When patients get caught up in "which program is better" or are told to "ignore what the staff in the other program said," the formerly seamless patient movement comes to a jarring halt.

Patient flow is best measured by the subjective experience of the patient. However, most measures of patient satisfaction focus on single programs and fail to address issues relating to ease of movement among organizational components. A strategy to enhance patient flow would incorporate such dimensions into patient satisfaction measures.

Another integrative mechanism for patient care processes is the systemwide milieu. The milieu or context of therapeutic activity is traditionally defined by the particular program the patient occupies. Patients experience a new milieu or culture every time they enter a different program. When an integrative perspective is adopted, attempts are made to provide continuity as the patient moves through the system. Consistency in therapeutic approach is a primary avenue for supporting a systemwide milieu. Placement of core mission and values statements in all program settings is another vehicle for promoting a systemwide milieu. Uniform logos, forms, personnel name badges, and other environmental characteristics can also support a systemwide milieu that pulls elements together harmoniously.

Creating a seamless delivery system is one of the chief aims of integration. The resultant efficiency and clinical continuity can contribute substantially to the overall success of the organization.

Personnel Resources

Within traditional systems, personnel tend to be viewed as the coveted "property" of each particular program or entity. There is little movement of staff among components of the system. Often individuals may be very unfamiliar with other system elements. Personnel policies and compensation practices may be tailored to different programs in different ways.

In such systems staff strongly identify with the program. A common bond unites the team members around their shared vision and attitudes. A high degree of cohesion is likely to exist, and to team members it may feel like it is "us against the world."

These conditions do strengthen individual programs and departments in many ways. However, programs with these characteristics cannot effectively function as an organized system of care. For an organization to succeed, the needs of the individual program cannot consistently take precedence over the broader needs of the system.

In an integrated delivery setting, personnel are viewed as resources of the entire organization, albeit as invaluable resources that must be regarded with respect and consideration. Placement of personnel in particular programs is understood in terms of the best fit for the system and the patients within those programs. Isolation of staff in one part of the system is not generally beneficial for either the employees or the patients. To make program boundaries more permeable, cross-training is provided and mobility is encouraged.

Models for *continuum-based staffing* have been described that attempt to extend personnel beyond traditional program boundaries (Lefkovitz 1995). The model preserves the concept of *core staff* to provide continuity and stability within the program. However, some of the staff may spend 20% or 30% of their time in other levels of care within the continuum. These arrangements can break down barriers among programs, enhance patient flow, and improve staff morale.

The issue of staff identity is a central concept in the integrated setting, as already noted. In an integrated system, the fact that staff tend to identify more with a broader mission that extends beyond their own particular program permits the type of staff movement that is clinically and financially beneficial.

Therefore, the basic integrative mechanism associated with personnel resources is to "redefine the team." The example from my system given earlier in this chapter provides a good example of the power of redefined staff identification. By redefining the team, we can rapidly bring down boundaries and barriers in the service of those treated. Chapter 10 provides a more in-depth look at these issues as well as the implications of integration for various mental health disciplines.

Facility Resources

In traditional systems, "bricks and mortar" often function to divide teams and promote turf-oriented thinking. Like the Berlin Wall, physical boundaries and dedicated space can separate people; they can symbolize barriers to coordination, cooperation, and a shared vision. In an integrated continuum, space is treated much less exclusively. In fact, opportunities are sought to make efficient use of space and contribute to the seamlessness of patient movement. This may involve collocation of programs or contiguous arrangements that permit some overlap of functions.

The issue of collocation of programs has been controversial in behavioral health. This has been especially true with respect to partial hospitalization and inpatient services. The earlier literature (Lefkovitz 1993) cautioned against such collocation as being inherently dangerous for the development of the partial hospitalization program. Dedicated space for this program was strongly advocated. It was felt that the unique identity and culture of the program could not be nurtured in the context of an inpatient setting. In contrast, more recent articles speak to the benefits of collocation (Lefkovitz 1995). Collocation stimulates better communication among the staff of involved programs. Transfer among programs becomes easier for patients because of familiarity with the setting. Finally, the flow of referrals may be enhanced because of the higher visibility of collocated programs to one another. Despite this, the issues that prompted concern in the earlier literature must still be addressed. Each level of care must still maintain certain boundaries that define its respective, unique functions. This need may be dealt with by some combination of dedicated and common space. Instead of duplicating all space for the partial hospitalization program, for example, it may be possible to assign a "home base" located in or contiguous with the inpatient program. Additional group room and activity space can then be shared with the inpatient program. Although, admittedly, this arrangement may somewhat dilute the cohesion within the program, it may serve the patients better in facilitating their journey through the entire system of care.

Programming Resources

Clinical programming flows directly from the philosophical foundation and orientation of a program. The structure and design of clinical programming should reflect the needs of the population served. The menu of activities, as well as the sequencing, pacing, and leadership, should be carefully designed to provide a helpful and targeted therapeutic experience for the patient.

The specificity of the objectives within each level of care has given rise to unique and tailored programs in most settings. Certainly, in traditional systems of care, each program exclusively arranges for its own clinical programming needs, with the possible exception of centralized departments such as activity therapy. This results in highly focused programs that are very specifically suited to the needs of the population served. Such programming also helps to nurture cohesion and program integrity.

At the same time, however, highly tailored programming may introduce barriers to patient movement. Also, scarce and precious organizational resources may be lost through duplication of efforts. Therefore, programming represents another organizational dimension that can be viewed within an integrative context. When the integrative mechanism of continuum-based programming is used, resources traditionally restricted to one program can be opened up to others. In an integrated behavioral health continuum, efforts are made to extend programming resources beyond traditional boundaries where appropriate. Proper integration of programming among levels of care can facilitate ease of flow among programs, help ensure philosophical consistency, and enhance cohesion within the broader continuum.

Preserving the integrity of each level of care is an especially sensitive issue that requires attention when such actions are considered. The same principles applied to facility and personnel resources also apply here. There must be an appropriate balance between the shared and the specific program components. All levels of care require a core program of clinical pursuits targeted to the specific needs of the patient population. Like dedicated space, these components should be reserved for patients in that level of care. However, some other activities may be shared by individuals across a broader segment of the continuum, enhancing both patient flow and efficiency. Table 2–4 provides some guidelines regarding the applicability of various types of groups across the continuum.

Recently the principles of integrated programming have found broader application. At contiguous junctures in the continuum, such as inpatient, partial hospitalization, and intensive outpatient program services, experimentation with this concept is taking place. "Programs within programs" reflect one example of this model. For example, intensive outpatient programs are being developed within the context of partial hospitalization programs, with some elements of shared programming.

Another example of shared programming involves making certain components of one program available to patients in other programs. For example, a menu of partial hospitalization groups, typically nonprocess, psychoeducational, or activity types, can be made available to the outpatient population. These groups can augment the outpatient modality and provide specific targeted therapies. A sufficient combination of groups, along with individual sessions, can represent a "bundled intensive outpatient" experience. Although typically there is concern about the influence of "outsiders" on the milieu of the program, there is usually little actual impact. With proper group selection, such individuals are accepted by the program as "guests" and typically pass through the program without adversely affecting cohesion.

Clinical Information

In health care all pertinent information about the patient is documented in the medical record, which serves as a vital vehicle for communication and coordination among care providers. It also represents an official transcript of the care provided to the patient for purposes of reimbursement, regulatory compliance, and legal protection. It is not uncommon, however, for information about the patient to become separated from the care of the patient. Often information does not follow the patient's movement through the system. In these instances vital information is not available to the care provider. An outpatient therapist may not see the inpatient record, the physician in the residential program may not have access to the partial hospitalization record, and so on.

The flow of clinical information represents the lubricant of integrated service delivery. In an integrated system, there should be a uniform documentation process that allows clinical information to efficiently move with the patient. Flow of clinical information helps facilitate continuity of care, reduce

TABLE 2–4. Continuum-based programming opportunities

Group	Opportunities for integration
Process group psychotherapy	Limited opportunities for integration at the more intensive range of the continuum. Possible opportunities at the middle and lower ranges. The capacity of patients to participate in and benefit from process groups is highly linked to level of functioning. May be possible to blend intensive outpatient program and partial hospitalization process groups but probably not partial hospitalization and inpatient groups.
Psychoeducational groups (theme-specific groups)	Good opportunities for blending across the continuum, but content must be applicable to all within the group. Certain groups may apply across the continuum. The issue of relevancy is key, however, and may restrict applicability to certain parts of the continuum. For example, a group on basic self-care skills may be appropriate for a group of inpatients but not for outpatients. Similarly, a group on assertiveness training may find more applicability in outpatient and partial hospitalization settings than in an acute inpatient unit.
Activity therapies	Range of opportunities from limited to good. Both the content and process of the activity may be restricting factors. For example, basic activity exercises that may be appropriate to inpatient settings may be experienced as demeaning in other settings. Highly interactive and complex activities that are appropriate to less intensive levels of care might be experienced as confusing and threatening to less functional patients.
Family education	Excellent opportunity for integration across the continuum. Although families do benefit from information about each program, they benefit even more from an awareness of the bigger picture. There is much overlap in helpful family education content across levels of care.

duplication of efforts, prevent repeated treatment errors, and build a better understanding of the patient's needs. The primary integrative mechanism supporting the flow of clinical information is the continuous medical record.

This record consists of a set of processes to ensure that clinical information is available when and where it is needed. It typically consists of a low-technology set of procedures that efficiently monitors the location of the chart and supports its rapid movement when needs arise. The logistic challenges of maintaining such a system are great in a geographically diverse system.

The electronic medical record represents a more sophisticated integrative mechanism for achieving continuous flow of clinical information. Such systems make clinical information immediately available to all care providers, within both the behavioral health and the medical domains. However, "many health care providers, including those in behavioral health, are moving slowly into this realm" (Kloss 1997, p. 29). The challenges of an electronic medical record are quite daunting. Costs are relatively high, many health care professionals are leery of computers, functionalities are not well developed, customization must be done, and information systems are fragmented. However, it is just a matter of time before technology effectively addresses those issues. New information platforms, voice recognition software, electronic billing, and diminishing hardware costs will eventually make the barriers disappear. These issues are explored further in Chapter 11.

EVALUATING SERVICE DELIVERY INTEGRATION

Service delivery integration can be an organizational challenge of great complexity. It can be a daunting task to evaluate areas of greatest need to determine where to start. It may also be difficult to discern the progress that has been made. A few instruments have been developed for the purpose of evaluation. Gillies et al. (1993) created a System Integration Scale for use in their landmark Health Systems Integration Study. Findings derived from the study were reported in a subsequent article in which they presented an "integration scorecard" (Devers et al. 1994). However, these instruments were not designed for behavioral health settings and tend to focus exclusively on multihospital/physician integration efforts.

I have developed an evaluative instrument based on the model outlined herein. The instrument, known as the Integrated Continuum Assessment Scale (see chapter appendix), is intended to be applicable either to single organizations or multicomponent behavioral health systems. Although it has been applied to a number of settings, normative information is not yet available. However, the scores provided can be used to highlight needed areas of focus and progress over time.

SUMMARY

A vision for service delivery integration involves an understanding of how static components of organizational life can be transformed into dynamic forces that extend across the entire system of care. Integrative mechanisms can be brought to bear on almost any element of structure or process within the organization. The frontiers of service delivery integration are just being opened up to exploration, and new integrative mechanisms still await discovery.

In this chapter I examine a variety of organizational dimensions and components within this context. The model for service delivery integration they represent provides a vehicle for system redesign that truly allows the whole to be greater than the sum of its parts.

REFERENCES

Bower KA: Clinically integrated delivery systems and case management, in Clinical Integration: Strategies and Practices for Organized Delivery Systems. Edited by Tonges MC. San Francisco, CA, Jossey-Bass, 1998, pp 179–198

Bowers MR: Product-line management in hospitals: an exploratory study of managing change. Hosp Health Serv Adm 35:365–375, 1990

Conrad DA, Dowling WL: Vertical integration in health services: theory and managerial implications. Health Care Manage Rev 15:9–22, 1990

Devers KJ, Shortell SM, Gillies RR, et al: Implementing organized delivery systems: an integration scorecard. Health Care Manage Rev 19:7–20, 1994

Evashwick C: The Continuum of Long Term Care. Albany, NY, Delmar Publishers, 1996

Gillies RR, Shortell SM, Anderson DA, et al: Conceptualizing and measuring integration: findings from the health systems integration study. Hosp Health Serv Adm 38:467–489, 1993

Hamm FB: The Galatea model: addressing individualized treatment. The Counselor March:18–21, 1993

Kiser LJ, Lefkovitz PM, Kennedy LL, et al: The continuum of ambulatory mental health services. Behav Healthc Tomorrow 2:14–16, 1993

Kloss LL: A guide to purchasing software packages. Behavioral Health Management Jan:29–31, 1997

Lefkovitz PM: Planning and implementing a short-term partial hospitalization program. Behav Healthc Tomorrow 2:35–39, 1993

Lefkovitz PM: The continuum of care in a general hospital setting. Gen Hosp Psychiatry 17:260–267, 1995

Scott K: Integrating clinical service lines. Health System Leader 3:4–11, 1996

Shortell SM: Transforming Health Care Delivery: Seamless Continuum of Care. Chicago, IL, American Hospital Association, 1994

Shortell SM, Gillies RR, Anderson DA, et al: Creating organized delivery systems: the barriers and facilitators. Hosp Health Serv Adm 38:447–466, 1993

Shortell SM, Gillies RR, Anderson DA: The new world of managed care: creating organized delivery systems. Health Aff 13:46–64, 1994

Shortell SM, Gillies RR, Anderson DA: Remaking Health Care in America. San Francisco, CA, Jossey-Bass, 1996

Appendix

Integrated continuum assessment scale

Integrated continuum assessment scale

For each item below, indicate the current status within your system by entering a score from 1 to 5 in the column to the left. Three descriptive statements with values of 5, 3, and 1 are provided to assist you in your ratings. Intermediate ratings of 2 and 4 may also be used as appropriate.

Score	Item	Ratings	
	1. Organizational alignment	5	All system components and processes fall under a formal, centralized administrative structure. A systemwide mission statement, vision statement, and strategic plan exist.
		3	Most system components and processes fall under a single centralized administrative structure, or system components are operationally independent but linked by a process for coordinated planning and problem solving.
		1	System components fall under independent administrative structures without a formal process for coordinated planning or problem solving.
	2. Financial alignment	5	Uniform financial management processes exist throughout system. Financial incentives are fully aligned among components. Systemwide financial targets are emphasized. Little competition exists among components.
		3	Uniform financial management processes exist among most functions/components. Financial alignment among programs is present but limited. Competition exists among components. Both system and component financial targets are emphasized.
		1	Financial management processes vary among components. Financial incentives are not aligned. Aggressive competition exists among components. Component financial targets are emphasized.
	3. Management of information	5	Centralized information management processes support full integration of registration, master patient index, billing, finance, reporting, and decision support functions across all system components.
		3	Information management processes are linked in a manner that allows for coordination of some functions. However, information is not integrated uniformly throughout the system.
		1	Independent information, billing, and other systems serve various components of the system. No efforts are made to coordinate information resources with one another or across system components.

Integrated continuum assessment scale *(continued)*

Score	Item	Ratings	
___	4. Access to system	5	Centralized access to all system components is available 24 hours per day, 7 days per week, via a team of neutral, specially trained professionals with no allegiance to any point on the continuum.
		3	Centralized access to all components within the system is available 24 hours per day, 7 days per week via professionals who are organizationally aligned with one or more service delivery points on the continuum.
		1	Access to the system is not centralized. System components establish their own procedures. Access to system components is available on a limited hours basis.
___	5. Levels of care	5	A highly comprehensive array of services is available including at least seven of the following eight levels of care for targeted population(s): Inpatient Residential 23-hour observation Partial hospitalization Intensive outpatient Outpatient Home care Wellness
		3	Multiple levels of care are available including four or five of the above for targeted population(s).
		1	One or two levels of care are available for targeted population(s).
___	6. Program boundaries	5	Program boundaries are flexible. System is service driven and patient focused. Program boundaries are delineated clearly enough to support integrity but permeable enough to meet a variety of clinical and financial needs. Staff identify primarily with clinical mission and secondarily with system component or professional discipline.
		3	Program boundaries are somewhat flexible. Most personnel identify primarily with system component or professional discipline and secondarily with clinical mission. Flexibility with respect to boundaries is seen on occasion.

Integrated continuum assessment scale *(continued)*

Score	Item	Ratings	
___		1	Boundaries around programs and/or professional disciplines are rigidly defined and vigorously defended. Strong identification exists at system component or professional discipline level. Isolation and turf-based rivalries may be seen among system components.
	7. Coordination of care	5	Uniform processes for coordination of care are present throughout the system, for example, case management. Philosophical consistency exists among system components. Clinical consistency is promoted through critical pathways or shared clinical protocols. Uniform quality management processes are in place. The treatment "milieu" extends throughout the entire system.
		3	Uniform processes for coordination of care or clinical consistency exist in some parts of the system, for example, pathways or shared clinical protocols. Philosophical consistency exists among most system components but not all. Case management processes are not clearly defined. Duplication of efforts may be evident in gathering clinical information.
		1	Uniform processes do not exist for coordination of care in any parts of the system. Transfers are treated as new admissions. Clinical information is generally regathered. Patient transitions are frequently accompanied by confusion and disorganization.
___	**8. Personnel resources**	5	Human resources policies and procedures are applied uniformly across system. Many staff are cross-trained and flow freely among system components and levels of care, with appropriate attention paid to integrity, continuity, and stability of system components.
		3	Human resources policies and procedures are applied uniformly across system components and levels of care. Some staff are cross-trained and there is occasional movement across system components and levels of care. Staff mobility is mostly limited to covering for absences in other system components.
		1	Human resources policies and procedures are not applied uniformly across system. Staff are assigned to one area and do not provide services for other programs.
___	**9. Facility resources**	5	Sharing of space across programs and levels of care to enhance efficiency and clinical integration of services is seen throughout system. Appropriate attention is paid to integrity and unique needs of programs.
		3	Most system components operate out of dedicated space. Limited examples of sharing to enhance efficiency and clinical integration are present.
		1	All system components operate out of fully dedicated space.

Integrated continuum assessment scale (*continued*)

Score	Item	Ratings	
___	**10. Programming resources**	5	Programming and therapeutic resources of programs are made available to one another across the system and levels of care. Sharing of such resources is carried out in a manner that facilitates patient movement across the continuum. Process groups are likely to be level of care specific, whereas structured or activity groups may be combined. Attention is paid to integrity, continuity, and stability of distinct levels of care.
		3	Programming and therapeutic services are occasionally extended across levels of care. However, most therapeutic programming is targeted to a specific system component.
		1	All programming and therapeutic services are targeted to specific system components. No programming resources are extended across the continuum.
___	**11. Flow of clinical information**	5	Uniform documentation procedures are present throughout system. Continuous medical record exists, through electronic or other means, allowing full movement of clinical information with patient.
		3	Uniform documentation procedures are present throughout system. Procedures are in place for key selected components of the clinical record (typically copies) to flow with the patient.
		1	Clinical documentation forms and procedures are not standardized within the system. Very limited clinical information follows the patient, typically limited to that shared in telephone contacts.
___	**Total score**	**Scale**	
		45–55	Highly integrated continuum of care
		30–44	Integrated continuum of care
		20–29	Traditional, departmentalized services
		11–19	Segmented, autonomous components

Source. Copyright 1997, 1999 by Paul M. Lefkovitz, Ph.D.

3

Barriers to Service Delivery Integration

Paul M. Lefkovitz, Ph.D.

Despite the natural human tendency to affiliate with others, ubiquitous forces exist that serve as powerful barriers to service delivery integration. These barriers are operative in all organizations. Although a proper vision establishes a road map for effective service delivery integration, it is necessary to be mindful of the detours, potholes, and other hazards that may impede the path.

Shortell (1994) and colleagues (1993) identified a number of barriers that operate within integrated delivery systems. These barriers include failure to understand the new core business of health care, inability to overcome the hospital paradigm, inability to convince the "cash cow" to accept system strategy, inability of board members to understand the new health care environment and their responsibilities, ambiguity of roles and responsibilities throughout the system; inability to "manage" managed care, inability to execute the strategy, and lack of strategic alignment.

In this chapter I explore a related set of barriers believed to exist in all behavioral health settings. Efforts to integrate service delivery at any level will involve confronting these barriers. To bring about effective integration, it is necessary to understand these barriers and to have a strategy for minimizing their impact on the desired objectives.

Two types of barriers are examined: systemic and attitudinal. *Systemic barriers* are operative at the organizational level and relate to inherent challenges or flaws in integrative design or execution. *Attitudinal barriers* flow from individuals and their collective views. In combination, they represent a potentially fatal virus when attempts are made to enhance the health of an organization through service delivery integration.

SYSTEMIC BARRIERS

A number of systemic dimensions are explored in this section, including leadership barriers, component fragmentation, incompatible financial incentives, competitive programs, physician integration, and geography. These dimensions touch a broad spectrum of organizational life and influence dynamics at multiple levels. However, because the personality of an organization tends to reflect its senior leadership, the discussion will begin there.

Leadership Barriers

Successful integration efforts require vigorous, persuasive, and visionary leadership. Because integration, by definition, embraces all aspects of the organization or organizations involved, lack of effective support at the very top can represent a significant barrier. A lack of passion for integration or of commitment to its strategies is one type of leadership barrier. This is most frequently seen in multisystem alliances brought about by "merger fever." If the primary rationale for integration is a reflexive or defensive one with respect to following trends in the local marketplace, the desire for meaningful integration may be missing.

Lack of commitment at the very top may also impede efforts within single organizations pursuing clinical integration. Often, clinical integration is championed by midlevel program directors or the chief clinical officer. They may succeed in obtaining a sincere expression of support from the chief executive, but without the chief executive's dedicated commitment and involvement, it may be impossible to bring about the necessary organizational/financial redesign and alignment to support clinical integration efforts.

Also, on occasion, executive leadership may be committed to integrated service delivery but lack the proper perspective to bring about the necessary paradigm shifts within the organization. The absence of a robust systems-oriented perspective can be a major obstacle to conceptualizing the decision-making structures and lines of communication needed to support integrative efforts.

Finally, the absence of certain leadership skill sets may represent a barrier. A micromanaging leadership style that places the top executive at the "hub of the wheel" for all organizational decisions would interfere with natural integration efforts. In an integrated delivery model, the parts of the system relate directly and efficiently to one another. A leader who impedes such communication and problem-solving processes can inhibit the integrative process.

Component Fragmentation

Component fragmentation refers to a lack of alignment among organizational components, both clinical and nonclinical. The fundamental importance of organizational alignment is discussed in Chapter 2. It is not uncommon, however, for attempts at integration, particularly along clinical lines, to take place in the absence of alignment.

A vivid example of component fragmentation was found in a behavioral health organization that operated within a midsize urban general hospital setting. According to the organizational table, mental health inpatient services reported to one hospital vice president, chemical dependency services reported to a second, and the partial hospitalization program reported to a third. As a result, this hospital lacked a common vision for behavioral health care. Different champions had initiated the various services over the years, resulting in the unusual reporting relationships. Not surprisingly, the behavioral health services were viewed as highly fragmented and uncoordinated. Repeated attempts at meaningful integration of care processes were fraught with conflict and ultimately doomed to failure.

As this example illustrates, component fragmentation is marked by the absence of a common vision for service delivery. Multiple visions contribute to competing strategies within the organization. "Silos" of operation develop to support the various strategies and vie with one another for available resources. Clearly, component fragmentation is one of the most fundamental barriers to integration.

Incompatible Financial Incentives

The importance of financial alignment is also discussed in the previous chapter. Financial incentives consistent with the goal of service delivery integration set the tone for successful operational redesign. They also help ensure enduring motivation to support those ideals on an ongoing basis. Yet financial incentives that are incompatible with the objectives of integration abound in the behavioral health industry.

For example, third-party payment practices have historically supported traditional, nonintegrated delivery models. Inpatient and outpatient care represented the mainstay of insurance benefit design for many years. Coverage for other alternatives was generally lacking. Inadequate coverage has been a potent barrier to the development of continuum-based delivery models. Throughout the 1970s and 1980s the case for equitable coverage for alternatives such as partial hospitalization was often presented in the professional literature (Fink et al. 1978; Goldberg and Goldwater 1977; Guillette et al. 1978).

It was not until the advent of managed care that a more flexible reimbursement posture began to emerge. Coverage for partial hospitalization became more common throughout the 1980s and 1990s, initially through "flexing" of inpatient coverage and more recently through established benefit design and case management. Yet coverage for other modalities, such as residential care, home care, and outpatient detoxification, has continued to remain inconsistent and generally rather restricted.

The spirit of the traditional bifurcated inpatient and outpatient delivery model will continue to prevail until third-party reimbursement practices more genuinely support the use of a comprehensive continuum of care (Lefkovitz and Knight 1999). Although significant progress has been made in recognizing partial hospitalization, financial disincentives continue to impede broader development of the continuum of care. This barrier is likely to remain a factor until current benefit structures are challenged. Rather than forcing patient need to conform to a restrictive list of approved treatments, benefits ideally should be matched to documented patient need in a flexible and individualized manner.

Already some managed care companies embrace a model that allows for a more creative use of the full continuum. Care is approved on the basis of its fit with demonstrated clinical need, even though the resultant plan may reflect a creative combination of therapies that defy categorization in the list of contracted services. Also a number of providers that accept significant financial risk in managed care plans have developed internal case management processes that are more flexible in matching patient need to services provided.

Perhaps voices within the industry can join to advocate for new reimbursement approaches that would reduce financial disincentives to continuum-based service delivery. In the absence of industry-wide reform, the individual provider can reduce the impact of these disincentives through proactive pursuit of participation in risk-based managed care plans. In such plans control over clinical processes shifts to the provider. The judicious use of the full continuum may serve to assist the provider in delivering tailored and, in the long run, highly efficient clinical services.

Incompatible financial incentives also exist in various forms within organizations. For example, in the traditional organization or system, components commonly compete with one another for financial resources. Such competition reinforces the silos of operation and "us/them" thinking. When one part of the system profits at the expense of another part or of the entire system, incompatible financial incentives operate as a barrier to integration. Most commonly this is seen in the form of competition for patients within the system. Competing programs will often vie for patients in support of adequate census and financial performance. Placing the financial needs of the program ahead of the clinical needs of patients compromises the quality of care and the broader viability of the system.

Other incompatible financial incentives can be observed in systems. For example, in environments in which capitation is common, fee-for-service reimbursement to physicians and others may encourage behavior that unnecessarily prolongs care and adds to costs. In such settings it will be helpful to shift financial incentives to reward efficiency and quality rather than quantity.

Because adequate financial support is necessary for an organization's survival, incompatible financial incentives are a key barrier to address. Maintaining a focus on desired clinical and financial objectives within the integrated system could help reduce the effect this barrier has on desired outcomes.

Competitive Programs

Competitive programs within an organization are primarily operative in systems brought together under some form of horizontal collaborative structure. The histories and missions of the various components have typically evolved independently of one another and may overlap. However, competitive programs may also be seen in single organizations in which planning efforts have been decentralized or not well conceptualized. For example, in one psychiatric hospital setting, two different partial hospitalization programs were developed to serve essentially the same population. One operated under the hospital's partial hospitalization division and the other was developed by the inpatient unit as a transitional resource. Competitive markets may also exist in settings without proper market segmentation. Home care programs and partial hospitalization programs are sometimes observed as competing with one another. Both provide an alternative to inpatient care and may serve similar target groups.

Meaningful integration may be impossible as long as internal competition exists. A centralized planning process is necessary to successfully address such issues. For components brought together as part of a merger or other collaborative structure, it may be necessary to address competitive programs through full assimilation of the components. A new organizational structure may need to be established that eliminates any functional or operational barriers among the components, essentially creating a different, larger entity. Schreter (1998) described a helpful process for carrying out such reorganization efforts. His recommended steps included formulating a mission statement and strategic plan as well as creating an organization capable of achieving the goals. He also spoke to the importance of creating a detailed organizational chart, developing a provider network, building administrative capacities, and paying attention to fundamental business practices. Although his intended focus was the individual hospital, the steps he outlined would be applicable to a multihospital/agency setting.

It may also be beneficial to formally scrutinize the markets of the various entities to better understand the nature of any overlap. On close examination it may be discovered that the core businesses are more distinct than was first apparent. If this proves to be so, it may be possible to shrink or refocus the scope of services of each entity around its unique core competencies. A new system would therefore emerge that maintains the original breadth of its collective components but minimizes or eliminates internal competition.

It may also be necessary to bring about appropriate market segmentation to reduce inherent competition. Lack of segmentation can be brought about by an innocent lack of coordination and planning. It can also be the result of having an overzealous program leader who may overstep his or her boundaries. When this occurs, establishing a clear mission for each component along with specific admission criteria will usually help reduce competition.

Physician Integration

Tonges (1998) identified physician integration as one of the three essential components of an organized delivery system. The expansive role that psychiatrists have traditionally played in behavioral health delivery makes it essential that proper integration take place. Models for physician–hospital integration have received frequent attention in the professional literature (Derzon 1988, Shortell 1988). However, as Shortell et al. (1995) pointed out, "the *hospital–* physician relation is the *wrong* unit of analysis. The more relevant unit of analysis is the physician's relation to, and position within, an integrated *system* of care" (p. 145). This observation offers insights into some of the primary barriers to physician integration.

Psychiatrists have traditionally functioned as independent professionals in relating to hospitals. Thinking of oneself as an interdependent player in a *system of care* may be a rather uncomfortable leap for many. Issues of autonomy and control may therefore be barriers to integration. Also, in the past some hospitals and psychiatrists have experienced conflictual relations. Efforts to achieve a new degree of integration may be met with distrust and even enmity.

The models for integration that exist may also represent a barrier. Many are extremely complex and difficult to operationalize. Some involve financial risk on the part of physicians, which may be unacceptable to those involved. Other models fail to provide a meaningful enough role for physicians in governance. Recently it appears that many systems and physicians are viewing direct employment as an appealing vehicle for physician integration.

Another barrier to physician integration relates to recent antitrust legislation. Stark I and II regulations as well as Internal Revenue Service rulings have placed significant restrictions on the types of financial arrangements that can be entered into by physicians and hospitals. Therefore, although financial alignment is one of the key factors in achieving a common vision for integration, regulatory restrictions may serve as a significant barrier. It goes without saying that any efforts to achieve financial alignment between physicians and hospitals must be pursued with the most stringent of attention to legal and ethical standards.

Chapter 10, which deals with staffing an integrated service system, addresses other issues and barriers related to the unique role of the psychiatrist.

Geography

The challenges of establishing and maintaining meaningful operational integration increase as systems of care become more and more geographically dispersed. Geographic dispersion, particularly as it extends to different communities, brings a number of special challenges. Organizational processes must be reasonably uniform to support efficiency and compliance with regulatory bodies that call for one standard of care. Such uniformity requires some degree of centralized planning. Yet community needs must also shape and mold the character of local service delivery. These conflicting forces must be reckoned with to find the proper balance between centralization and decentralization.

It is helpful to consider these challenges from at least three perspectives: organizational structure, policies and procedures, and communications vehicles. The organizational structure of an integrated system that is geographically dispersed must address the need for decision making at the local level. Relying solely on centralized processes will likely cause local community needs, resources, and decision making to be overlooked. Policies and procedures should be established that outline which types of decisions should be made centrally and which should be made locally. Communications vehicles such as electronic medical records, e-mail, faxes, video conferencing, and telepsychiatry can all serve to draw together and integrate geographically scattered components of the system.

ATTITUDINAL BARRIERS

The barriers explored thus far are systemic dimensions inherent in all organizations. In addition to these, a number of barriers flow from attitudinal dynamics among individuals within the organization. These attitudes and beliefs are often unspoken and generally go unrecognized. Hence they can be more insidious than systemic barriers and more resistant to change. Attitudinal barriers explored in the remainder of this chapter include 1) the inpatient unit as the hub of the wheel, 2) turfism, 3) conceptual orthodoxy, and 4) "either/or" thinking.

Inpatient Unit as the Hub of the Wheel

The traditional view of health care places the inpatient unit at the hub of the wheel. Mental health is no exception, particularly in hospital-based systems. This emphasis stems partly from the enormous financial clout that inpatient operations enjoy as a result of their financial contributions to the operations. There is also much historical tradition surrounding this view in health care settings, medical training, and industry dynamics. Shortell et al. (1993) spoke of the "inability to overcome the hospital paradigm" as a barrier to system development and asserted,

> It is time to pay due respect to the past—perhaps even grieve over it—but then to get on with inventing and managing the new delivery systems to meet the needs of the future. It is not simply recognizing that an ever-increasing volume of health care services are being delivered in nonacute settings but rather, recognizing that the hospital may not even be the logical starting place or center of system integration efforts. (pp. 452–453)

The tendency to view the inpatient unit as the hub of the wheel becomes a barrier when system planning is carried out by the inpatient unit. For example, in the 1970s the growth of partial hospitalization was significantly impeded because the potential contributions of the modality were examined from an inpatient perspective. The comparatively modest financial returns associated with partial hospitalization resulted in a lack of administrative support in many settings. Many programs that reached implementation status were based on an inpatient clinical model and organizationally placed under the direction of inpatient leadership. In several instances these factors compromised the uniqueness and effectiveness of the mode.

Efforts have been made to challenge and depart from the inpatient model. The most notable and perhaps radical example is the Day Hospital Inn (Gudeman 1985). That effort, however, simply replaced the inpatient unit as the hub with another level of care, partial hospitalization. Ideally, the hub should not be any particular level of care. At the center of a delivery system should be a uniform process for assessment, triage, and referral so that placement at the proper point on the continuum can readily be achieved. This key issue is addressed in the chapters covering access (Chapter 5) and level of care decisions (Chapter 6).

In an integrated continuum all levels of care are viewed in a dynamic interplay of functionality. A level playing field is established in which all services are regarded as vital to comprehensive care. Strategic and operational decisions are based on the system's overall effectiveness and efficiency without undue influence from any one particular level of care.

This ideal can be pursued in a number of ways. At the broadest level, the organizational structure can be reengineered so that the patient, rather than the hospital or inpatient unit, is placed at the hub of the wheel. One avenue for achieving this is to establish a service line organizational structure (Bowers 1990). Divisions representing target populations such as adults, youths, patients who are severely and persistently mentally ill, patients with a chemical dependency, senior adults, and so on would exist in lieu of traditional divisions organized around level of care, such as inpatient services, partial hospitalization services, and outpatient care. In this manner, services can organizationally be wrapped around the needs of the populations served, with all levels of care working collaboratively toward that end.

It is also possible to move away from the traditional dependence on the inpatient perspective through education and other activities. Strategic planning efforts that project a picture of the delivery system of the future help concretize the movement away from acute services. Providing an equitable forum for dialogue about non-inpatient activities can also be helpful in broadening the base for planning and decision making.

Capitation and other risk-sharing arrangements move the inpatient unit out of the position of cash cow. Although risk sharing through capitation within the industry seems to have fallen out of favor, further movement in that direction would serve to lessen reliance on the inpatient unit for financial subsistence.

Turfism

Turfism is characterized by overdefined and overprotected boundaries among system elements. Silos of operation essentially stand alone in pursuit of their own objectives without significant regard for other system components. Turfism is supported and nurtured by attitudes and values that place the importance or preservation of one's own program, department, or hospital ahead of others within the system. As such, competition is stimulated and threats to the existence of the organizational unit may frequently be perceived. At times open animosity among components exists. When turfism prevails as an attitudinal factor, it is difficult to stay focused on the overall goals of the system. Frequently, control is at the bedrock of all these dynamics.

Turfism is the very antithesis of integration; it is the rationale for isolation. All too often, turfism is defended in the name of patient quality. However, where turfism prevails, objectives are likely to be achieved in one organizational unit at the expense of another unit, the overall system, or the patient's well-being. For example, one partial hospitalization program adopted narrow and restrictive admission criteria that resulted in many patients being denied access to the program. These criteria were said to be necessary to ensure quality of care. From the program's perspective that was undoubtedly true; more restrictive criteria led to a more manageable and responsive patient population. However, the broader organization found that large numbers of patients were "falling into the cracks" without adequate care. It became necessary to address the boundary issues raised by the partial hospitalization program in a way that respected the program's integrity and at the same time better responded to the broader needs of the system and the patients.

A related issue concerns the practice of patient "dumping." As stated earlier in this volume (Chapter 2), accusations of patient dumping signal the likely presence of turfism. Such accusations are associated with heightened sensitivities around program boundaries. In an integrated system, programs work together creatively and collaboratively to find a care plan that best meets the patient's current needs and, in doing so, disputes about dumping are avoided.

Although turfism is an attitudinal factor, interventions can occur at the system level to gradually bring about change. Introducing a service line organizational structure, as mentioned earlier, can be very beneficial in reducing turfism because it emphasizes system thinking. A range of processes can be implemented to support service line thinking, short of a formal organizational overhaul (Charns and Tewksbury 1993). One helpful measure is to reduce competition for financial resources among organizational units. Isolation can be combated by introducing greater staff mobility as described in Chapter 10. Finally, system productivity can be emphasized over program performance by modifying monitoring and accountability processes.

Conceptual Orthodoxy

Conceptual orthodoxy refers to a fixed and often rigid set of beliefs that guide one's work and philosophy of care. Conceptual orthodoxy frequently accompanies turfism and is usually cultivated in an environment of isolation. However, this barrier is unique in that it is generally based on a formal approach or conceptual model. In organizations it is not uncommon for various units to draw their inspiration from different sources. However, where inconsistencies among perspectives exist, continuity may suffer as patients move through various parts of the system.

Subtle inconsistencies between programs may exist in the form of shifts in focus and content that the patient can usually assimilate. Other inconsistencies may be less subtle. For example, to move from a cognitive approach in a partial hospitalization program to a psychodynamic approach in an outpatient setting may be unsettling to a patient. The inconsistency itself is perhaps not as important as the way it is presented to the individual. The change in orientation can be offered in the context of a different form of work that is appropriate to the patient's current needs, with some further detail provided about the objectives of the new approach.

When staff members are driven by conceptual orthodoxy, however, they may adopt a disdainful and destructive approach. There have been reports of patients being told that other members of the staff were not properly trained or were using an "inferior" approach. This type of devaluation certainly undermines the overall course of treatment, particularly if the patient should ever need subsequent care in the "inferior" program. Conceptual orthodoxy can lead to antagonistic relationships between departments and make trust impossible.

A good example of conceptual orthodoxy may be found in the chemical dependency arena. For many years the 28-day program was rather rigidly viewed as the only vehicle for effective care. Attempts to develop alternatives, such as intensive outpatient programs, were met with out-and-out hostility by many veterans of chemical dependency treatment. Even today, now that the 28-day program is a thing of the past, subtle tensions continue to exist between proponents of inpatient care and other forms of rehabilitation.

The best remedy for more flagrant examples of conceptual orthodoxy is to challenge them as examples of disrespect. For more subtle forms, intellectual insulation can be combated through educational efforts. Ensuring staff familiarity with new approaches and technologies helps prevent this type of thinking. Opportunities to engage in sincere dialogue about differing conceptual models can also be beneficial.

In an integrated system there will generally be efforts to bring about some uniformity in clinical approaches while respecting individual styles. Clinical pathways, standards of care, and other models can be adopted to provide balance between tolerance for diverse conceptual approaches and uniform clinical processes throughout the system.

EITHER/OR THINKING

To explain either/or thinking, it is helpful to start with the observation that people seem to have a natural tendency to simplify rather than to expand options. In mental health care, either/or thinking has been dominated by the inpatient–outpatient dichotomy in a black-and-white way for many years. This dichotomy left little room for other treatment alternatives. Yet once partial hospitalization emerged in the 1960s, instead of embracing a "third" option, writers began to ask if partial hospitalization could "replace" inpatient care. Some early writers expressed the hope that partial hospitalization could obviate the need for state hospitals (Glasscote et al. 1969). Most research during this period focused on the degree to which partial hospitalization could serve as an effective "alternative" to inpatient care (Herz et al. 1971; Zwerling and Wilder 1964). Relatively little emphasis was placed on how partial hospitalization could take a meaningful place alongside inpatient and outpatient care in the continuum of services.

A similar process occurred in the 1980s in the public sector, when the community support model captured the imagination of funders and providers. Many harbored the belief that community support or psychosocial rehabilitation models could "replace" partial hospitalization for patients who were seriously mentally ill. Again there was no consideration of how the two modalities could work together to provide a more effective continuum of care. Either/or thinking seemed to prevail in this period, as entire state systems significantly reduced or terminated financial support for partial hospitalization programs in favor of community support and clubhouse models. Partial hospitalization became scarce in the public sector until Medicare recognized the modality and it enjoyed a resurgence of development (unfortunately, recent problems with Medicare reimbursement have reversed that resurgence).

Once again the process of either/or thinking is affecting the modality of partial hospitalization. Writers and observers began asking in the early 1990s whether the newly emerging intensive outpatient programs could "replace" partial hospitalization (Hoge et al. 1992). Indeed, it is now clear that some managed care programs are shifting their support from partial hospitalization to intensive outpatient programs or traditional outpatient treatment (Lefkovitz and Knight 1999). In reality all of these levels of care should be available within a truly comprehensive system of care. As illustrated in Chapter 8, each level of care serves a distinct purpose. Quality of care is compromised and inefficiencies result when there is a gap in the continuum. However, this fundamental aspect of the nature of the continuum can become obscured in the reductionism of either/or thinking.

Although new technologies can occasionally truly replace old ones, more often they better serve to complement one another. In fact, calling one level of care an *alternative* to another is an archaic misnomer and an expression of either/or thinking. It is more accurate to speak of the *right* level of care, rather than an *alternative* level of care. In an integrated system there is full support for the richness of choice and the diverse range of services that can efficiently and effectively address the multiplicity of patient needs.

SUMMARY

The path to effective service delivery integration is blocked by many hazards. In every system of care, barriers give rise to turfism, isolation, and disharmony among its components. However, it is possible to reduce the impact of those barriers. In this chapter a number of dimensions have been explored with that end in mind. Consideration of these powerful factors and the steps that can be taken to reduce their impact should help operationalize the ideals of integrated service delivery.

REFERENCES

Bowers MR: Product line management in hospitals: an exploratory study of managing change. Hosp Health Serv Adm 35:365–375, 1990

Charns MP, Tewksbury LS: Collaborative Management in Health Care. San Francisco, CA, Jossey-Bass, 1993

Derzon RA: The partnership between physicians and hospitals: operations for improvement. Frontiers of Health Services Management 4:4–19, 1988

Fink EB, Longabaugh R, Stout R: The paradoxical underutilization of partial hospitalization. Am J Psychiatry 135:713–716, 1978

Glasscote RM, Kraft AM, Glassman SM, et al: Partial Hospitalization for the Mentally Ill. Washington, DC, Joint Information Service, 1969

Goldberg FD, Goldwater M: Obtaining state legislation for insurance coverage of day hospitalization. Hospital and Community Psychiatry 28:448–450, 1977

Gudeman JE, Dicket B, Hellman S, et al: From inpatient to inn status: a new residential model. Psychiatr Clin North Am 8:461–469, 1985

Guillette W, Crowley B, Savitz SA, et al: Day hospitalization as a cost-effective alternative to inpatient care: a pilot study. Hospital and Community Psychiatry 29:525–527, 1978

Herz MI, Endicott J, Spitzer RL, et al: Day versus inpatient hospitalization: a controlled study. Am J Psychiatry 127:1371–1382, 1971

Hoge MA, Davidson L, Hill W, et al: The promise of partial hospitalization: a reassessment. Hospital and Community Psychiatry 43:345–354, 1992

Lefkovitz PM, Knight M: Is there a middle ground? Behav Healthc Tomorrow 8:7–8, 1999

Schreter RK: Reorganizing departments of psychiatry, hospitals, and medical centers for the 21st century. Psychiatr Serv 49:1429–1433, 1998

Shortell SM: The evolution of hospital systems: unfulfilled promises and self-fulfilling prophesies. Med Care Rev 45:177–214, 1988

Shortell SM: Transforming Health Care Delivery: Seamless Continuum of Care. Chicago, IL, American Hospital Association, 1994

Shortell SM, Gillies RR, Anderson DA, et al: Creating organized delivery system: the barriers and the facilitators. Hosp Health Serv Adm 38:447–466, 1993

Shortell SM, Gillies RR, Devers KJ: Reinventing the American hospital. Milbank Q 73:131–160, 1995

Tonges MC: Clinical integration in organized delivery systems, in Clinical Integration: Strategies and Practices for Organized Delivery Systems. Edited by Tonges MC. San Francisco, CA, Jossey-Bass, 1998, pp 3–17

Zwerling I, Wilder J: An evaluation of the applicability of the day hospital in the treatment of acutely disturbed patients. Isr Ann Psychiatry Relat Discip 2:162–185, 1964

4

Design of Integrated Delivery Systems

Anthony M. Trachta, M.S.W.
David F. Raney, M.D.

The first three chapters build a case for system redesign, present a model for integrating service delivery, and review barriers impeding progress toward improved efficiency and effectiveness. In this chapter we address those aspects of organizational structure, both internal and external, that require consideration in creating integrated delivery systems (IDSs).

REDEFINING THE SYSTEM

Clearly, IDSs can be designed to meet a number of related and simultaneous goals. Often survival is the most visceral goal for providers who organize integrated systems; they hope that size will help protect against external threats. Many also see an opportunity to improve the system of care. To sustain an organization through the redesign process, goals must extend beyond survival to improvements in clinical outcomes, fiscal and operating efficiencies, and alignment between clinical and fiscal incentives.

The current changes in health care provide an opportunity for systems-knowledgeable clinicians to shape care and to define new and more functional models of service delivery. Knowledge of patient care and what would make it better should become a critical focus of the changing system. Clinical goals include better coordination of care across a complete continuum, improved clinical information sharing, and improved quality management.

Obviously, however, system change must incorporate many other factors. It is important to emphasize that viewing the business opportunity as a means to improve clinical care is fundamentally different than viewing IDSs primarily as a business opportunity. Knowledge of regulation, how to work well in the industry as it is currently constituted, and financial issues across various human services is a necessary means to the end of redefining the system. The promise/hope of risk bearing (especially risk bearing that crosses multiple funding streams, thus eliminating cost dumping) is that both high quality and cost effectiveness will actually be favored in this financial model. However, rules change, financial incentives are fickle, and only an eye on long-term goals can keep a group energized toward achieving an improved system.

As stated earlier, there is hope that the financial and clinical incentives will be well aligned in these new systems and that, in fact, new financial models will actually facilitate higher-quality care. It is hoped that the same strategic and operational changes will improve both clinical care and fiscal stability. However, as means toward those ends, responsiveness to payors and to payor opportunities becomes an important goal. Behavioral health IDSs can potentially relate to a broad variety of payor sources including private insurance payors, public insurance payors, direct governmental contracts for mental health services, and direct contracts with business. In addition, human services IDSs may have relations with multiple governmental payor sources beyond those that behavioral health providers traditionally consider. These include moneys from various funding streams including mental retardation, juvenile justice, children and youth services, and housing authorities. Aligning the IDSs with potential payors is challenging. The differences between public- and private-sector systems of care in many markets can be profound. Although some providers successfully work in both the public and the private sectors, many do not. Although the public and private sectors require different services to provide a quality continuum of care, working with both the public and the private sectors has advantages clinically and financially. On a clinical level, many patients move between these payor sources or are dually eligible. In addition, familiarity with the services used in the public sector can inform providers about the services needed for more ill private-sector patients. From a financial standpoint, the ability to span payors provides flexibility for the IDS and also makes it a more attractive partner for many providers.

Major challenges must be met to align clinical and fiscal models of service delivery in today's environment. As a result many organizations are proceeding cautiously while awaiting the maturing of the marketplace and the design of appropriate financial incentives. One potential approach is to begin to create the most logical clinical system now, finding strength by melding the cultures of providers with overlapping missions. The organization would then be prepared to maximize the benefit to patients as more fundamental evolution of the system is possible.

Embracing Change: Leadership

Most administrators of behavioral health programs and services would agree that system reengineering is necessary. Most funding sources, whether commercial, state, federal, or foundation, see the creation of continuums of care and IDSs as attractive ways to accomplish a cost-effective, quality-oriented approach. Certainly, most clinicians are eager to embrace the principles of continuum-based integrated care, as are consumers. So we pose the question—why is redesign not happening more quickly? Where are we in the developmental process of moving toward IDSs? What can be done to move things ahead? Is there a way to be on track with rational health care planning and delivery? We believe that although advocacy, lobbying, legislation, and health care finance reform are all essential processes and should be encouraged to evolve, change must also go on—one agency, organization, provider, consumer group, hospital, or program at a time. How does this happen?

There is a natural inertia in the provider system that needs to be overcome. Fee-for-service financial models naturally have encouraged certain approaches on the part of providers. The advent of managed care has forced us all to look around for alternative approaches, if only to survive. Most administrators in behavioral health came up through the clinical and supervisory ranks; many are self-taught and have invested enormous personal time and energy to rise to leadership positions. Most are value driven and honestly strive to make things better for their organizations and the stakeholders. Most are very passionate about their work and thus may also be resistant to change. The same energies that helped them rise to the top of their profession may also be diverted to "hunkering down" against change.

If leaders focus on change as the enemy from without, they may miss the opportunity to create a full continuum of behavioral health services and to forge linkages with related human services. Although it is important to continue to make organizations more cost effective, the climate in which the delivery system operates needs to evolve. Organizations must adopt a better awareness of market forces in the industry and involve their staffs, stakeholders, and boards in a process of growth, linkage, new product development, and business planning. Through strategic planning, a continuous quality improvement approach should be adopted, initiating a never-ending process of change toward better service delivery.

Leaders must get out of the office and fearlessly soak up the environment, then relay the information in helpful ways to their constituents. Goals should be set and met regarding the number and types of linkages to be formed, not only with like entities but also with multiple payors and funding sources. Network inclusion and formation needs to be a "top of mind" agenda item in management and planning forums with specific data requirements to enable decision making. Payors respond to providers who are involved in proactive planning and are willing to implement pilot projects for general and special populations.

Successful IDSs will demand strong skills from leadership in collaboration, strategic planning, and conflict resolution (Longest 1998). In our experience, functional integration is a developmental journey that requires careful attention to positive interpersonal interaction between the members and an unwavering focus on the goal of an improved system. The ability to make and enact difficult decisions on a systemic level is also necessary.

Balancing between local autonomy and the need for coordination will be an ongoing challenge. Given the historical autonomy focus of health care providers, achieving this balance may become a central issue (Ummel 1997a). Balancing the needs of the members with those of the overall system can be an art form. Choosing which functions to centralize is critical. Strategic planning, contracting, information systems, case management, quality assurance, and utilization review logically cut across the system.

In addition to providing strong helmsmanship within the organization, leaders must take an active role in changing external system dynamics. Several issues require involvement and advocacy from IDS leaders. One is the inertia within payor systems. Since the 1990s, virtually all holders of commercial insurance plans have been subjected to the rigors of managed care. In behavioral health, rates have fallen dramatically. Simultaneously, providers have been forced, often by contract, to diversify their portfolios to drive down costs and improve access. It is clear, however, that evolution in benefit plans lags far behind the rapidly changing delivery system. Many benefit plans remain close to the traditional fee-for-service, inpatient/outpatient model. Insurers blame this on employers who want to lock in cost-saving rates through extended contracts. In addition there are the substantial ongoing difficulties in coordinating across the funding streams that have long separated behavioral health from welfare, housing, justice, and other sources of human services. The public behavioral health delivery system, in its traditional role as a backstop for patients who have exceeded benefits, is evolving a managed care perspective that will limit access to extended care.

It will be critical for leaders to understand and work with local and regional direction and to have an understanding of national trends and successful as well as unsuccessful experiments. A learning-oriented stance in which one expects to modify strategy regularly and continuously will work most effectively. Given that changes in funding will have unpredictable time frames, local variation, and an experimental nature, it is important to steer in a clear and steady direction guided by clinical principles and an overarching vision.

Focusing on Internal Processes

Strategic Planning

For many leaders and organizations, strategic planning consists of a yearly marathon of writing documents that often are not used or referred to again until updating is needed. Until recently strategic planning was often done by organizational leaders without input from middle management or professional and support staff. For system reengineering, strategic planning has taken on a new form and is now seen as a more organic, evolving process that is inclusive, open, and dynamic.

Because the new, dynamic strategic planning mandates a substantial amount of decision making at the program and operational levels, the question of who should be involved at what levels of the organization needs consideration. Often there are individuals with ideas, skill, and creativity who are not in the management pool but could be considered for inclusion. Most human service professionals are eager to try to make things better and have thought and dreamed about systems of care that are more efficient and effective. They should be encouraged to become involved, because they often are the implementers of change when it occurs and can lend essential buy-in. Involvement can also serve the purposes of increasing the understanding of market forces and their effect on service planning and provision and of reducing dissatisfaction and burnout among staff whose daily activities of service provision can be draining and constraining.

Ideally, strategic planning in service organizations should be multidisciplinary, including physicians, nurses, social workers, paraprofessionals, psychologists, support staff, and consumers. Planning affects the future of the entire organization and is both internal and external in nature; multidisciplinary groups can assist in both revising internal structure and maintaining a clearer view of the external environment. That view, important for identifying potential partners of quality and integrity, can be very helpful. Multidisciplinary planning also helps to create a common planning language.

The next step involves the formulation of well-understood and agreed-on goals. One compelling reason to engage in the strategic planning process is to reorganize the delivery of clinical services to provide a full continuum of care. However, not every organization is of sufficient size and positioning to accomplish this alone. Thus, planning can focus on integration of services, new program development, closure of underused programs, or joint venturing. In the remainder of this chapter we focus not only on the internal steps needed to upgrade an organization's delivery system but also on the considerations necessary to establish linkages to other organizations.

Internal Restructuring

To ensure the success of an IDS, most organizations must first do some internal restructuring, looking at what services are offered and how they fit together. Effective treatments are the cornerstone to successful patient outcomes and survival in the marketplace. Therefore, the strategic planning group must dedicate some of its efforts to examining the strengths and weaknesses of its product lines. The group must ask itself a number of questions:

- What array of services is offered?
- Is the program in demand by patients and payors?
- Is the program delivering high-quality clinical outcomes?
- Are there easily accessed linkages to other programs?
- Are patients and families satisfied with the services?
- Can a program be enhanced by modification or linkage?
- Is the program cost effective?
- Are the needs of special populations being met effectively?

Many modern organizations have found that adopting "service lines" that combine sets of services that naturally work together because of age, diagnosis, or payor categories is an efficient, convenient way to start the process (Charns et al. 1998). It is useful to survey service line leadership about what is actually being offered so that gaps and duplications can be identified. A simple spreadsheet can be created to serve as a guide in ongoing strategic planning and can be shared with potential partners as needed. Analysis of internal structure will reveal the status of the organization in relation to its desire to integrate with other providers. As is often the case, single organizations, regardless of size, will find unsatisfactory answers to many of these questions. They will then be faced with deciding how to move forward—either doing it by themselves or seeking partners.

Determining How to Proceed

Because of the pace of consolidation, organizations more often have to consider how to integrate: whether to develop their own new services, create completely new business entities, join with partners (joint ventures), or complete mergers with other providers to achieve their goals. This is often called the "build versus buy" decision and mandates several factors for consideration (see Table 4–1).

It is evident that the organization's planning group must be careful to weigh as many of these decisions as possible before recommending a course of action. Depending on the state of the marketplace and the resources of the organizations, it is often desirable to consider more than one strategy. It may be very time consuming to set up a joint venture with another organization for a small

TABLE 4–1.   Build versus buy decision making

	Cons	Pros

Building	Takes time
	Requires a steep learning curve
	Can be expensive
	Can duplicate services
	Requires additional human
	  resources
	Can be politically risky
	Can be financially risky
		Gives ownership
		Gives control
		Potentiates a better fit
		Creates opportunities for staff
		Requires less legal/consultation
		  expense

Buying	Requires a process Can be labor intensive Can be expensive Can make enemies Can strain corporate cultures Requires more legal/consultation expense	Adds to the continuum quickly Brings existing capability Can be financially rewarding Creates a collaborative atmosphere Allows multitasking

project when time dictates entering a new product in the market quickly and cleanly. On the other hand, the time invested in such a strategy may favorably dispose the parties to work together on larger and potentially more beneficial ventures later. The balance seems to lie in the ability of organizations to build relationships of trust based on good business sense while staying tuned in to ever-changing market conditions. All of this must occur while the organization's core business is maintained. Not an easy feat to accomplish!

Focusing on External Processes

Several competing models are evolving for structuring an IDS; unfortunately it is not yet clear which models are most effective. In general the promise of integrated systems has not always been met; the reasons for this are unclear. One study suggests that horizontally integrated hospital systems improve marketing but otherwise do not materially affect the system's efficiency (Dranove et al. 1996). Walston et al. (1996), citing experience in other industries, raised questions about the benefits of owned vertical integration in health care. However, true functional integration has been hard to achieve in health care IDSs, and some authors have recommended caution in moving to this model (McCarthy 1997; Slenack 1997).

Despite some continued uncertainty about the benefits of integrated systems, they are clearly proliferating. A study published in *Hospital and Health Networks* (Solovy 1997) reviewed the top 100 integrated health systems. Of note was the wide variability in size (revenues from $112 million to $4.5 billion), number of business units (5–300), and number of covered lives for which they were at risk (5,000–2.5 million). There were 630 such systems in 1997, accounting for $250 billion in revenue, 8.6 billion outpatient visits, and 271 million hospital admissions. Although this is a snapshot of the medical side, the scope of consolidation and integration in health care is quite impressive and suggests that the trend is increasing (Solovy 1997). This same study suggested that systems go through degrees of integration, although there seems to be no hard-and-fast time frame for this process. Table 4–2 outlines the five levels of integration.

In mental health, specifically, a variety of models for structuring IDSs evolved in the 1980s and 1990s. The first of these, *horizontal integration*, calls for the connection of two or more systems that provide similar types of care. An example of this would be the integration of several community mental health centers with broad geographic coverage. Because these centers are mandated to provide five levels of core services, there is great similarity among them. The goal of this type of affiliation is to better coordinate care across a region and within the levels provided by each organization. This model was very popular in the early 1990s, presenting organizations with a relatively low-risk method to gain managed care business. Our experience in dealing with horizontally integrated organizations, however, is that the organizations often remain fairly independent, with separate administrations, supervisory styles, and levels of quality, providing substantial challenges to quality clinical integration.

Vertical integration, defined as an attempt to create a continuum of care encompassing all levels of service delivery, offers another approach. In this model various organizations and individual providers come together to combine strengths in service delivery and to fill gaps. Connecting hospital inpatient programs, partial hospital programs, intensive outpatient programs, emergency services, long-term care, and care management services may achieve greater access and cost efficiencies and may also contribute to enhanced quality. Providers can reduce their isolation and attain greater strength to deal with payors and competitors. There are many challenges as well. Often organizations that differ in size and primary mission have widely differing approaches to information systems, contracting, billing, and collections. Whenever hospital-based organizations are in the mix, there are always issues of medical staff inclusion and alignment with primary and specialty medicine. Credentialing can also be complicated, and responsibility for its completion can be unclear. The stage of integration achieved depends on how many of these issues are addressed and resolved. Although fraught with complications, vertical integration has the potential of offering the array of services and access that payors want and patients need.

TABLE 4–2. Levels of integration	
Category 1: Horizontal	Coordinated care among similar providers Decreased costs, increased productivity Plans for vertical integration Few centralized functions
Category 2: Vertical integration, inpatient/outpatient	At least two levels of service Some integration in administrative functions
Category 3: Vertical integration, partly centralized	Full range of care via several providers Owned or under contract Administrative functions mostly centralized
Category 4: Vertical integration, mostly centralized	Full range of services via different kinds of providers Headquarters and staff separate from hospital or health maintenance organization Centralized administrative functions
Category 5: Full integration	System provides full range of care Administrative functions performed for the entire system, possibly in the form of a parent company

Source. Solovy 1997.

Experiments regarding the types of human services integrated systems will naturally occur based on local market conditions, financially integrated models, virtual integration, and regional health systems, to name a few. Financially integrated models require substantial capital for acquisition and integration costs. Achievable with less capital investment, virtual integrated systems bound together by contract may be as effective or more effective than financially integrated systems. However, both models are likely to evolve. Behavioral health integrated systems connected to regional medical systems are evolving. A model for this may involve the behavioral health system as a subsystem of a regional health system (Nauert 1997).

Forming Alliances and Coalitions

If the era of managed care has taught us anything, it is that health care provider organizations, even large, well-financed ones, are fearful of standing alone and expecting to survive. Consolidation is the watchword of the health care industry, and organizations are wise to study their markets for opportunities to partner. It is not so easy, however, to bring organizations together in ways that bring value and improve quality and access.

Often service line leaders will be the most knowledgeable in terms of the quality and reputation of any potential partner. They should be encouraged to solicit feedback from those staff members who actually deal with other organizations regularly, make and receive referrals from them, receive clinical information and reports, and have knowledge of client outcomes. Beyond that, the following aspects are important to consider:

- Strength in the market
- Available continuum of care
- Single point of access
- Willingness to assume risk
- Dynamic management
- Information systems' capability and capacity
- Commitment to the community
- Knowledge of local environment
- Value system
- Financial capacity to take risk
- Management capability
- Outcomes/clinical pathways capability
- Access to physician resources
- Network of primary care and medical services
- Training/education resources
- Access to expert consultation
- Consumer relations
- Future commitment to the market region

Often these issues determine the viability of a partnership more than does mere history or previous business relationships. As we have watched consolidation in the health care industry, we have observed that the partnerships being formed are often curious and surprising. It is not unusual for organizations that were formerly "mortal enemies" to do business together or even merge. If asked to prioritize the top three considerations from the list above, we would rank values alignment, management capacity, and access to medical resources highest, but the order of priority may be difficult to ascertain. If organizations are comfortable with the criteria for partnering, creating new business entities presents an exciting and potentially financially positive opportunity.

Although there is no "cookbook" for forming and maintaining alliances and coalitions, there are goals, principles, strategies, and tactics to be considered. The goals of value, quality, and access are joined by added strength in the market and cost containment. Among the principles trust, fairness, quality improvement, and reduction of duplication rank high. An appreciation and understanding of the culture of each of the member organizations forming the system are likely to be helpful (Ummel 1997b).

Strategies and tactics often cause organizations' efforts at consolidation to fail. Traditional behavioral health and human services organizations, while trying to join the new health care market, may be forced to rethink their status as independent operators and consider co-owning or comanaging new and expanded programs or services. Without experience in these areas, and facing the threat of assimilation by larger, well-financed corporate medical entities, behavioral health organizations are at risk for harmful business decisions that have negative effects on clients, staff, and funding.

Successful collaboration involves examining the processes for information exchange, which is often taken for granted in organizations. It is important to create several documents for use in alliance building. Because of the nature of the behavioral health services marketplace, organizations need as many "guarantees" as possible that they will not compromise sensitive information as they choose and plan with partners. Therefore, agreements that cover confidentiality, joint planning, and intent are essential to the process. The agreements should be prepared and/or reviewed with legal representation so that they not only provide safeguards but also motivate the parties involved to consider the seriousness of the activity. Joint planning agreements and letters of intent bind organizations to an agreed-on process, even when the conclusion is not yet clear.

In any collaboration of separate organizations, careful attention must be given to the legal and regulatory issues. Antitrust issues vary depending on the size and complexity of the marketplace. As information is shared and entities move toward greater clinical/fiscal integration, organizations are at greater risk of unknowingly violating laws enacted to protect the right to fair competition. Ongoing consultation to ensure compliance with antitrust laws can save potential partners from last-minute legal problems as deals are ready to close.

It is important to find and involve fiscal specialists who can identify and support financial plans necessary to make the partnership work from a business perspective. Every potential partnership should have a business plan, a due diligence process, and an agreed-on repository of the information gathered. These internal considerations and processes not only provide a structure on which to operate, they create a greater sense of security for those who are ultimately in a position to approve the partnership.

Considering Mergers and Joint Ventures

There are aspects particular to joint venture and to merger discussions. They include the following:

Joint Ventures

- Projects that would add to capabilities of all involved must be prioritized.
- Clinical and fiscal strengths must be brought together.
- Current and future funding sources must be identified.
- Control issues must be put on the table.
- Project champions must be identified.

Mergers

- Functionality is the goal.
- Structure follows function.
- They must be done for the right reasons.
- The continuum must be built.
- Consumers must be helped.
- Capability must be added.

The considerations above are merely a short list of what must be thought through when entering the world of joint ventures and mergers. The variety of forms and functions of joint ventures alone can be confusing and inhibiting. Conflicts over portions of equity, governance, staffing, clinical standards, and access can, if not addressed early in the process, become barriers to implementing the best-designed, most clinically sound, market-sensitive products.

Mergers can take several forms, including full acquisition, combining assets, and systems mergers that maintain degrees of separateness. They require a sense of timing and prioritization and are fraught with control issues, board issues, subcorporation management issues, and even the corporate name. In health care, mergers can disrupt traditional means of service delivery and set organizations up for rates of accelerated growth that outstrip their capacity to manage. Often consolidation predicts individual downsizing before individual capabilities can be measured and strikes fear in the hearts of staff whose job security is sometimes at stake. Leaders should anticipate and be prepared to deal with these issues.

CONCLUSION

Although these and other considerations are crucial to ensure the successful creation of new systems of care, the most critical element remains the vision to think and plan boldly and honestly and to be well prepared to enter the brave new world of integrated care.

REFERENCES

Charns MP, Parker VA, Wubbenhorst WH: Clinical service lines in integrated health care delivery systems. Working paper, series #24; Center for Health Management Research. Berkeley, CA, University of California–Berkeley, July 1998

Dranove D, Durkac A, Shanley M: Are multihospital systems more efficient? Health Aff 15:100–103, 1996

Longest B: Managerial competence at senior levels of integrated delivery systems. J Healthc Manage 43:115–135, 1998

McCarthy R: Do integrated delivery systems do it better? Bus Health, Sept 1997, pp 39–44

Nauert R: Managed behavioral health care: a key component of integrated regional delivery systems. J Health Care Finance 23:49–61, 1997

Slenack K: Making integrated healthcare work. Hospital News Aug:3–4, 1997

Solovy A: The health care 100. Hospital and Health Networks 71:34–36, 38–50 1997

Ummel S: Pursuing the elusive integrated delivery network, I: overcoming our obsession with autonomy. Healthcare Forum Journal, March/April 1997a, pp 13–17

Ummel S: Pursuing the elusive integrated delivery network, II: five high-impact steps toward an integrated delivery network. Healthcare Forum Journal, May/June 1997b, pp 73–76

Walston S, Kimberly J, Burns L: Owned vertical integration and health care: promise and performance. Health Care Manage Rev 21:83–92, 1996

5

Access to the System of Care

Margaret Moran, R.N., M.S.H.A.
Laurel J. Kiser, Ph.D., M.B.A.

In the United States many people believe that access to health care information and treatment is a basic right of all human beings, but for many uninsured and underinsured Americans this is an ideal rather than a reality. Thus issues related to obtaining adequate health care are critical to every stakeholder in today's health care industry. In fact, when asked to identify crucial health care issues, stakeholders consistently list access to care among the top three tiers in importance.

For patients, access to adequate health care involves recognizing the need for care and then finding available services and the resources to cover their costs. For payors, access to services typically translates into utilization costs. For employers, providing timely access to health care for employees has an effect on absenteeism, morale, productivity, and ultimately profitability. For the integrated system of care, taking clinical and fiscal responsibility for the health of a specified population necessitates providing adequate services to cover population needs and managing the demand for health care.

Inherent in the definition of *integrated delivery systems* (IDSs) is the notion of population-based care and the way it alters the role and responsibility of provider systems vis-à-vis access. Population-based care requires that provider systems develop an understanding of need at the population level and assume responsibility for both the wellness and the illness care of that population. Thus, in this chapter we define access for IDSs and outline mechanisms for controlling need, demand, penetration, and utilization.

Understanding Access

Definitions of *access* are as varied as the interests of the various stakeholders. The National Alliance for the Mentally Ill formally defines access as "the ability to obtain desired health care. Access is more than having insurance coverage or the ability to pay for services. It is also determined by the availability of services, acceptability of services, cultural appropriateness, location, hours of operation, transportation, and cost" (Malloy 1995, p. 302).

Although consumers generally have little interest in a formal definition of access, they elaborate a working definition in other ways. For example, consumers comment on access by discussing their frustrations with nonapprovals, benefit limitations, increased out-of-pocket expenses resulting from increasing copayments and deductibles, and lack of claims payment. Consumers also complain about long waits for appointments, inconvenient locations and hours of operation, limited access to specialists and sometimes to their primary care physicians (need to see a nurse practitioner first), poor customer service (busy lines), and limited time for discussions with payors or treaters regarding their particular situation.

Payors define access in four ways. First, they define it through the structuring of benefit plans, including restrictions and limitations. Second, they define it as a process for ensuring compliance with benefit restrictions, such as gatekeeper requirements, utilization management processes (e.g., precertification and concurrent review), or case management. Once a patient enters the system, payors quantify access through standard measures such as penetration/ utilization rates (see next section). Third, payors—acting as purchasers of care—define access according to providers' responsibilities. For instance, access can be defined in terms of span of coverage (i.e., 24-hours/day, 7-days/ week, 365-days/year services), geographic availability, triage, and emergency evaluation protocols. Finally, payors define access for their consumers through customer service standards such as telephone abandonment rates and on-hold time measurements.

Employers, as the primary purchasers of health care, define access by establishing many of the rules that govern the use of services. Employers play a major role in determining who has access to what types of health care. They assume control of access by determining which employees are eligible for health care benefits, by determining the package of health care benefits available for their employees, and by establishing processes through which employees can access those benefits.

Facilities and provider systems define access in just as many ways. The Institute of Medicine defines access as the extent to which those in need of mental health and substance abuse care receive services that are appropriate to the severity of their illnesses and the complexity of their needs.

Concern over access for providers has been limited historically to management of referrals and referral sources. Traditionally, providers thought of access as the way into their system (i.e., referrals, triage, scheduling appointments). However, access to services was also dependent on the level of care criteria required to make placement decisions, the development of relationships with payors, and the timeliness of utilization management/managed care organization approvals. Additionally, complaints from patients and families helped providers understand the access issues that affected patient satisfaction with services rendered.

To take clinical and fiscal responsibility for a specified population, an IDS must be concerned about controlling access at the population level rather than at the individual patient level. Population-based care shifts the mandate for providers from developing and maintaining active referral networks and filling beds or slots for care to assessing the needs of the population; evaluating benefit and management structures; and delivering the quantity, variety, and intensity of services that match the determined level of need.

An IDS assuming clinical and fiscal responsibility for the mental health of a specified population has an added responsibility to control the flow of enrollees who access services. Processes of care must facilitate timely access to appropriate treatment for those who need services (determined by some predetermined criteria) and must restrict access for those who seek care but do not meet the necessary criteria or who, through prevention, could avoid the need for care altogether. Without such management of access, the logical rationing of care necessary for maximizing financial resources would be lacking.

In summary, an IDS must view access from a different perspective than traditional providers do. Therefore, we suggest the following working definition of *access to IDSs*:

> An efficient, effective, multistep, reiterative process through which systems of care manage individual and population needs. This process involves assessing need; providing input into benefit plan design and external monitoring; providing a centralized process by which individuals enter the system and obtain the medical care needed to remedy a situation affecting the quality of their lives, according to the language of their particular health insurance policy; developing a service array matched to assessed needs; providing services to reduce need and demand and to improve population health; and evaluating the results.

Access and Population-Based Care

To develop processes that appropriately control the flow of individuals who access services, IDSs must understand the following concepts (see Table 5–1): need, excess need, caseness, prevalence rates, demand, excess demand, penetration rates, and utilization rates (American Psychiatric Association Monograph 1997; Dorwart and Epstein 1992; Fries 1994).

TABLE 5–1.   Terms commonly used in an integrated delivery system

Term	Definition
Need	"Clinical manifestation of illness that meets established criteria and indications for medical treatment" (Dorwart and Epstein 1992, p. 13). "Illness burden" (Fries 1994) that equates to worry, pain, suffering, loss of abilities, loss of functioning, direct costs (costs of care), and indirect costs (e.g., lost days at work) of an illness for the population
Excess need	Illness burden associated with preventable illness
Caseness	Individual classified with an illness
Prevalence rates	Rate at which a disorder is diagnosed in a specific sample
Demand	Requests for health care
Excess demand	Requests for inappropriate medical services or services that are not likely to provide relief, failure of self-management (e.g., use of emergency department for general care) Demand – medical necessity = excess demand
Penetration rates	Number of individuals who contact the system seeking services during a given period of time, expressed as a percentage of the entire covered group
Utilization rates	Number of individuals who use a particular service during a given period of time, expressed as a percentage of the entire covered group

How are these concepts relevant? Fundamental to the continuum model of integrated service delivery is the matching of population need to services offered. Obviously, then, understanding and measuring need, excess need, demand, and excess demand is essential to the delivery of an adequate quantity and variety of services.

Within health care, we use several concepts to help quantify *need*. First, we determine caseness by assigning a diagnostic classification to those individuals who meet specific illness-related criteria. Within traditional systems under indemnity payment plans, caseness—the presumptive criteria for medical necessity—is the key to access to services. Caseness equates with the medical necessity criteria requiring a patient to have a current psychiatric diagnosis. In contrast, IDSs extend access to the system of care to individuals before they are diagnosed with an illness in the hope that targeting those at high risk or with premorbid conditions will reduce the number of individuals actually diagnosed (i.e., caseness). Second, using this classification system, we can determine the *prevalence*, or the rate at which each diagnosis occurs within a given population. By putting these two concepts—caseness and prevalence—together, we can determine at the individual and population level who demonstrates the need for care.

Unfortunately, there is only a theoretical correspondence between need and *demand*. Individuals vary greatly in their demand for health services, even when their health status is similar (Fries 1994). This variation in demand is affected by several factors in addition to need, including perceived efficacy of health care, previous experience with health care, systems of belief, and health confidence. Typically, a small percentage of the population (20%) uses a great proportion of the total services (80%). Given this loose correspondence, IDSs develop processes and mechanisms for managing demand within the population.

Penetration rates indicate the number of covered individuals who seek either information or services from the provider system. The goal for most payors is to minimize this number, whereas the goal of IDSs is to maximize it and then to provide appropriate services for all—information, education, decision assistance, prevention and wellness programs, self-help programs, assessment, and triage—through an array of treatment modalities. Maximizing penetration rates need not translate into higher utilization rates. In fact, IDSs hope to alter utilization patterns so that the majority of individuals who penetrate the system receive information, education, prevention, and wellness care, with the most intensive and expensive services reserved for those having the greatest need.

What Enhances and What Inhibits Access?

Many factors influence access to health care; some enhance access and others inhibit it. It is necessary to understand the many contributors and inhibitors that influence access to the health care system before mechanisms to control need, penetration, or use can be developed and implemented.

Access contributors include the knowledge all parties have about benefits, the presence of staff members who are knowledgeable and helpful, the number and types of services available, and having convenient locations and timely appointments as well as more appropriate benefit structures. *Access inhibitors* include delayed referrals, inappropriate diagnoses and treatment, provider incentives for underutilization, provider choice restrictions, and inadequate benefit structures. Table 5–2 includes a list of access contributors and inhibitors.

ASSESSING POPULATION NEED

The importance of assessing population need cannot be underestimated. An accurate picture of the prevalence of risk and resilience factors as well as the disorders present in the population is necessary for assuming responsibility for a specified population, both for clinical and fiscal reasons. Before negotiating any at-risk contract, it is important to assess and understand these factors for the specific population under consideration. IDSs assuming risk for a population must base development of their service array on an analysis of prior uti-

TABLE 5–2.   Access contributors and inhibitors

Access contributors	Access inhibitors
Knowledge of benefits by all parties	Delays in referrals from primary care physicians
Adequate and appropriate benefit structures	
Adequate resources	Primary care physicians' lack of behavioral health knowledge and experience
Centralized system	
Service availability/convenient hours	
Signage	Traveling long distances because of managed care organization restrictions
Qualified staff	
Cultural competence	Denial of services
Advocacy	Special interest restrictions (age, substance abuse)
Reasonable copays and deductibles	
Knowledge of medical necessity criteria	Shifting responsibility for mental health/substance abuse among several systems (criminal, family, medical, safety)
Eligibility	
Timely appointments	
Convenient locations	
Program evaluation (audits and shopper calls)	Lack of confidentiality
	Inappropriate diagnosis/treatment
Respectful communication	Provider choice restrictions
Good listening and synthesizing skills	Negative past treatment experience
Knowledge of community resources	Provider incentives
	Delays in approvals
	Services not available/limited capacity/ delayed appointments
	Inadequate review staff
	Stigma
	Poor listening and communication skills
	Inadequate benefit structures
	Gatekeeping
	Inconvenient hours
	Unable to advocate for own treatment

lization rates and a projection of future utilization rates for this specific population. Additionally, IDSs must base contract rates (case rates or per member/per month) on the specifics of that population. A variety of techniques are available for assessing population need:

- *Analyzing prior rates of penetration and utilization available from the previous provider or from the payor.* When analyzing these data it is important to understand whether the care was managed or unmanaged and what kinds of services were available. For instance, in a population moving from fee-for-service reimbursement with an unmanaged environment to capitation, it is possible to discount utilization for inpatient care, especially if the IDS offers a comprehensive continuum of services including partial hospitalization and intensive outpatient services.

- *Making actuarial assessments of population need.* These estimates are based on epidemiological statistics modified for region. However, they typically are not calculated on specific information regarding a particular population.

- *Obtaining information from community-based providers.* Community-based providers have much of the information needed to assess the mental health and substance abuse needs of a specified population if they have been involved in delivering that care already. Through years of experience they have a good understanding of the prevalence rates for specific disorders within their communities as well as use rates for their service systems. This basic knowledge can be augmented by reviewing national and regional prevalence rates from epidemiological studies and studies of risk and resilience factors regarding mental health and substance abuse.

- *Conducting population-based needs assessment.* IDSs may want to conduct a population-based needs assessment before assuming responsibility for a specified population. Such assessments take a random sampling of individuals included in that population and conduct surveys regarding demographics, lifestyle, general health, and behavioral health concerns.

INPUT IN BENEFIT PLAN DESIGN AND EXTERNAL MONITORING

The health care insurance industry uses varying benefit design strategies to reduce costs. These strategies lower costs by restricting access to health care and service delivery (see Table 5–3). Benefit manipulations that decrease utilization include benefit limitations such as days-per-service limits (i.e., 30–60 days per year inpatient) or dollar-per-service limits (i.e., $500–$1,500 per year outpatient). In addition, benefits are managed by imposing exclusions for certain diagnoses, lifetime maximums, varying copays and deductibles, and maximum out-of-pocket expenses. The health care industry also manages benefits to contain costs through gatekeeping and establishing medical necessity criteria.

Some examples of the effects of benefit structures on penetration and utilization will help illustrate the power of these management strategies. Suppose that an employer and its insurance company wanted to decrease costs for behavioral health care. To accomplish this the employer decides to implement a $20 per visit copay. What result might the employer expect? One study dem-

TABLE 5–3.   Benefit structures used to manage access

No benefits (penetration)
Deductibles (penetration)
Preexisting condition (caseness)
Copays (penetration, utilization)
Yearly limits—number of visits, dollar amounts (utilization)
Lifetime limits—number of visits, dollar amounts (utilization)

onstrated that a copay of $20 resulted in a 16% decrease in likelihood of use (penetration) but no change in visit rate (utilization), whereas a $30-per-visit copay resulted in no additional change in penetration but a 9% decrease in visits per year. The most striking result is that these changes in penetration and utilization were found regardless of the need for service (Simon et al. 1996).

Benefit structures also influence use of services along the continuum. Benefit structures that exclude payment for certain treatment modalities/levels of care or restrict the number of days/visits allowed affect providers' ability to offer a comprehensive array of services. Evidence clearly supports the effect that such changes in benefit design have on both admissions and length of stay with restrictions associated with significant decreases in both use of service and days used (Patrick et al. 1993).

On the other hand, benefit plans that include equitable coverage for a comprehensive system of care, including intermediate-level services, change the pattern of use. Within such systems, "hospitalization [is] related more closely to functioning; the availability of intermediate levels of care let clinicians reserve hospital care for the most severe cases" (Bickman et al. 1996, p. 80). In general, there is little examination of and insufficient data on the impact of these manipulations, particularly on patients. Thought is rarely given to where patients will receive treatment if services are restricted through benefit design by the behavioral health care system. Unfortunately, these strategies typically create short-term savings with cost shifting to other systems (e.g., general medical, public, criminal, school). These approaches also ignore the societal impact of untreated mental illness and chemical dependency (Geraty et al. 1994). However, the powerful incentives inherent in benefit structures necessitate that IDSs have input into benefit plan design if they are to be held clinically and fiscally responsible for the health of a specified population.

Gatekeepers and Gatekeeper Models

Gatekeeping refers to the need for special authorization by an agent for the payor. Gatekeeper models are characterized by an individual, usually a clinician, who controls the access to health care services for members of a specific group. In many health maintenance organization settings, this gatekeeper is the primary care physician or his or her staff. In other health care delivery systems (and in health maintenance organizations in which behavioral health services are contracted out), the gatekeeper is often the case manager of the behavioral health organization (Callahan and Merrick 1997). Gatekeepers may assume responsibility for controlling access to the system of care at all three levels: penetration, caseness, and utilization.

Primary Care Case Management

Primary care case management is a gatekeeper model in which a primary care physician (e.g., physician or nurse practitioner) serves as a case manager, providing assessment and nonspecialty treatment in addition to authorizing specialty referrals (Stroup and Dorwart 1997). This model includes the coordination of general health, mental health, and substance abuse services. Use of the primary care physician as a gatekeeper to mental health and substance abuse services raises serious concerns for some stakeholders. These concerns center on data that indicate primary care physicians underdiagnose behavioral health disorders and that this underdiagnosis leads to undertreatment (Croze 1994).

Utilization Management

Utilization management, which evolved from utilization review, is a set of techniques used on behalf of purchasers of health benefits to manage costs through case-by-case assessments of the clinical justification (medical necessity) for proposed medical services (Faulkner and Gray 1996). The utilization management process consists of precertification, concurrent review, case management, and sometimes discharge reviews. Utilization management is typically handled over the telephone by nurses or master's-level licensed clinicians. The primary function of utilization management is to control use of services.

Employee Assistance Programs

Employee assistance programs (EAPs) are designed to assist employees, their family members, and employers in finding solutions for workplace and personal problems (United HealthCare Corporation 1994). EAP programs began in the 1950s with a primary emphasis on substance abuse. Today EAP counselors are often a covered employee's initial contact with the system for behavioral health and substance abuse concerns and referrals. As such, EAPs function as a bridge between human resources in the workplace and the "front end" of a managed behavioral health system. EAPs primarily function to control caseness and utilization. They do so by providing an initial assessment of the problem and often by providing short-term counseling before referring for specialty care.

Point-of-Service Plans

Point-of-service (POS) plans attempt to combine risk-based management processes with freedom of choice. POS plans typically increase the options through which a covered individual can access services; however, these added options are subject to financial penalties or higher premium dollars. In POS plans covered individuals can choose to see either providers who are in the network or providers out of the network, and they have direct access to specialists.

IDSs must be aware of any external gatekeeping processes being imposed on them by contractors or employers. This is particularly relevant in carve-out arrangements or when an EAP is involved. In these cases, the boundaries between the gatekeeper system and the IDS need to be clearly stipulated before the IDS finalizes the behavioral health services contract. Additionally, the IDS needs to work closely with the gatekeeper system (primary care physicians/EAPs) to provide education; coordinate access issues; and develop protocols for who treats what, when a member is to be referred for specialty care, and so on. Ideally, in a fully integrated system, the IDS subsumes most gatekeeper functions.

Medical Necessity Criteria

In addition to gatekeeper systems, medical necessity criteria are used to control utilization and to ration care by establishing boundaries between what should be funded with medical dollars versus social/legal/education dollars. Until the funding streams for these different services are consolidated, medical necessity criteria play an important role in determining how the medical dollar is spent. Although there is no industry standard, medical necessity criteria should be consistent with medical and clinical standards of care. These criteria typically include 1) current DSM diagnosis/classifiable medical illness; 2) level of risk, including dangerousness and immediacy; 3) level of functional impairment, including medical needs, self-care, vulnerability, activities of daily living, and developmental appropriateness; 4) past treatment or failed treatment at a lower level of care; and 5) ability to benefit and compliance.

Medical necessity criteria are written for each level of care for which coverage is provided and as such become *de facto* admission criteria for a specific service. Thus, medical necessity criteria can effectively prevent or restrict access to services. They can also create significant problems for providers if, in fact, the medical necessity criteria used do not match the actual admission criteria for a treatment program because of the potential that patients will be placed in danger.

As with gatekeeper functions, IDSs must be aware of any external medical necessity criteria being imposed on them by contractors or employers. In these cases, the IDS must demand adequate input into the development and implementation of the medical necessity criteria used so that these criteria are consistent with the delivery system. Again, in a fully integrated system, establishing medical necessity criteria is a responsibility assumed by the IDS. Medical necessity criteria written by the IDS correspond with the model of behavioral health services used, which in this case is the continuum of behavioral health services.

ACCESS SYSTEMS

Portals of entry to the health care system can be either centralized or decentralized. Each model has its own characteristics and warrants further investigation.

Decentralized Access Model

A decentralized access system has multiple entry/access points. Individuals access the system through various points of entry: emergency rooms, clinics, outpatient programs, medical services, and so on. This type of system has several disadvantages: there is no central repository for information, which is needed for requests for proposals, outcome studies, and reporting; patients may be "bounced" around and referred to the wrong service; and frustration often results that may lead to lost business and contracts. A decentralized access model promotes an array of negative outcomes that includes confusion, misinformation, untimely treatment, and dissatisfaction.

Centralized Access Model

A centralized access system (CAS) provides a more effective portal of entry because it is a single point of entry (access) system with reception, information, triage, and assessment capabilities that facilitates access by payors, consumers, and referents. A schematic representation of this model is shown in Figure 5–1.

An effective CAS comprises specific elements to ensure optimal availability, timeliness, clinical staff, clinical programs, systems, and management support and training. These elements combine to allow for telephone and face-to-face evaluation and disposition, eligibility verification, and scheduling capabilities. Figure 5–2 depicts the specific categories and requirements.

The most important feature of a CAS is ease of access, which is highly valued by all constituencies. Another valuable feature is the capacity to monitor patients' adherence to scheduled appointments. This capacity ensures that patients are hooked into the system and do not fall into the cracks. This is not

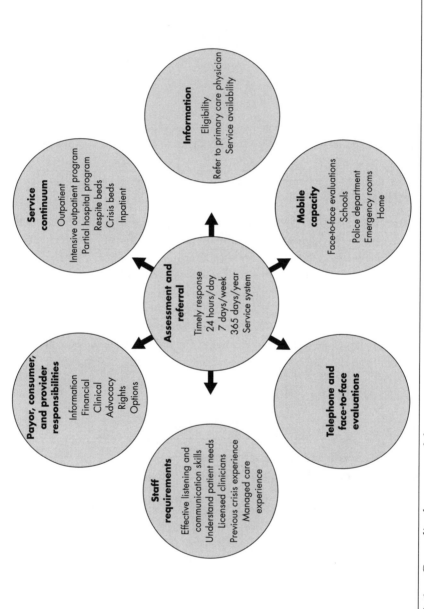

FIGURE 5–1. Centralized access model.

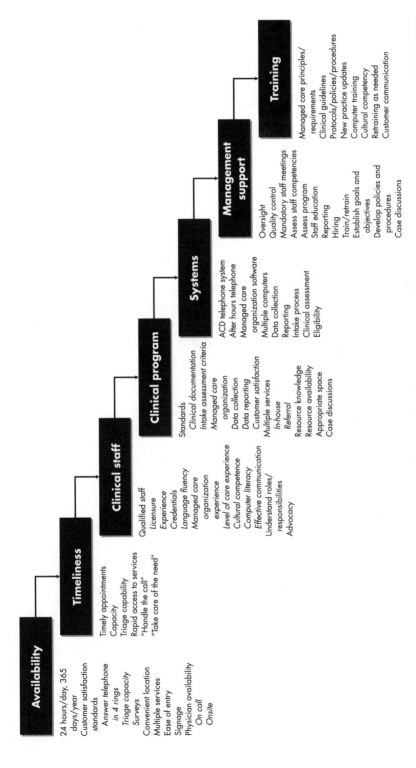

Availability

24 hours/day, 365 days/year
Customer satisfaction standards
Answer telephone in 4 rings
Triage capacity
Surveys
Convenient location
Multiple services
Ease of entry
Signage
Physician availability
On call
Onsite

Timeliness

Timely appointments
Capacity
Triage capability
Rapid access to services
"Handle the call"
"Take care of the need"

Clinical staff

Qualified staff
Licensure
Experience
Credentials
Language fluency
Managed care organization experience
Level of care experience
Cultural competence
Computer literacy
Effective communication
Understand roles/responsibilities
Advocacy

Clinical program

Standards
Clinical documentation
Intake assessment criteria
Managed care organization
Data collection
Data reporting
Customer satisfaction
Multiple services
In-house
Referral
Resource knowledge
Resource availability
Appropriate space
Case discussions

Systems

ACD telephone system
After hours telephone
Managed care organization software
Multiple computers
Data collection
Reporting
Intake process
Clinical assessment
Eligibility

Management support

Oversight
Quality control
Mandatory staff meetings
Assess staff competencies
Assess program
Staff education
Reporting
Hiring
Train/retrain
Establish goals and objectives
Develop policies and procedures
Case discussions

Training

Managed care principles/requirements
Clinical guidelines
Protocols/policies/procedures
New practice updates
Computer training
Cultural competency
Retraining as needed
Customer communication

FIGURE 5–2.   Optimal elements of a centralized access center.

only a value-added service but a cost-effective component as well. A critical outcome of the centralized system is the repository of important clinical and demographic information created by tracking demographics, diagnosis, referral type/name, time of entry, primary care physician, and wait times. The CAS must have the ability to collect and report on specific data elements such as diagnoses, length of stay, diversion (where patients were referred) percentages, referral patterns, timeliness of appointments, and service needs (such as bilingual/bicultural and service unavailability issues).

Functions of a Centralized Intake Service

Initial Assessment

The CAS becomes the service that conducts all initial evaluations for individuals entering the system of care. These evaluations may involve telephone, office-based, and/or mobile capabilities. Initially, CAS staff members screen calls to determine the urgency of the request and schedule an evaluation within the time frames established for seeing patients: Regular, face-to-face contact, within 3–5 working days; Urgent care, within 24–48 hours; Emergent care, within 1–4 hours. According to current industry standards, master's-degreed, licensed professionals conduct these initial assessments with oversight by doctoral-level (Ph.D., M.D.) professionals.

The goal of the initial assessment is to collect patient information about current problems, signs and symptoms of psychiatric disorders, current level of functioning, and previous mental health or substance abuse treatment. The clinician synthesizes this information to assign a diagnosis and to make an initial level of care placement decision. In some IDSs, the initial assessment goes well beyond this and involves a comprehensive assessment that culminates in an episode of care or treatment plan.

Some CASs combine assessment and referral with care management. In this model, a specific individual monitors a patient caseload. This is an ongoing process, with the care manager remaining involved from the patient's admission through his or her discharge from the system. The care manager also helps the patient negotiate movement along the continuum.

Psychiatric Assessment and Case Review

Not all consumers seeking behavioral health services require a psychiatric evaluation, but some do. In these cases, information from the psychiatrist is necessary before a placement decision can be made. Additionally some complicated cases require input from multiple disciplines before a placement decision can be made. Thus, the CAS has a psychiatrist available for initial evaluations on a regular basis.

Case staffing is another important component of an assessment and referral service. Having a multidisciplinary team of professionals, including a psychiatrist, review a percentage of cases weekly is a useful approach. Cases selected for review can be a random sample or those that meet specified criteria, such as emergency referrals, medically complicated cases, and frequent users of services.

Medical Clearance

At times acute psychiatric symptoms are related to general medical illness. For example, the signs and symptoms of a panic attack can be associated with cardiac dysfunction. Medical complications are frequently associated with substance abuse and geriatric mental health emergencies. Part of the decision making in such cases involves ruling out medical complications and obtaining medical clearance for patients before they are placed in a behavioral health service. Thus, consultation/liaison with general medical personnel should be an established part of a CAS.

Crisis Services/Acute Intervention

The CAS usually includes a crisis system designed to provide patients with responsive urgent and emergent behavioral health assessment and triage, level of care assessment, and authorization of services. In addition, this crisis system offers some acute interventions as prevention for hospital care. Crisis services are usually in place to cover patients on a short-term basis while they are in crisis and require intensive intervention. These services cover patients in crisis who are new to the system of care as well as those who are already receiving treatment.

Crisis services typically include five community-based components:

1. Crisis telephone services, which act as an entry point to services and are staffed 24 hours/day, 7 days/week
2. Walk-in intervention, for which CAS or in-house staff members are available or on call (e.g., hospital emergency department)
3. Mobile crisis outreach, which consists of multidisciplinary teams at an out-of-office environment
4. Observation services and/or beds that are integrated into or available to the CAS unit
5. Crisis residential services, which are protective, supervised settings such as shelters, therapeutic foster care, small group homes, and stabilization units that are within the system or are readily available.

Level of Care Determination and Triage

Results of the initial evaluation provide information on the patient condition variables (signs and symptoms, level of functioning, risk/dangerousness, commitment to treatment, and available social supports) used to define levels of care. CAS clinicians working with the consumer determine what specific program or services will best meet that consumer's needs by matching his or her needs with service characteristics. Chapter 6 discusses decision analysis and decision support tools; the focus here is on clinical decision making.

It is important for the CAS staff to have a working knowledge of each level of care available as well as the many combinations of programs and services that can be bundled in a treatment plan. CAS staff members need to know the specific admission criteria for each program and have a feel for the types of patients that are most successful and least successful in each program. Because CAS staff members are highly influential with regard to who goes where, the CAS typically is a separate unit without direct affiliations with any of the services offered. Once a level of care placement determination is made, the CAS clinician schedules an admission to that service. Centralized scheduling is an important ingredient for the successful streamlining of this process.

DEVELOPMENT OF SERVICES ARRAY

At minimum, systems of care have emergency services, outpatient programs, intensive outpatient programs, respite care, crisis stabilization, holding beds, and inpatient services. What they usually do not have are services across the entire continuum; services for all age groups (i.e., child, adolescent, geriatric); specialty services (e.g., eating disorders, substance abuse, dual diagnoses); or services for special populations, such as case management and transitional living services for clients with severe and persistent mental illness.

More sophisticated systems (IDSs) develop these services through affiliation, joint ventures, and merger relationships. These relationships can take care of some of the deficiencies that a system might have in providing services for clients in their particular population who have geographic, bicultural, and special service needs.

IDSs, following an assessment of population needs, design a service system geared to meet those specific needs. IDSs organized by service lines may develop multiple delivery systems specifically geared toward the segment of the population covered by the service line (e.g., child and adolescent, geriatric, substance abuse). Figure 5–3 shows the array of services potentially needed for a comprehensive service system.

Network Composition and Geographic Access

As an IDS develops its delivery system, important decisions about network composition and geographic access need to be made. In addition to determining the array of services necessary to meet the needs of the covered population,

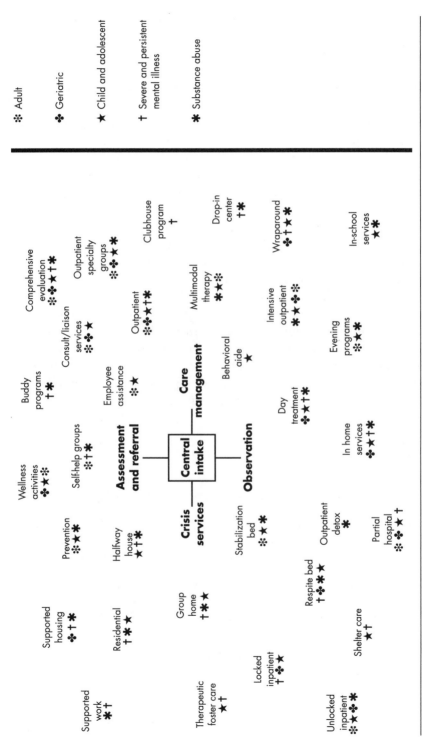

FIGURE 5–3. Service array. This is a partial listing of the many types of programs that may exist within a service system.

the IDS must determine the number of providers (behavioral health clinicians) and the number of specialists (child and adolescent, geriatrics, substance abuse) needed per enrollee. These ratios are based on estimates of penetration and caseness within the population. Some managed care organizations suggest that provider networks be composed of 25% psychiatry, 35% psychology, and 40% master's-level counselors. As integrated systems better define professional roles and responsibilities (see Chapter 10), the proportions of providers needed from the various disciplines will be easier to determine.

Geographic proximity of services to consumers in the covered population is another dimension of access. Distance traveled for care can either enhance or inhibit access. Certainly the more frequently treatment modalities are used, such as daily for partial hospital programs, weekly for outpatient care, or once or twice yearly for 24-hour-care facilities, the more convenient the service needs to be. Standards for travel times are being set in accreditation documents and large contracts; for example, case management, outpatient, intensive outpatient, partial hospital, mobile crisis, respite, and pharmacy/lab services are all within a 30-minute radius, whereas inpatient and 24-hour residential services are within a 60-mile radius of the covered population.

Planning for practice sites, both short-term and long-term, is different for systems concerned with population-based care than it is for traditional provider organizations. Variables such as demographic trends, geographic barriers, and commuting patterns of the covered population require study and future trends projection for appropriate planning.

Cultural Competence

IDSs providing population-based care must consider the needs of ethnic minorities and other special populations, such as rural consumers, in a systematic way. Special consideration of these groups is necessary because

> Ethnic minorities in the United States may (a) experience a disproportionate burden of health illnesses and disease compared with White Americans, (b) encounter the greatest number of barriers to accessing health and mental health services, (c) have the fewest financial resources to obtain appropriate services, and are subsequently overrepresented in the numbers of Americans who are insured or uninsured, and (d) may experience lower quality of care when they do receive health and mental health services. (Abe-Kim and Takeuchi 1996, p. 276)

To provide more culturally sensitive services, Abe-Kim and Takeuchi (1996) recommended a review and, perhaps, a reconfiguration of the processes that link organizational/structural factors, procedural variables, and outcomes for these populations. A specific review of benefit design, utilization management processes, gatekeeping procedures, medical necessity criteria, assessment and referral processes, and staff training needs to be done to ensure that cultural biases are not operational and restricting access to services for select groups of consumers.

SERVICES TO REDUCE NEED AND
DEMAND AND IMPROVE HEALTH

Demand Management

Demand management is the term used in economics for the processes and mechanisms implemented by a system "that ultimately result in the reduced demand for, use and corresponding costs of goods and services" (Gorsky et al. 1997, p. 8). Demand management is one of those concepts borrowed from business and industry that have important implications for health care delivery.

> We need to improve life-styles and avoid preventable illness, principally chronic illness, to reduce the need for medical services. The lifetime medical costs of those with good health habits are less than half the costs of those with poor health habits. We need to improve decision assistance, health education, and objective guidance so that individual decisions are consistent and enlightened in terms of expected health outcomes, in order to develop a collective individual restraint and to restrain demand. (Fries 1994, p. 150)

Methods for demand management include improvement of consumer decision-making skills. Media campaigns directed toward all individuals covered by the contract provide education regarding high-frequency concerns and questions. Topics for such campaigns might include stress and anger management; warning signs for common disorders, such as depression; and promotion of education, prevention, and wellness services. Other demand management programs include introduction of health advisors/advice nurses, self-management guidelines, and decision assistance services such as warm lines—telephone services that provide counseling and consultation and teach consumers to analyze their situations and seek appropriate services.

Improving Health Status

Managed health is a new concept for health care systems subsuming the functions of health promotion and disease prevention. The concept behind managed health is to prevent illnesses from occurring and to empower individuals who are ill to manage their disease processes better. To reach this desired outcome, IDSs make specific tools available to individuals to guide them in their quest for wellness. These tools include health risk assessments, selected screening programs, outreach to high-risk groups, health confidence boosters, behavioral health promotion, health education (information provided through various media such as the telephone and the Internet), lifestyle changes, and drug-free workplace environments.

IDSs can also build in financial incentives for meeting personal health goals. By appropriately structuring deductibles and copays, IDSs can provide rewards for healthy lifestyles, use of prevention and wellness programs, self-management, and compliance with treatment recommendations. Several examples illustrate this approach. Lower deductibles and copays can be established for individuals who score higher on behavior risk inventories (e.g., habits, stress management, exercise). Costs for education, wellness, and prevention programs can be covered by the plan. Copays can be reduced or waived with compliance.

Because of these initiatives, individuals will finally participate in their health decisions long before they become ill. Those who are or become acutely ill will have better tools (knowledge base) to assist in making decisions and managing their illness.

EVALUATING ACCESS

We have some indicators to measure access to health care, including

- Population health status
- Admissions per 1,000 population/members
- Average length of stay
- Number of times the telephone rings before it is answered
- Length of waiting times for appointments/delays in emergency department
- Patient satisfaction surveys
- Patient encounters per 1,000 covered lives
- Patient days per 1,000 population/members
- Number of visits per covered lives
- Length of wait times and abandonment rates
- Geographical location (within a radius of 25–30 miles)

However, despite all this information, many unanswered questions remain. For example, how do we know that access is appropriate and that systems of care meet the needs of patients? Is a penetration rate of 10% meeting the needs of the population or is 20% a truer estimate? Systems need to be developed to answer these questions. Only then can we truly measure access and understand where the deficits are and thus help individuals begin the treatment process they need to live healthier lives.

REFERENCES

Abe-Kim JS, Takeuchi DT: Cultural competence and quality of care: issues for mental health service delivery in managed care. Clinical Psychology: Science and Practice 3:273–295, 1996

American Psychiatric Association Monograph: The Psychiatrist's Guide to Capitation and Risk-Based Contracting. Washington, DC, American Psychiatric Association, 1997

Bickman L, Foster EM, Lambert EW: Who gets hospitalized in a continuum of care? J Am Acad Child Adolesc Psychiatry 40:74–80, 1996

Callahan JJ, Merrick EL: Designing public sector managed care systems, in Managed Mental Health Care in the Public Sector, A Survival Manual. Edited by Minkoff K, Pollack D. Amsterdam, B.V., Netherlands, Harwood Academic Publishers, 1997, p 45–57

Croze C: Network collaboration can produce integrated care. Behav Healthc Tomorrow 3:41–44, 1994

Dorwart R, Epstein SS: Economics and managed mental health care: the HMO crucible for cost-effective care, in Managed Mental Healthcare: Administrative and Clinical Issues. Edited by Feldman J, Fitzpatrick RJ. Washington, DC, American Psychiatric Press, 1992, pp 11–25

Faulkner and Gray: Appendix, in Medical Utilization Review Management Directory. Washington, DC, Faulkner and Gray, 1996, p 451–453

Fries JF: Health care demand management. Med Interface 7:56–58, 1994

Geraty R, Bartlett J, Hill E, et al: The impact of managed behavioral healthcare on the costs of psychiatric and chemical dependency treatment. Behav Healthc Tomorrow 3:18–30, 1994

Gorsky B, Beskin N, Parkinson D, et al: Improving Demand, Performance and Health Risk Management: Integrating Mass and Cluster Risk Management Within Worksite, Managed Care, Clinical and Community Settings. Elmhurst, IL, HPN WorldWide, 1997

Malloy M: Mental Illness and Managed Care: A Primer for Families and Consumers. Arlington, VA, The National Alliance for the Mentally Ill, 1995

Patrick C, Padgett, DK, Burns BJ, et al: Use of inpatient services by a national population: do benefits make a difference? J Am Acad Child Adolesc Psychiatry 32:144–152, 1993

Simon GE, Grothaus L, Durham ML, et al: Impact of visit copayments on outpatient mental health utilization by members of a health maintenance organization. Am J Psychiatry 153:331–338, 1996

Stroup TS, Dorwart RA: Overview of public sector managed mental health care, in Managed Mental Health Care in the Public Sector, A Survival Manual. Edited by Minkoff K, Pollack D. Amsterdam, B.V., Netherlands, Harwood Academic Publishers, 1997, p 6

United HealthCare Corporation: The Managed Care Resource: The Language of Managed Health Care. Minnetonka, MN, United HealthCare Corporation, 1994

6

Designing Level of Care Criteria

John S. Lyons, Ph.D.
Melissa E. Abraham, M.S.

Rapid changes in the behavioral health care system have had dramatic effects on decision making about the setting and intensity of mental health treatment. These concepts, setting and intensity, are the components of "level of care." Decisions about where to provide treatment and how much treatment to provide within a particular time frame are the clinical decisions most closely linked to the costs of behavioral health care. In the assertive purchaser period of the late 1980s and the 1990s, these decisions came under great scrutiny because they hold the key to successful cost containment in the public sector and to profitability in proprietary managed care.

Although there is little evidence that the number of admissions to psychiatric hospitals has declined, the average duration of stays in the hospital has become increasingly short (Mechanic et al. 1998). Though uncommon only two decades ago, 2- and 3-day psychiatric hospital stays have become routine. Formerly routine stays of several weeks have become rare, except in state-operated psychiatric hospitals. Partial hospital programs sprang up as alternatives to acute psychiatric hospitalizations only to be replaced by intensive outpatient programs that are intended to be less programmatic and more sensitive to individual variations in need. Twenty-three-hour crisis beds and in-home crisis services have also been advanced as alternatives to full or partial hospitalization (Yohanna et al. 1998).

Concern about the high costs of acute psychiatric services has led to a more pressing interest in understanding the clinical predictors of level of care decision making. Without a structured clinical method of determining a client's level of care, triage decisions can seem arbitrary. Often, the "micro-certainty, macro-uncertainty" hypothesis is supported (i.e., staff are very confident in the appropriateness of their personal recommendations), but the types of services recommended across a system of care are highly variable (Baumann et al. 1991; Hendryx and Rohland 1997). Guidelines can easily improve the consistency of decision making, but guidelines that direct individual service recipients to the optimal level of care based on their specific needs require a larger body of empirical knowledge than is currently available.

Even when a method is in place to enhance the accuracy of level of care decisions, there may be considerable variation in what is done. In one study of clinician reliability in judging the appropriate level of care using agency guidelines, interjudge reliability was close to zero (Bickman et al. 1997). However, if guidelines are thoughtfully constructed and carefully implemented, they have the potential to improve the likelihood of clinically appropriate decision making.

Decision support tools that can facilitate high-quality utilization management and quality improvement are important. To date, several such tools have been developed and evaluated using the decision analysis method (Lyons et al. 1997b). The primary objective of decision analysis is to identify key clinical information needed to 1) determine the nature and setting of treatment (i.e., level of care), 2) predict resource utilization, and 3) predict differential anticipated outcomes. Thus the information necessary for understanding decision making should allow one to facilitate and monitor treatment planning, evolve utilization management within a context of service need, and adjust anticipated outcomes for varying severity and complexity of cases. In this chapter we describe the methods necessary for effective decision analysis approaches relevant to level of care decisions and review existing measures and methodologies.

A focus on decision making in service delivery requires unique measurement and methodological approaches as compared with traditional approaches for measurement. The major difference between decision analysis and traditional outcomes approaches is that the former focuses on the clinical information needed to determine the nature and setting of treatment, and the latter focuses on assessing clinical factors that change as the result of mental health intervention. The combination of decision analysis with effectiveness measurement ultimately will allow us to identify what decision processes are associated with optimal outcomes.

Chase et al. (1996) distinguished three approaches to decision analysis. *Normative decision analysis* tends to be formal and mathematical, assuming that the decision maker is fully rational. In normative approaches formal models of decision making would be generated *a priori* based on clinical theory. When possible, this is an ideal approach to decision analysis in clinical settings. However, it is necessary to have a fully elaborated clinical model of the decisions to be made. *Descriptive decision analysis* attempts to understand how clinicians actually make decisions in practice. There is no assumption of a rational decision process; rather, the attempt is to identify how decisions are actually made. *Prescriptive decision analysis* is the application of normative and descriptive approaches in an effort to improve decision-making practice. Descriptive decision analysis is one approach, in the absence of clear theory, for building an understanding of what might be the ideal clinical model of decision making. Practice guidelines and decision support tools are forms of prescriptive decision analysis (Chase et al. 1996).

DEFINING LEVEL OF CARE

Before any meaningful discussion about models of predicting level of care or supporting decisions in clinical practice, it is necessary to agree on a conceptualization of level of care. In general, *level of care* has been defined as a continuum of intensity (e.g., Kiser et al. 1999; Kramer et al. 1990). However, in behavioral health care, intensity can vary across at least two dimensions.

It is useful to conceptualize the therapeutic milieu as having dimensions of intensity of service. This would be consistent with others' demarcations of intensity of residential services. However, the intensity of specific behavioral health care interventions is independent of the therapeutic milieu. This service intensity reflects the frequency and type of treatment. Table 6–1 depicts the relationship of common services to these two types of intensity: milieu intensity and service intensity. However, one should keep in mind that the typological name given to a treatment facility or program can vary and the characteristics of different facilities overlap greatly. For example, a particular day treatment program may have a lower intensity of service provision than does a particular group home.

Review of Table 6–1 suggests that efforts to understand the appropriate placement of an individual require the assessment of residential and treatment needs. Thus one of the complexities of research in this area is the necessity of including both predictors of milieu intensity and predictors of service intensity in level of care guidelines and decision support models. This may be one of the reasons there are few comprehensive models of level of care that incorporate the full array of available services. Rather, the work to date has focused on elaborating decisions between two levels of care (e.g., hospitalization or not, residential placement or not). This pattern of replacing one type of care with another in a categorical fashion is antithetical to the continuum of care and does not adequately move toward integration (see Chapter 3).

Decision analysis approaches in outcomes management are unique both from a measurement and a methodological standpoint. In terms of measure-

TABLE 6–1. Conceptualization of levels of care on dimensions of milieu and service intensity with examples of services for each level

Milieu intensity	Service intensity	Examples
High	High	Psychiatric hospitalization
High	Medium	Residential treatment
High	Low	Board and care
Medium	High	Partial hospitalization, assertive outreach
Medium	Medium	Wraparound services, skills training
Medium	Low	Group home
Low	High	Day treatment, psychosocial rehabilitation
Low	Medium	Intensive outpatient
Low	Low	Traditional outpatient, primary care

ment the goals of decision analysis are fairly static, as the measurement generally takes place at one point in time. With regard to level of care, these decisions often are reconsidered at different points during an episode of care, especially transitions and evaluations (see Chapter 7); however, each decision point is relatively independent. The first step of successful measurement is to identify those clinical characteristics that should be related to the target decision.

The unique aspect of level of care definitions in psychiatry is that they generally represent an assessment of risk: the likelihood of an untoward outcome at a less intensive level of care. For adults, the primary risk factors are suicide, violence to others, and profound self-care impairment (Allen 1997). For children and adolescents, additional risks may include elopement, crime and delinquency, and sexually abusive behavior (Lyons et al. 1997a). Ironically, the risk criteria were first advanced as the conditions of involuntary admission to protect the civil rights of persons with mental illness. In the managed care environment these have become medical necessity criteria.

The "least restrictive alternative" principle, which historically protected individual rights, has turned into a debatable and poorly understood rationale for lowering the intensity (and therefore costs) of services (Johnston and Sherman 1993). *Medical necessity* is a concept that lacks universal acceptance in the manner it is applied because there are so many different perspectives on what the term means (Hein 1997). Both physicians and their patients, as well as insurers or employers, must negotiate, often with frustration and animosity, to obtain the services they feel they need. There is a danger that level of care decisions will be made based on the cost containment perspective of the payor rather than on a determination of what is clinically necessary for the consumer.

In behavioral health care one of the complexities of analyzing decisions concerning level of care is that the clinical characteristics that inform decision making are more relevant at higher levels of care. In addition, rapid changes in the service system have resulted in outcomes expectations for services at all levels. For example, the rapid reduction in length of hospital stays has moved the focus from symptom relief to risk reduction, crisis stabilization, and resource mobilization (Coleman et al. 1996). Thus, there is generally insufficient time during inpatient stays to provide treatment intended to ameliorate the symptoms of psychiatric disorders beyond those that place the person or others in danger of harm.

For the highest levels of milieu intensity, the presence of risk behaviors is the most important clinical consideration. The level of actual risk, however, is offset at least somewhat by the qualities of the individual's current living environment. For example, one would be comfortable treating an individual with suicidal ideation in an intensive outpatient program if he or she lived with family members who were knowledgeable about the person's problems and could provide a sufficient level of monitoring, support, and/or supervision. Once risks are stabilized, the discharge decision making is influenced more by consideration of the severity of symptoms and impairments in functioning (Deane et al. 1995). If risks cannot be stabilized, then there is a need for continuing the intensive level of either milieu or service. This is a common problem in child welfare because foster parents who can successfully manage children with significant risk behaviors are difficult to find. Referring wards of the state from psychiatric hospitals to residential treatment is common (Lyons et al. 1998).

Most risks, particularly suicide and dangerousness, influence decisions about both milieu and service intensity. These relationships can be somewhat independent for self-care risks. For example, self-care impairments, particularly those determined by the individual's executive cognitive functioning, can influence milieu intensity but may be less important for considerations about service intensity (Royall et al. 1993). Thus, board and care or other residential placements might be guided by chronic self-care impairments that make it dangerous for a person with severe and persistent mental illness to live independently.

Decisions about service intensity sometimes can be made independently of those about milieu intensity. For example, regardless of a person's living arrangement, consideration may be given to his or her suitability for psychosocial rehabilitation. Rehabilitation programs are designed to improve functioning (Anthony 1996). Therefore, this level of service intensity is indicated when a person with severe and persistent mental illness has significant but addressable functional impairments. Anderson and Lewis (1999) reported that only a subset of people living in intermediate care facilities for those who are mentally ill use the workshops and other rehabilitative services. Not surprisingly, these are often the least severely ill among those living in these intensive milieu service settings.

For individuals who have symptoms and subjective distress but are not a danger to themselves or others and have no significant functional impairments, traditional outpatient mental health services are indicated. This population represents the vast majority of individuals with behavioral health care needs. However, it is a definition in the negative. In other words, we can define persons who need more than outpatient services, but it becomes difficult to define who actually needs outpatient services, specifically. It may be possible to determine what characteristics are most associated with the ability to successfully benefit from psychotherapeutic and psychopharmacologic interventions. However, the research attempting to identify these characteristics is by no means definitive. Determining when outpatient behavioral health care is medically necessary is an exceptionally complex endeavor.

It is important to note that the characteristics included in a decision analysis approach should be clinical. Inclusion of demographic variables, although common in research, is inappropriate for purposes of decision support. For example, when Longres and Torrecilha (1992) analyzed out-of-home placements they found that race was a factor in these decisions. The implication of this finding is not that race should be included in the decision model. Instead, it provides evidence of problems of cultural competence. If a provider has equivalent decision-making processes that result in equivalent outcomes across members of different cultural groups, then we can be more confident that the provider is competent to serve people of the different cultures represented. If, on the other hand, one group has significantly different decision-making processes or outcomes, more evaluation is needed to determine whether deficits in cultural competence exist. Once established, clinical models of decision support can be used to assess cultural and gender competence, but these and similar variables should not be included in the decision model. For example, the proportion of African Americans hospitalized in the face of a model that predicts an alternative (e.g., in-home services) should be the same as this proportion for Caucasians.

METHODOLOGY OF DECISION ANALYSIS

The methodological approaches to decision analysis include the use of multivariate statistical models, decision support algorithms, and cutoff scores. The choice of which methodological approach to pursue will influence later decisions on implementation and applications.

Multivariate Statistical Models

Within the multivariate statistical models category of approaches, several different statistical models have been used. The most common strategy is to use logistic regression to predict the target decision (note that discriminant function analysis can be used in an identical fashion). Once the regression equation is established, it is possible to assign predicted group membership to any new case.

We have used this method on a number of occasions for modeling decisions about admission to the psychiatric hospital (Lyons et al. 1997a, 1997c). Once established, a logistic regression can be used to calculate the probability that a case with particular characteristics would be hospitalized (or not). Using this technique, we have demonstrated that inappropriate admissions have worse in-hospital outcomes than do appropriate admissions (Lyons et al. 1997c).

Because these approaches are quite powerful statistically, it is crucial to cross-validate any models on new samples before using them in clinical practice. Logistic regression will take advantage of sample specific covariation to identify a model that is optimal for that particular sample. This model may not be valid for different samples.

Cutoff Scores

Some decision support tools, particularly those based on classic psychometric test theory (e.g., Nunnally 1976), require the decision maker to complete a questionnaire and score it. Decisions are made based on a certain cutoff score. The key to understanding the utility of cutoff scores is to establish the score with the optimal sensitivity and specificity. Sensitivity refers to the ability of the cutoff score to identify a true case. The specificity refers to its ability to identify a true "non-case."

The receiver operating characteristic curve is one method used to determine the maximum validity for a cutoff score (Murphy et al. 1987). On a graph, the complement of specificity (i.e., 1-specificity) is graphed against the sensitivity of the instrument at each possible cutoff score, producing a curve that can be used to determine 1) the cutoff score that results in the optimal sensitivity and specificity compared to an appropriate gold standard and 2) the overall discriminative performance of the instrument as measured by the area under the curve.

Decision Support Algorithms

A third approach to providing decision support is to establish guidelines or algorithms that involve more complex profiles of characteristics. The advantage of algorithms is that they do not require statistical applications nor do they require the reduction of a potentially complex set of variables into a single number. The disadvantage of the approach is that it tends to be more complicated in its application. Generally, the specification of a decision algorithm requires Boolean logic.

Table 6–2 provides an example of a decision support algorithm for use in level of care decisions concerning children and adolescents. This algorithm is

TABLE 6–2.	An example of a decision support algorithm using the Severity of Psychiatric Illness–Child and Adolescent Version

Level I. Psychiatric hospital
  A. Presence of a level of symptoms consistent with a serious emotional disorder.
  B. Presence of an acute risk behavior (e.g., suicide, danger to others, impulsivity)
  C. Presence of problems of caregiver capacity

Level II. Residential treatment center
  A. Presence of a level of symptoms consistent with a serious emotional disorder
  B. Presence of at least one recent risk behavior
  C. Presence of problems with caregiver capacity

Level III. Individualized services in community placement (wraparound)
  A. Presence of a level of symptoms consistent with a serious emotional disorder
  B. Presence of at least historical or recent risk behaviors
  C. Absence of any caregiver problems

Level IV. Outpatient services only
  A. Presence of some symptoms of a psychiatric disorder
  B. Absence of acute risk behaviors
  C. Absence of any caregiver capacity problems

Level V. Family therapy with caregiver(s) only
  A. Absence of symptoms of psychiatric disorder
  B. Absence of risk behaviors
  C. Presence of problems with caregiver capacity

based on the Severity of Psychiatric Illness—Child and Adolescent Version (CSPI; Lyons 1998). The CSPI is a decision support and outcome monitoring tool that assesses three multi-item dimensions: symptoms, risk behaviors, and caregiver capacity. The decision support model uses various profiles across these three dimensions. Each dimension is rated on a 4-point scale. A score of 0 represents "no evidence": under these conditions no action is required on that dimension. A score of 1 represents a subthreshold problem that should be watched because preventive services might be indicated but no direct action may be needed. A 2 represents a level that requires action, such as a diagnosable serious emotional disorder. A score of 3 represents a level that requires immediate or intensive action, for example, under suicide potential a 3 is given when there has been both a recent attempt and current ideation. As demonstrated in Table 6–2, the individual items of the CSPI are then used in profiles rather than added up into a total score to provide decision support to case managers and other providers.

DECISION SUPPORT TOOLS

The process of making level of care decisions can be systematized using any of the methods discussed above. Several researchers have devised tools that efficiently assess the information required to make these decisions. Some have used utilization history or global demographic characteristics to make the decisions. However, neither of these methods functions well to provide appropriate information about an individual patient's needs. Instead, using the patient's clinical characteristics is much more informative and gives a comprehensive assessment of needs. Table 6–3 shows instruments we selected that feature clinical characteristics and emphasize more comprehensive, objective, and substantiated information in deciding level of care. The instruments described tend to adhere to a philosophy of care across a continuum. This listing is intended to provide examples of a few of the instruments that are available, not to be an exhaustive review of all methods and combinations of instruments used in practice.

PRINCIPLES FOR THE DEVELOPMENT AND CHOICE OF LEVEL OF CARE DEFINITIONS AND DECISION SUPPORT

There are some basic guiding principles to consider when developing, selecting, and using a level of care decision support tool (see Gray and Glazer 1994; Sowers 1998; and Chapter 7, this volume). The following provides a summary of some of the more important considerations:

1. Decision support should not be an expert system. There will always have to be a human element involved in the decision making. In other words, decision support tools are *aids* to clinical decision makers, they should not replace them.
2. Decision support tools for level of care should not be diagnostically driven. There is little evidence that diagnoses influence service or milieu intensity. Diagnoses primarily influence the type of treatment.
3. The inputs into any decision support tool must be quantifiable.
4. A need to be comprehensive must be balanced with a need to be brief. Our guidelines have always been that clinicians cannot be expected to use consistently any form that takes more than 5 minutes to complete. Therefore, efficiency of form and informational content are primary objectives.
5. To the extent possible, the level of care model should be based on the clinical needs (and strengths) of the person and not on his or her history of service use. This is particularly important in a rapidly changing service system in which the previous use of a service has a different meaning than does current use.

TABLE 6–3. Decision assistance tools

Instruments designed to assess needs and determine appropriate level of care

1. **Camberwell Assessment of Needs** instrument from the London Institute of Psychiatry (Phelan et al. 1993)

This instrument is designed to assess clinical as well as social needs of people with serious mental illness. There is both a clinical and a research version. The clinical interview format covers 22 areas, including items such as self-care, physical health, psychotic symptoms, safety to self, safety to others, child care, and social benefits. The instrument determines the severity of the problem in terms of *no problem, no problem or moderate problem due to continuing intervention,* or *serious problem.* In addition, it rates the adequacy of the help only as either yes or no. This instrument has demonstrated high inter-rater reliability (Hansson et al. 1995).

Commentary: This instrument can assess particular needs, but is not especially equipped to match to specific levels of care. Instead, it allows only for approximate anchor points of level of care.

2. **New York Level of Care Survey and derivations**

The Level of Care Utilization System for Psychiatric and Addiction Services, developed by the American Association of Community Psychiatrists (1996). Based on the original New York State Level of Care Survey, this amended method defines dimensions of patient evaluation of functioning, dangerousness, history, etc. It also defines different levels of care, such as outpatient and secure residential, that are described in terms of the resources they have available. A proposed method of scoring is offered to facilitate decisions of placement and level of care.

Commentary: This instrument integrates substance use and other mental health conditions. Thus far, the method is still in the process of being evaluated (Sowers 1998).

3. **Missouri Level of Care** (Massey et al. 1989)

This instrument was designed to improve residential treatment placement prediction by taking into account the state's available facilities. This was based on the idea that the population and service characteristics of, and even terminology used for, treatment facilities vary across states and regions. The Missouri Level of Care is a 79-item questionnaire, originally based on the New York State Level of Care Survey (see above), based on Missouri's continuum of care, with items that address specific functioning abilities, behavior problems, and care requirements, including items such as level of family support and patient motivation. The instrument yields the probability of appropriate placement in each of several facility types as well as identifying the most appropriate placement for the client. In general, a study of the instrument demonstrated that the instrument can identify the best one or two facility types for patients (Kramer et al. 1990). Later analyses of the Missouri Level of Care have come up with seven factors in its composition: community living skills, self-care, nuisance behavior, sociability, need for skilled nursing, proclivity for violence, and control of anger (Massey et al. 1989).

Commentary: This instrument illustrates how specific aspects of the environment (such as local service delivery systems, resources available) can be implemented into a measure, making it more useful for the population served.

TABLE 6–3. Decision assistance tools (*continued*)

4. **American Society of Addiction Medicine/Dimension Rating System** (May 1998)

The patient placement criteria published by the American Society of Addiction Medicine (ASAM; 1996) represent the dimensions of behavior used to make decisions for substance-abusing patients. The procedure is used to match treatment modalities (four levels of care) to assessment of symptom severity in six domains associated with positive treatment outcomes. The ASAM criteria were implemented and modified into a new instrument by May (1998) and published as the Dimension Rating System. This instrument has anchored responses to six dimensions: withdrawal, biomedical, biomedical, motivation, recovery potential, and quality of recovery environment.

Commentary: This ASAM criteria-based tool has been shown to be useful in programs that emphasize 12-step facilitation (May 1998), but perhaps is not as useful in other types of programming (e.g., Project MATCH, Project MATCH Research Group 1997).

5. **Severity of Psychiatric Illness** (Lyons 1998a; 1998b)

There are three versions of this instrument, one for adults in acute care settings, an expanded version for adults in community mental health settings, and one for children and adolescents (5–18 years old). The adult acute care version has been widely used and validated (Lyons 1998a; Lyons et al. 1997c; Lyons et al. 1995). The child and adolescent version gathers information on current and historical clinical characteristics, such as emotional disturbance, conduct or behavioral disturbance, and impulsivity (Lyons 1998b; Lyons et al. 1997a). An empirically constructed guideline for level of care decisions based on the severity of the items is provided. The community mental health version is an expansion of the acute care instrument that includes dimensions relevant to service planning in community settings. It is now being piloted at four sites. Early findings suggest that it is reliable and valid.

Commentary: This instrument uses clinical characteristics as opposed to utilization history. It has very high face validity and is easy to use reliably. It can be used either prospectively or retrospectively. It has built-in audit potential to monitor the quality and consistency of decision making.

Use of two or more instruments or particular method to determine level of care.

Some investigators have tried to assess how well various instruments (such as functioning assessment or clinical rating tools) together might help in making level of care decisions or how a system using various types of measures might be implemented to structure level of care decision making. Here, brief examples of these methods are given below:

TABLE 6–3. Decision assistance tools *(continued)*

1. Using a global clinical assessment, the **REHAB (Rehabilitation Evaluation of Hall and Baker;** Baker and Hall 1986) scale, and a clinical rating instrument, the Brief Psychiatric Rating Scale—Expanded Version (BPRS-E), as measures of potential for discharge and rehabilitation, Ruud et al. (1998) used logistic regression to determine how to predict global assessment of level of care. The REHAB scale includes assessments of functioning, such as behavior, self-care, speech skills, and community skills (Baker and Hall 1986). Only some of the BPRS-E (Lukoff et al. 1986) subscales were used in this study (hostile-suspiciousness, thought disturbance, anergia, and activation). The authors concluded that it was impossible to make placements decisions based on the REHAB alone but REHAB in combination with the more clinical BPRS-E may offer a better opportunity to obtain good placement information for recipients (Ruud et al. 1998). The REHAB general behavior scale, along with age, predicted 88% of the classification of need for institutional care or not. The REHAB instrument, then, helps identify patients who can potentially be placed in the community, whereas the BPRS-E may help identify those who are still in need of psychiatric institutional care (Ruud et al. 1998).

2. The **Level of Need-Care Assessment (LONCA)** method (Uehara et al. 1994) was developed in *Washington State* as a way of allocating resources for mental health services. Using a variety of tools, it follows several steps to link resources to needs. First, consumer needs in specific domains of functioning are measured. Then, the minimal but appropriate type and intensity of services are specified, and consumers with similar need and cost profiles are clustered. A rather complex system underlies each of these steps. In fact, the method's complexity may make it less useful for clinical decision making (Sowers 1998).

3. **Level of Care Utilization System for Psychiatric and Addiction Services (LOCUS)** (Version 2000; American Association of Community Psychiatrists 2000); and **Child and Adolescent Level of Care Utilization System (CALOCUS)** (Version 1.5, American Association of Community Psychiatrists/ American Academy of Child and Adolescent Psychiatry 2000)

   The LOCUS is a multidimensional assessment designed to assess service needs and guide the matching of clients to six levels of resource intensity and recommended level of care. Evaluation parameters, defined on a scale of one to five, include risk of harm, functional status, comorbidity, recovery environment, history, and engagement. Each of the six levels of care are described by four flexible service categories, including care environment, clinical service, support services, and crisis resolution and prevention services. Reliability and validity of the instrument have been favorably demonstrated (Sowers et al. 1999). The child and adolescent version of the instrument (CALOCUS) has similar structure and may be used with populations with developmental as well as psychiatric disorders. It is primarily used for initial level of care placement decisions but may also be used in service planning and outcome monitoring.
   Commentary: The LOCUS instruments provide thorough assessments of level of care needs and are therefore somewhat more complex and time consuming than some instruments. Because they were developed using a multidisciplinary consensus process, however, they have high clinical utility and relevance.

6. The ideal decision support tool is consistent with practice guidelines and medical necessity criteria and has implications for service planning and anticipated outcomes. Thus the validation of a level of care decision support tool requires not only that it predict actual decisions but that it predict differential outcomes when its recommended decisions are not followed.

7. Successful implementation of decision support tools requires the buy-in of all stakeholders. Over time the ease of use and value of the information provided will determine whether the tool is successful.

Clinical Illustration of the Use of a Level of Care Decision Support Tool

To illustrate the process of developing and implementing a decision support tool, we discuss the use of the CSPI measure with statewide crisis assessment services for child welfare in Illinois. The CSPI is a 26-item tool that allows for the description of mental health needs of children (5 years of age and older) and adolescents. Originally, the CSPI was developed for a needs-based planning project regarding residential placements (Lyons et al. 1998). This planning was expanded to include crisis assessment and psychiatric hospitalization services (Lyons et al. 1997a).

In Illinois all wards of the state who are in crisis and may need psychiatric hospitalization are seen by a crisis worker under the auspices of a statewide screening, assessment, and support services (SASS) program that is contracted to local mental health provider agencies. SASS workers assess the children or adolescents in their natural environments and determine whether psychiatric hospitalization is warranted and if not, what types of intensive community-based services are needed to stabilize the children. The goal of SASS is not to reduce hospital use but rather to ensure that the mental health needs of wards are met with the appropriate level of care.

Originally, the CSPI was used in a retrospective review of SASS files in Cook County. This review suggested that about 70% of hospitalization decisions were predictable based on the level of risk (i.e., suicide potential, dangerousness to others, and impulsivity; see Lyons et al. 1997a). This review also demonstrated that home or relative placements were much more willing to manage deflections than were foster parents or even residential treatment settings. This review was used to 1) establish the validity of the CSPI for this service population, 2) develop some benchmarks for comparison, and 3) build enthusiasm for the use of the CSPI prospectively.

In the next step, SASS crisis workers were trained in the reliable use of the CSPI and asked to complete this measure after all screenings. The completed forms were sent to a central location for data processing. Initially, no reports were generated. This was intentional because we wanted the workers to get used to completing the forms but to have no consequences associated with the scores. After the CSPI was used in this manner for about 9 months, a full service reporting system that included the CSPI was implemented. Since that time data on all cases have been submitted monthly. From these data, reports are generated that provide analyses of decision making. Specifically, cases are identified (using logistic regression models) that are either low-risk admissions (i.e., possible inappropriate use of hospital) or high-risk deflections (i.e., possible inappropriate failure to use the hospital). Thus, the decision model provides an analysis of each case benchmarked against the performance of all SASS workers statewide. Each SASS agency is asked to explain cases that do not fit the decision making of their statewide peers.

When we first started giving feedback, we got an interesting response. Some SASS workers apparently thought that decision misses meant they needed to fill out the CSPI differently (rather than think differently about identified cases). It took some convincing to help them understand that the goal was not to sanction questionable decision making but rather to initiate a dialogue about complicated cases. The only sanction has been that it is necessary to complete the CSPI for the agency to get credit for serving the child. Agency service logs influence future levels of funding. To manage the risk that workers would begin to "game" the CSPI, we initiated a random audit procedure. Because this measure can be used retrospectively or prospectively with equivalent reliability and validity, we are able to randomly select six cases each year from each agency and complete the CSPI based on clinical data in the file. This provides a check for gaming and assesses needs for additional training in the reliable use of the measure. In general, results of these audits suggest that the form continues to be used reliably.

There are several salient points regarding this case example. First, care was taken to involve stakeholders in the original design of the instrument and document its utility with the target population. This was important in building credibility for the approach. Second, the actual decision support has never been proactive. In other words, crisis workers do not complete the CSPI and check what they should decide with regard to hospitalization. We have consistently believed that to do so is not clinically appropriate. Rather, the decision support is accomplished in a quality improvement model well after actual service delivery and benchmarked on the decision making of peers. This process also reduces the chance of untoward consequences and enhances the credibility of the approach. Finally, although used after the fact, the data do not grow too old before their inclusion in the reports. Agencies and workers receive feedback within a maximum of 8 weeks of actual service delivery.

SUMMARY

In the behavioral health care service sector, the decision about level of care is the single most important determinant of the costs of a service episode. It is also quite likely a significant determinant of both the short- and the long-term clinical outcome of a case. Because of these circumstances, building clinical models for cost-effective decision making is a priority within the mental health service system. As a foundation for understanding the clinical rationale for these decisions, level of care options can be clarified along two dimensions of service intensity and milieu intensity. Recent research and developments within managed behavioral health care have demonstrated that aspects of these decisions are quite rational and predictable. Further decision support tools can be used to improve the consistency of decision making and identify opportunities for quality improvement. When used properly, they can lessen the influence of eccentricities and politics in clinical decision making (Gray and Glazer 1994).

To date, the majority of work has focused on decisions about the use of hospitalization. Much more work is needed to identify the clinical models that extend across the full array of service and setting options within the mental health services system of care. The primary consequence of developing reliable and valid level of care models and instruments that support these models is that they help us ensure that people with mental illness receive the type of services they need in the settings best suited for good outcomes. The secondary consequence of this work is that it develops and documents the sound clinical reasoning behind the use of services in the behavioral health care industry. Such documentation is critical for the long-term success of behavioral health care providers in our evolving age of accountability.

REFERENCES

Allen J: Assessing and managing risk of violence in the mentally disordered. J Psychiatr Ment Health Nurs 4:369–378, 1997

American Association of Community Psychiatrists: Level of Care Utilization System for Psychiatric and Addiction Services. Pittsburgh, PA, American Association of Community Psychiatrists, 2000

American Association of Community Psychiatrists/American Academy of Child and Adolescent Psychiatry: Child and Adolescent Level of Care Utilization System. Pittsburgh, PA, American Association of Community Psychiatrists, 2000

American Society of Addiction Medicine: ASAM Patient Placement Criteria for the Treatment of Substance Related Disorders, 2nd Edition. Chevy Chase, MD, American Society of Addiction Medicine, 1996

Anderson RL, Lewis D: Clinical characteristics and service use of persons with mental illness living in an intermediate care facility. Psychiatr Serv 50:1341–1345, 1999

Anthony WA: Integrating psychiatric rehabilitation into managed care. Psychiatric Rehabilitation Journal 20:39–44, 1996

Baker R, Hall JN: User's Manual for Rehabilitation Evaluation of Hall and Baker. Aberdeen, UK, Vine Publishing, 1986

Baumann AO, Deber RB, Thompson GG: Overconfidence among physicians and nurses: the "micro-certainty, macro-uncertainty" phenomenon. Soc Sci Med 32:167–174, 1991

Bickman L, Karver MS, Schut LJ: Clinician reliability and accuracy in judging appropriate level of care. J Consult Clin Psychol 65:515–520, 1997

Chase J, Crow RA, Lamond D: Overview and critique of judgment and decision making in health care: social and procedural dimensions. J Eval Clin Pract 2:205–210, 1996

Coleman RL, Hunter DEF, Vartelas H, et al: Quality management in mental health, II: managing risk of dangerousness. Am J Med Qual 11:227–235, 1996

Deane FP, Huzziff R, Beaumont G: Discharge planning: levels of care and behavioural functioning in long-term psychiatric inpatients transferred to community hospitals. Community Mental Health in New Zealand 9:18–27, 1995

Gray GV, Glazer WM: Psychiatric decision making in the 90s: the coming era of decision support. Behav Healthc Tomorrow 3:47–54, 1994

Hansson L, Bjorkman T, Svensson B: The assessment of needs in psychiatric patients. interrater reliability of the Swedish version of the Camberwell Assessment of Needs instrument and results from a cross-sectional study. Acta Psychiatr Scand 92:285–293, 1995

Hein K: Medical necessity: making sense out of nonsense. Journal of the American Board of Family Practice 10:222–226, 1997

Hendryx MS, Rohland BM: Psychiatric hospitalization decision making by CMHC staff. Community Ment Health J 33:63–73, 1997

Johnston JM, Sherman RA: Applying the least restrictive alternative principle to treatment decisions: a legal and behavioral analysis. The Behavior Analyst 16:103–115, 1993

Kiser LJ, Lefkovitz PM, Kennedy LL, et al: The Continuum of Behavioral Health Care Services. Alexandria, VA, Assocation for Ambulatory Behavioral Healthcare, 1999

Kramer HB, Massey OT, Pokorny LJ: Development and validation of a level-of-care instrument for predicting residential placement. Hospital and Community Psychiatry 41:407–412, 1990

Longres JF, Torrecilha RS: Race and the diagnosis, placement, and exit status of children and youth in a mental health disability system. Journal of Social Services Research 15:43–63, 1992

Lukoff D, Liberman RP, Nuechterlein KH: Symptom monitoring in the rehabilitation of schizophrenic patients. Schizophr Bull 12:578–602, 1986

Lyons JS: Severity and Acuity of Psychiatric Illness Manual: Adult Version. San Antonio, TX, The Psychological Corporation, Harcourt Brace Jovanovich, 1998a

Lyons JS: Severity and Acuity of Psychiatric Illness Manual: Child and Adolescent Version. San Antonio, TX, The Psychological Corporation, Harcourt Brace Jovanovich, 1998b

Lyons JS, Colletta J, Devens M, et al: The validity of the Severity of Psychiatric Illness in a sample of inpatients on a psychogeriatric unit. Int Psychogeriatr 7:407–416, 1995

Lyons JS, Kisiel CL, Dulcan M, et al: Crisis assessment and psychiatric hospitalization of children and adolescents in state custody. Journal of Child and Family Studies 6:311–320, 1997a

Lyons JS, Howard KI, O'Mahoney MT, et al: The Measurement and Management of Clinical Outcomes in Mental Health. New York, John Wiley and Sons, 1997b

Lyons JS, Stutesman J, Neme J, et al: Predicting psychiatric emergency admissions and hospital outcomes. Med Care 35:792–800, 1997c

Lyons JS, Mintzer LL, Kisiel CL, et al: Understanding the mental health needs of children in residential treatment. Professional Psychology: Research and Practice 29:582–587, 1998

Massey OT, Pokorny LJ, Kramer HB: The development of factor-based level of functioning scales from a level of care instrument. J Clin Psychol 45:903–909, 1989

May WW: A field application of the ASAM placement criteria in a 12-step model of treatment for chemical dependency. Journal of Addictive Diseases 17:77–91, 1998

Mechanic D, McAlpine DD, Olfson M: Changing patterns of psychiatric inpatient care in the United States, 1988–1994. Arch Gen Psychiatry 55:785–791, 1998

Murphy JM, Berwick DM, Weinstein MC, et al: Performance of screening and diagnostic tests; application of receiver operating characteristic analysis. Arch Gen Psychiatry 44:550–555, 1987

Nunnaly J: Psychometric Theory. New York, John Wiley and Sons, 1976

Phelan M, Slade M, Dunn G, et al: Camberwell Assessment of Need. London, England, London Institute of Psychiatry, 1993

Project MATCH Research Group: Matching alcoholism treatments to client heterogeneity: Project MATCH post-treatment drinking outcomes. J Stud Alcohol Jan:7–29, 1997

Royall DR, Mahurin RK, True JE, et al: Executive impairment among the functionally dependent: comparisons between schizophrenic and elderly subjects. Am J Psychiatry, 150:1813–1819, 1993

Ruud T, Martinsen EW, Friis S: Chronic patients in psychiatric institutions: psychopathology, level of functioning and need for care. Acta Psychiatr Scand 97:55–61, 1998

Sowers W: Level-of-care determinations in psychiatry. Harv Rev Psychiatry 5:286–290, 1998

Uehara ES, Smukler M, Newman FL: Linking resource use to consumer level of need: field test of the Level of Need-Care Assessment (LONCA) method. J Consult Clin Psychol 62:695–709, 1994

Yohanna D, Christopher NJ, Lyons JS, et al: Characteristics of short-stay admissions to a psychiatric inpatient service. J Behav Health Serv Res 25:337–346, 1998

7

Movement Along the Continuum of Care

Eunice Hartman, R.N., M.S., C.S., C.N.A.A.

Previous chapters focused on the *structure* of an integrated delivery system (IDS), including issues related to the design and structure of a full continuum of care, establishing a central point of access and level of care criteria. The next challenge for an organization is to address the *processes* of integrating care delivery across the continuum of services. In this chapter I present eight strategies for developing an integrated, consumer-focused culture throughout the continuum and facilitating continuity of care as clients move among levels of care.

STRATEGIES FOR ESTABLISHING EFFICIENT COORDINATION AND INTEGRATION OF CARE

Strategy 1: Education and Training

Helping employees understand, accept, and embrace the changing paradigms of treatment in today's behavioral health market is a challenge all provider organizations face, especially newly integrated systems of care. An organization must make a concerted and consistent effort to provide the training required to ensure that professionals have the knowledge and tools they need to be successful in the changing environment. Education and training should facilitate employees' understanding of the need for integrated systems in today's market and of managed care and continuous quality improvement concepts. Giving staff the information and tools required to understand the changing models of care as well as an opportunity to participate in the design of efficient processes of care across the continuum empowers them as crucial players in designing and implementing needed changes in service delivery.

Communication and education about internal aspects of the system are also critical. To change existing cultures, clinical staff members need to develop a system alliance that overrides the program alliance. Thus, the mission and the vision of the IDS need to be articulated and understood throughout the continuum of care. Staff members need to understand how their roles and their programs contribute to the organizational mission and how the organization fits into the bigger picture of behavioral health care delivery. Staff members should be integral participants in the development of and be thoroughly trained in the level of care criteria, policies and procedures, clinical pathways, and disease management protocols for the IDS. The importance of communicating logistical information about all of the programs and services in the system should not be overlooked—information such as contact persons, hours of operation, telephone numbers, addresses, specialty services, and the range of services provided within each program needs to be emphasized. Additionally, both program and employee performance standards that reflect the organization's values can help staff members achieve success in this new playing field.

Strategy 2: Joint Planning Across the Integrated Delivery System

As organizations form strategic alliances or partnerships to develop integrated continuums of care, key staff members from each organization/program should be involved in developing or selecting the tools that will be used throughout the continuum. Joint planning facilitates the development of an "integrated culture" and a uniform language across the levels of care. Integrated work groups should be designated to develop or select level of care criteria for all levels of care in the delivery system (see Chapter 8); program performance specifications that meet or exceed the purchasers' requirements; clinical policies, procedures, and protocols that define processes for integrated treatment planning and the movement of clients within the continuum of care; standard assessment, outcome, and satisfaction measures and tools (see Chapters 11 and 15); clinical pathways; and disease management protocols.

Strategy 3: Developing Clinical Policies and Procedures

As an IDS is developed, one of the first priorities is to establish an integrated continuum work group (representing each level of care) to develop the policies and procedures that will be used for all clients throughout the system. Policies and procedures should address issues such as how integrated treatment planning will occur, what the standards for documentation will be, how frequently level of care assessment will be documented, how the clinical record will be integrated, what processes will be in place for referral and transfer to other levels of care (including what documentation will accompany a transfer), what criteria and processes will be used for coordinating with physical health providers, and what criteria and processes will be used for coordinating with human service agencies.

Policies and procedures set standards across the delivery system, but do not address the specific care processes of a population or diagnostic group, per se. However, as clinical pathways are developed, systemwide standards can be incorporated into them. For example, a policy and procedure may be developed that addresses the system's standards for the timing of aftercare appointments. This standard may be reflected in a clinical pathway for the treatment of adults with depression as well as in a pathway for the treatment of children with attention-deficit/hyperactivity disorder.

Strategy 4: Implementing Integrated Treatment Planning

To develop a client-focused, integrated treatment plan that addresses an episode of illness across the continuum of care is both a clinical and a technological challenge. Efficiency can be gained when all staff members work from an integrated, centralized treatment plan with consistent problems and goals being addressed across the continuum of care. The assessment and treatment plan can be updated and progress toward goals noted, instead of duplicating planning and assessment processes at each level of care. Integrated treatment planning provides a sense of continuity for the client, avoids duplication of effort by staff, and decreases the possibility that clients will receive conflicting messages about their treatment.

When a consumer enters a system of care, the initial assessment, preliminary treatment plan, and level of care determination are made through a central access system. During this initial phase of treatment, an integrated treatment team with representatives from the entire continuum of care can be assigned to coordinate treatment planning for the full episode of care. The value of having integrated treatment planning meetings is intrinsic. This planning should include a multidisciplinary team, the consumer (and his or her family or significant others), the primary behavioral health care provider, and representatives from specified programs along the continuum of care as well as involved physical care providers and other human service agencies. For persons with severe and persistent mental illness or addictive disorders, providers from recovery levels of care should also be included. From this team, some IDSs also identify a primary therapist or care manager who facilitates the coordination of services. Other organizations designate a psychiatrist who follows the consumer across all levels of care.

Strategy 5: Developing Level of Care Criteria and Clinical Pathways

Level of care criteria define the structure of the continuum, or what services are appropriate for a given consumer. By mapping out best practices, clinical pathways describe the process of delivering care both within a given level of care and across the continuum. The objective is to establish a professional standard. Chapter 8 is devoted entirely to a discussion of level of care criteria; the focus in this chapter is on understanding and developing clinical pathways.

Understanding Clinical Pathways

The level of care needed by a consumer is based on the assessment of his or her needs and acuity, using level of care criteria. Clinical pathways describe the standards for the processes of care within each level of care. A primary goal is to improve the quality of care and the efficiency of care delivery.

A clinical pathway is a map that describes the course of treatment for clients or consumers with a similar diagnosis. It describes the optimal sequencing and timing of therapeutic interventions for a specific disorder. The purpose of clinical pathways is to bring increased standardization to the processes of care, that is, they serve as tools to manage clinical processes and to maximize the quality of care. Some other terms for the management of clinical processes are *best practice guidelines, practice parameters, clinical guidelines, clinical protocols, clinical algorithms,* and *clinical benchmarking.*

Pathways describe standards, interventions, time and frequency, responsible staff, and outcome measures based on essential elements of treatment at each level of care. They contain specific timelines for interventions to occur as well as the processes for transition to the next level of care. For example, a consumer may meet the level of care criteria for medically monitored detoxification by virtue of having symptoms of withdrawal, a history of substance addiction, and so on. A clinical pathway for this level of care would describe frequency of vital signs evaluations; dosage and frequency of medications for detoxification; and frequency of group, individual, and family therapy (therapy schedules) as well as nutritional assessment, intervention, and education. Clinical pathways should be inclusive of clients' assessment of their own treatment needs, their attitude, their engagement, and their ability to participate in and assume responsibility for their recovery. Essential elements of treatment that should be addressed in a clinical pathway include comprehensive assessment and evaluation, establishing the diagnosis, developing the treatment plan, providing treatment, coordinating care, measuring progress and outcomes, reviewing the treatment plan, and planning the discharge. Table 7–1 presents an overview of these essential elements.

TABLE 7–1.   Components of a treatment pathway

Perform comprehensive assessment/ evaluation	Level of care assessment History and physical examination Psychiatric evaluation Mental status examination Laboratory tests
Establish diagnosis	Observation Process of "rule outs"
Develop treatment plan	Integrated multidisciplinary team Client/family participation Components of care
Provide treatment	Treatment modalities Laboratory tests/consultations Medication Psychoeducation Psychosocial rehabilitation Vocational rehabilitation Peer support Physical health
Coordinate care	Care management Human service agencies Other behavioral health providers Physical health providers Housing Family/significant others Community supports
Measure progress and outcomes	Level of care assessment to guide transitions Measurement tools, type and frequency
Review treatment plan	Integrated, multidisciplinary team Client/family participation Process and frequency
Plan discharge	Barriers to aftercare Physical health services Social services
Facilitate transition and do follow up	Outcome and satisfaction measurement Follow-up

Developing Clinical Pathways

The process of developing level of care criteria and clinical pathways is an invaluable learning experience for any organization. Involving staff in developing criteria and pathways provides an opportunity to begin to challenge assumptions, break down barriers that may exist between various components of the system, and decrease the variances that exist in the delivery of services. Table 7–2 outlines the developmental process.

The first step in developing clinical pathways is to select the diagnostic groups for pathway development. It is not possible to do everything at once, so this process should be kept simple, and uncomplicated pathways should be done first. Diagnostic groups such as depressive disorder, bipolar disorder, schizophrenia, anorexia, and panic disorders are good places to start.

The next step is to identify the team of people to write the pathway. Clinical pathways should be developed by a multidisciplinary group of senior clinicians that is representative of the full continuum of care, with input from clients, families, advocacy groups, and other subject area experts. The team should review numerous models of clinical pathways and select or design the format that will be used in developing pathways specific to its system of care.

TABLE 7–2.   Process for pathway development

Select diagnostic groups for pathway development

Identify a multidisciplinary group of clinicians representative of the continuum of services

Review current literature and other consensus documents

Select/design the format for pathways

Document current practice in each level of care, including timing of assessments, procedures, treatments, consultations, medications, diet, teaching, family involvement

Study internal and external processes: What is done? Why? Does it contribute value? Could it be done more efficiently? Are there barriers?

Solicit input from clinicians, consumers, family members

Ensure that pathways reflect the mission and objectives of the organization

Develop pathways

Define key measures of conformance and outcomes

Select tools for measurement

Secure approval by quality assurance committee and board

Test pathways

Measure variance to pathways

Review and revise

The work group next should document current practice at each level of care (including timing of assessments, procedures, treatments, consultations, use of medications, diet, teaching, family involvement). The group should study internal and external processes to determine what is done and why. Does the process contribute value and could it be done more efficiently? Are there barriers that contribute to delays and inefficiencies? The work group should solicit input from clinicians, clients, and family members as the pathways are developed.

Finally, the work group should improve current clinical pathways by incorporating information from the professional literature and current "best practices" literature into the existing practices. Examples of resources that might be used include *Practice Guidelines* developed by the American Psychiatric Association, the *Expert Consensus Guideline Series* developed by the *Journal of Clinical Psychiatry*, and the *National Institutes of Health Consensus Statements* (National Institutes of Health 1991). Another useful tool is the *Desktop Reference for Managing Chronic Behavioral Disorders*, which discusses integration of services, screening and assessment tools, treatment matching, pharmacological management, outcomes measurement, and relapse prevention. DeRubeis and Crits-Christoph (1998) identified empirically supported, efficacious psychosocial treatments for 10 adult mental health disorders: major depressive disorder, generalized anxiety disorder, social phobia, obsessive-compulsive disorder, agoraphobia, panic disorder, posttraumatic stress disorder, schizophrenia, alcohol abuse and dependence, and substance abuse and dependence. The body of literature to inform the development of clinical pathways is expanding every day, and empirical studies should be used to enhance the organization's current knowledge and experience.

Development of clinical pathways includes describing criteria that necessitate variance from the pathway and any issues or events that would signify the pathway is not indicated. Clinical pathways describe the course of assessment, diagnosis, and treatment for persons with similar diagnostic presentations. They are meant to provide guidelines for the treatment of a diagnostic disorder. They do not define treatment for each individual who has a diagnosis within this diagnostic grouping. Variances may include factors such as legal complications, medication side effects, and placement problems.

As each pathways work group proceeds, the group needs to ensure that the pathway reflects the mission and objectives of the organization. The work group should incorporate the level of care criteria into the pathway and determine the frequency of level of care assessments that guide the movement of clients, it is hoped, to less intensive levels of care. The group also needs to define key measures of conformance and select tools for measurement of outcomes; any systemwide standards should be incorporated into the pathways.

Before clinical pathways are implemented, each pathway should be reviewed and approved by a body such as the quality management committee, as determined by the IDS. Once a pathway is approved, the system can proceed with testing it by measuring and evaluating outcomes and variances from the pathway. Clinical pathways should be reviewed and revised at least annually and as current knowledge regarding preferred practices changes.

Strategy 6: Developing Disease Management Protocols

The terms *disease management protocols* and *clinical pathways* are sometimes used interchangeably, but they are not the same. The distinction is that disease management protocols encompass a broader approach to managing a specific illness. For example, clinical pathways describe and guide the treatment process for a person who is admitted to a system of care, whereas disease management protocols include a broader population approach, with education, prevention, and population screening techniques. Disease management protocols are especially applicable to organizations that have capitated contracts and can use a portion of shared risk dollars to invest in preventive strategies. A clinical pathway for the assessment, diagnosis, and treatment of the illness may be incorporated into the disease management model—that is, it is one component of a total disease management approach.

The development of disease management protocols was initially focused on medical illnesses. *Behavioral Disease Management Report* (Vega 1998) described an American Association of Health Plans (AAHP) report on breast cancer programs developed by several health maintenance organizations (HMOs). The AAHP report emphasized approaches to serve a patient's physical, emotional, and spiritual needs—the psychological implications of breast cancer. In 1999, Blue Cross and Blue Shield of Massachusetts collaborated with the American Psychological Association and the Linda Pollin Institute at Harvard Medical School to study the impact that psychological and social supports have on patients with breast cancer. The goal of this research is to determine whether intensive psychosocial interventions help women who are newly diagnosed with breast cancer. Psychological adjustment, health behaviors, knowledge of disease, involvement in health care, satisfaction, medical cost offset, immunologic function, and long-term outcomes will be measured. This type of empirical research can be used to guide the development of disease management protocols, both for physical and behavioral health.

An IDS has multiple opportunities to develop disease management protocols to guide efforts for education, screening, early intervention, and the integration of physical and behavioral health treatments. The process for developing disease management protocols is similar to that described above for clinical pathways.

Strategy 7: Developing Effective Care Management and Case Management Models

Each organization should evaluate the needs of the populations it serves and plan for care management services to address those needs. Many IDSs have a broad base population, that is, they treat consumers from both public- and private-sector contracts and consumers with episodic or short-term issues as well as consumers with long-term disorders (such as those with severe and persistent mental illness and chronic addictive disorders). To meet the needs of these divergent populations, IDSs have the opportunity to develop innovative care and case management models. The term *care management* is used to describe the role of coordinating treatment, benefits, and authorization for-payment of care, as needed. *Case management* is used to describe a direct service role, that of overseeing provision of the treatment plan, assisting the consumer in negotiating systems of care and/or entitlements, and assisting consumers with the day-to-day management of their responsibilities.

An IDS can create a tiered system of care management by combining components of centralized care management services, program-based care management functions, and community-based or targeted case management. Such a tiered system provides a conceptual framework that is flexible and can be easily adjusted to meet the changing needs of the system and population (e.g., a new contract includes a larger proportion of adults with serious mental illness, or a risk contract is secured by the organization). A tiered model of care management incorporates both care and case management roles, organized to gain efficiencies of scale by centralizing some care management functions (such as data gathering and outcomes measurement) while defining and coordinating program-based and individualized case management functions. A tiered system of care management can be organized in a number of ways.

Centralized Care Management Functions

The development of centralized care management functions is crucial in an IDS's preparation to manage risk-sharing or risk-bearing contracts. Centralized care management functions should truly be value-added services to the programs within the system—they should help programs reach their access, utilization, and quality targets. Care management functions provided by a central service might include service authorization and data collection for risk-based contracts as well as 24-hour screening and referral. This service might also provide care management supervision, strategic planning, psychiatric (and psychopharmacologic) consultation, outcomes measurement and quality management, provider profiling and network management, reporting and data analysis, and information technology development and management. This model allows for efficiencies of scale for subject area expert consultation to the system. Centralized care management can provide senior-level care managers to supervise and oversee program-based care managers. Additionally, centralized care management may schedule follow-up contacts with consumers to determine their status at designated points in time and to collect satisfaction and outcomes data.

Program-Based Care Management Functions

IDSs can expand on existing program infrastructure by adding program-based care management functions. These functions can be designed to oversee the use of clinical pathways and/or disease management protocols to improve standardization of care delivery throughout the system. In this model, the care manager serves as a contact person to facilitate access to indicated services during transitions between levels of care. Program-based care management functions may include follow-up and tracking for persons with an episodic illness on a relatively short-term basis—to ensure that aftercare services are available and sufficient to meet the needs of clients as they move back to their homes and work.

Community-Based or Individual Case Management Functions

Although models vary, most systems of care include the provision of longer-term (sometimes referred to as individualized, intensive, or targeted) case management for consumers with serious mental or addictive disorders. Criteria for the assignment of case management services are needed. *Case Management Practice Guidelines for Adults with Severe and Persistent Mental Illness* (Giesler and Hodge 1997) described three levels of intensity of case management with criteria for each of the levels. Regardless of the model of case management provided, an IDS system needs to assess and develop the processes for the linkage between centralized or program-based care management functions and individualized case management functions.

As with the development of tools for use across the continuum of care, planning for care and case management services should be driven from an integrated work group approach; use empirical data and best practice research to inform development; be inclusive of consumers, advocates, and subject area experts; be evaluated regularly on an ongoing basis; and be revised as current knowledge changes.

Strategy 8: Planning for Successful Transitions

Coordination of care with seamless movement requires helping consumers negotiate successful and expedient transitions between levels of care in the integrated continuum. Techniques to expedite transitions include

Introducing the Consumer to Setting and Staff
Introducing the consumer to the setting and staff allows the consumer to spend some time on site at the next level of care before a transfer. This often affords a level of comfort for the consumer. This process also is inclusive of consumers' input into whether they are ready to make the transition to a lower (or higher) level of care.

Identifying a Primary Caregiver
Consumers feel more supported in making a transition if they have an identified primary care provider. In some systems the psychiatrist may be the primary caregiver and provide medical management across all levels of care. In some systems there may be a primary therapist. Other systems may choose to have the care manager provide continuity for consumers as they move through the continuum of care. One model, as described earlier, is to have a fully integrated treatment team that stays involved in the consumer's care, whatever the setting in the continuum.

Introducing the Consumer to a Peer Liaison
Introduction to a consumer peer liaison is another way to establish support during transition. Consumer liaisons (buddies or peers) can assist the consumer with integration into the milieu and play an instrumental role in assisting in transitions between levels of care. This technique gives assisting consumers a sense of movement and self-worth as they progress in their own recovery (see Chapter 16).

Including the Consumer and Family in Planning
As in all treatment processes, the consumer and family or significant others (as indicated) should be included in the planning for transitions within the continuum. This should include identifying barriers to participation or access to services as well as barriers to the consumer's adherence to the treatment plan.

Providing Outreach and Crisis Planning
An outreach and crisis plan should be in place for the consumer throughout the episode of care and if treatment is terminated. This plan should be developed with input and agreement from the consumer (and family or guardian) and the treatment team. It should be clearly defined and include consumer directives that guide behavioral health treatment in an emergency (see Chapter 9).

Addressing Logistical Issues
Logistical issues such as transportation, child care, adequate prescriptions, and access to a pharmacy need to be addressed with consumers before they

are moved to less intensive levels of care that require more independence, time management, and management of life logistics.

The following case example illustrates how a patient can be helped to make successful transitions from one level of care to the next.

Case Example

M.B., a 24-year-old single mother of two small children, called the toll-free central number to the integrated system. She described suicidal thoughts, symptoms of severe depression, and fear of harming her children. She was at home alone with her children. She had had no previous psychiatric treatment. The central access line was able to help access the mobile crisis team and keep her on the line until the team arrived. The crisis team found M.B. to be overwrought, with vegetative signs of depression, and assessed her to be at extreme risk. Because of feelings of guilt, M.B. had not reached out to her extended family for help. The mobile crisis team arranged for a family member to take care of her children and transported M.B. for hospitalization. It was determined that M.B. was a member of an HMO and that the IDS was managing the behavioral health services for that HMO. The central access line approved the admission and documented the presenting clinical information in the centralized clinical record.

The inpatient assessment determined an initial diagnosis of postpartum depression. M.B. was assigned a program-based care manager from the inpatient unit and was placed on the appropriate clinical pathway (antidepressant medications were provided and there was coordination with her obstetrician/gynecologist and her children's pediatrician). Her progress was monitored using standardized tools and documented in the centralized medical record. The care manager was able to assist in arranging for M.B. to see her children and family members on day 2 of her hospitalization. It was determined, in conjunction with M.B., her family, and the treatment team, that if her progress continued as expected, she would transition to the partial hospital program on day 4 and would be able to be at home with her children in the evening.

On day 3 a program-based care manager came to the inpatient unit to explain the partial program to the patient. M.B. was then taken to visit the partial program and introduced to a peer liaison. Authorization for partial hospitalization was obtained from the centralized care manager. M.B. transitioned to the partial program on day 4, and her medications and treatment continued to be supervised by the psychiatrist from her treatment team. M.B. attended the partial program daily for 5 days and continued on the postpartum depression treatment pathway. Continued assessment indicated the need for parenting classes and a parenting support group as well as outpatient follow-up and medication management. The program-based care manager arranged her aftercare appointments and confirmed that transportation was in place. Follow-up calls were arranged with M.B. to determine that the aftercare plan was initiated. She was discharged to the outpatient department and home on day 9 of the episode of care.

On day 11 the program-based care manager contacted M.B. to determine whether she would attend her first outpatient appointment. M.B. reported that her mother had become ill and was not able to provide transportation to her outpatient appointment. She reported feeling increasingly overwhelmed and depressed. The care manager called the centralized care manager for authorization for home-based treatment. The central care management services contacted M.B.'s HMO and arranged short-term home health care through her pediatrician and a psychiatric visiting nurse to provide a medication visit in her home. Her outpatient appointment was rescheduled, and the care manager checked in with her daily. Within the next week, M.B.'s mother recuperated from her illness and was able to provide additional assistance. M.B. was able to attend her outpatient appointment and the parenting support group the following week. A crisis plan was in place that included a possible readmission for several days to the partial program or additional home health interventions if needed. It was determined that the centralized care manager would call M.B. at 30, 90, and 180 days to conduct outcomes and satisfaction interviews. These data would be added to the centralized record. The 24-hour central service had access to her medical record and her treatment and crisis plan and could contact her current outpatient provider or implement the crisis plan if needed.

SUMMARY

In this chapter I address the challenges faced by an IDS in developing effective processes for the movement of consumers along the continuum of services. Discussions included approaches for making the system client centered and for optimizing service delivery processes for the consumer, specifically, education and communication; integrated treatment planning and record keeping; the establishment of treatment guidelines, clinical pathways, and disease management protocols; the use of care management strategies; and techniques for successful transitions between levels of care. These strategies can be used to improve service coordination as consumers move along the continuum of care.

REFERENCES

Vega P: Breast cancer initiative emphasizes psychological aspects of disease. Behavioral Disease Management Report 2:2, 1998

DeRubeis R, Crits-Christoph P: Empirically supported individual and group psychological treatments for adult mental disorders. J Consult Clin Psychol 66:37–52, 1998

Giesler L, Hodge M: Case Management Practice Guidelines for Adults with Severe and Persistent Mental Illness. Ocean Ridge, FL, National Association of Case Management, July 1997

National Institutes of Health: Diagnosis and treatment of depression in late life. National Institutes of Health Consensus Statement Online, November 4–6, 1991, pp 1–27. Available online at http://odp.od.nih.gov/consensus/cons/086/086-statement.htm

8

Levels of Care

Michael A. Hoge, Ph.D.

Historically, behavioral health services have consisted of two modalities: inpatient care and routine outpatient care. Other modalities of intermediate intensity did exist, but their use remained rather limited, in large part because of private and government insurance programs that typically reimbursed for inpatient care, offered very limited coverage for outpatient services, and seldom reimbursed for other modalities.

This system of incentives and disincentives has changed significantly since the mid-1980s, mainly because of the introduction of managed care. Operating outside the constraints of traditional insurance policies, managed behavioral health care organizations have had the freedom and flexibility to reimburse a much broader range of services. Private and other government insurance programs have followed suit by expanding their range of covered services, driven in part by the dissatisfaction of business and political leaders with the rising cost of health care.

Although the merits of managed care and other efforts at health care cost containment can be debated, the landscape of behavioral health services has been dramatically altered. The broad array of treatment modalities exhibits such infinite variation that it can be confusing to providers, patients, and payors. Using the levels of care concept has emerged as a common approach to classifying and communicating the range of current modalities.

CONCEPT OF LEVELS

When only inpatient and outpatient modalities were in use, selecting a treatment for a specific patient essentially required determining whether a high-intensity (inpatient) or low-intensity (outpatient) clinical intervention was appropriate. This distinction of high versus low easily translated into the notion of *levels of care*. As the number of modalities expanded, professionals simply began to place these on a continuum between inpatient and outpatient, ranked roughly according to level of intensity.

At first blush these orderings suggest that available services fall on a simple linear continuum, with the intensity of services as the defining variable. However, careful examination of current service arrays reveals a far more complex reality (see Table 8–1). Modalities vary not only in intensity but also in function and in form. Each modality addresses one or more treatment functions such as screening and identification, crisis intervention, symptom reduction, stabilization, and relapse prevention. A modality may have some or all of its functions in common with other modalities. Modalities of similar intensity and function are likely to differ in form, perhaps distinguished by factors such as whether the care is delivered in an office or in the community and whether staffing is predominantly professional or paraprofessional. Finally, the average length of stay or duration of treatment for different modalities varies widely.

TABLE 8–1.   Key treatment variables

Treatment function
Screening and identification
Crisis intervention
Symptom reduction
Stabilization
Relapse prevention
Rehabilitation
Growth and development

Treatment intensity
High
Medium
Low

Treatment form
Setting (facility, office, community)
Format (individual, group, family)
Staffing (medical, professional, peer)

Treatment duration
Short term (brief)
Intermediate term
Long term

To complicate matters even further, the matching of an individual with a modality, which is addressed elsewhere in this volume (see Chapter 6), is influenced by numerous patient-related variables such as illness severity, acuity, chronicity, dangerousness, ability to contract for safety, and quality of available social supports. Thus, although the concept of levels of care is still used routinely, it has in practice come to represent the notion of a service matrix in which one or more treatment modalities are matched to an individual's specific characteristics and needs at a specific point in time (McFarland et al. 1997).

THREE APPROACHES TO LEVELS OF CARE

As stated by Srebnik et al. (1998), "levels of care are used implicitly whenever service providers design treatment plans to meet clients' needs" (p. 91). Beyond this implicit use of the concept, three general approaches have been used to more explicitly articulate the levels of care: 1) conceptual models, 2) utilization management and practice guidelines, and 3) decision support tools.

Conceptual Models

A number of experts have developed detailed level of care models. Drawing on published research and theory, they present frameworks for understanding the relationship between modalities. Such models are designed to educate professionals and guide those responsible for designing, funding, and managing systems of care.

As an example of this approach, in 1993 the Association for Ambulatory Behavioral Healthcare issued a position paper defining three levels of service between standard inpatient and outpatient care. The authors, Kiser et al. (1993), grouped modalities into levels by function and delineated the service characteristics and patient characteristics pertaining to each level. Since then Kiser et al. (1999) have extended their analysis to other levels as well.

Utilization Management and Practice Guidelines

As managed behavioral health care organizations became more sophisticated, they began to emphasize the continuum of care and the matching of patients to the most appropriate treatment. To support that work, these organizations developed increasingly detailed written guidelines that govern the staff's utilization management decisions and inform providers about the rules being applied in these decisions. Guidelines such as those published by MCC Behavioral Care (1996) and Merit Behavioral Care Corporation (1997) typically contain a level of care model and associated algorithms for matching patients to an appropriate level of care.

Largely in response to the growth and impact of managed care, professional organizations increasingly have been generating practice guidelines (American Psychiatric Association 1996). Drawing on research findings and expert consensus, these represent attempts to outline recommended approaches to the treatment of various disorders. Similar to the utilization management guidelines crafted by managed behavioral health care organizations, these practice guidelines contain either implicit or explicit level of care models and explicit guidelines or algorithms for matching patients to appropriate modalities. The placement criteria published by the American Society of Addiction Medicine (1991, 1996) are perhaps the best examples of that approach. The authors of these documents argued that they have provided a nomenclature for the continuum of addiction treatment. The most recent edition (American Society of Addiction Medicine 1996) expanded the levels of care identified in the initial edition (1991), reflecting the growing complexity of substance abuse services.

Decision Support Tools

A number of professionals have attempted to introduce a greater level of rigor into the process of defining levels of care and developing algorithms for matching patients to treatments. Gray and Glazer (1994) detailed the history of these efforts involving the development of checklists or rating scales. Ratings of patients and their environments serve as the input into algorithms that yield a recommended level of care or treatment modality. Like the utilization management and practice guidelines described earlier, the level of care models and placement algorithms are derived from research findings and expert consensus. However, their formal structure allows the reliability and validity of these tools to be evaluated (Srebnik et al. 1998). From the vantage point of this discussion, these decision support tools are noteworthy in that they must contain very explicit models and definitions of the levels of care.

CONTINUUM OF BEHAVIORAL HEALTH CARE MODEL

To further explore the concept of levels of care and the treatment modalities currently available, I have outlined below the Association for Ambulatory Behavioral Healthcare model developed by Kiser et al. (1993, 1999). Specific descriptions and a discussion of each level follow, accompanied by case examples illustrating modalities within the level. Tables 8–2 and 8–3 reprint the Kiser et al. (1999) summary of the service and patient characteristics associated with each level.

A few caveats are in order before proceeding. The modalities grouped within a level are functionally similar. An attempt has been made to highlight some

TABLE 8–2. Continuum of behavioral health care: service variables

	Service variables					
	Primary care	Outpatient	Multimodal outpatient	Intermediate ambulatory	Acute ambulatory	Inpatient/Residential
Service function	Provide screening, early identification, and education; medication management	Decrease in symptoms related to mild to moderate disorders; maintain severe stable disorders	Coordinate treatment to prevent decline in functioning when outpatient care cannot meet patient need	Stabilize patient, reduce symptoms, and prevent relapse	Provide crisis stabilization and acute symptom reduction; serve as alternative to and prevention of hospitalization	Provide 24-hour monitoring, supervision, and intensive intervention
Scheduled programming	Incorporated with visits for general medical care	Sessions scheduled as needed with maximum of 3 hours per week	Minimum of 4 hours per week	Minimum of 3–4 hours/day, at least 2–3 days/week	Minimum of 4 hours/day scheduled 4–7 days/week	24 hours/day
Crisis backup availability	Decision-assistance programs; established liaison with behavioral health specialty care, warm lines	On-call coverage	24-hour crisis and consultation service	24-hour crisis and consultation service	Organized, integrated 24-hour crisis backup system with immediate access to current clinical and treatment information	24-hour/day staffing with personnel skilled in crisis intervention
Medical involvement	Not applicable	Medical consultation as needed	Medical consultation as needed	Medical consultation	Medical supervision	Medical management
Accessibility	Regular appointments scheduled within 3–5 days	Regular appointments scheduled within 3–5 days	Capable of admitting within 72 hours	Capable of admitting within 48 hours	Capable of admitting within 24 hours	Capable of admitting within 1 hour

TABLE 8–2. Continuum of behavioral health care: service variables *(continued)*

	Primary care	Outpatient	Multimodal outpatient	Intermediate ambulatory	Acute ambulatory	Inpatient/ Residential
				Service variables		
Milieu	Relationship between provider and patient	Within the session and relationship between therapist and patient	Active therapeutic; primarily within home and community	Active therapeutic within treatment setting, home, and community	Planned, consistent, and therapeutic; primarily within treatment setting	Planned, consistent, and therapeutic within treatment setting
Structure	Minimal; afforded through scheduled appointments	Minimal; afforded through scheduled appointments	Individualized and coordinated	Regularly scheduled, individualized	High degree of structure and scheduling	High degree of structure, security, and supervision
Responsibility and control	Patient functions independently with support from family and community.	Patient functions independently with support from family and community.	Monitoring and support placed primarily with patient, family, and support system.	Monitoring and support shared with patient, family, and support system.	Staff aggressively monitors and supports patient and family.	Staff assumes responsibility for safety and security of patient.
Service examples	Regular medical checkup	Outpatient office visit Specialty group Psychotherapy	Aftercare Clubhouse programs	Psychosocial rehabilitation Day treatment programs Intensive outpatient program 23-hour respite beds	Partial hospital programs Intensive in-home crisis intervention Outpatient detoxification 23-hour observation beds	Acute inpatient unit Crisis stabilization bed

Source. Copyright 1999, Association for Ambulatory Behavioral Healthcare. Used with permission.

TABLE 8–3. Continuum of behavioral health care: patient variables

				Patient variables			
	Primary care	Outpatient	Multimodal outpatient	Intermediate ambulatory	Acute ambulatory	Inpatient/Residential
Level of functioning	At-risk, subclinical, or mild impairment	Mild to moderate impairment in at least one area of daily life	Moderate impairment in at least one area of daily life	Marked impairment in at least one area of daily life	Severe impairment in multiple areas of daily life	Significant impairment with inability to maintain activities of daily living without 24-hour assistance
Psychiatric signs and symptoms	At-risk, subclinical presentation, or mild symptoms related to behavioral health disorder	Mild to moderate symptoms related to acute condition or exacerbation of severe/persistent disorder	Moderate symptoms related to acute condition or exacerbation of severe/persistent disorder	Moderate to severe symptoms related to acute condition or exacerbation of severe/persistent disorder	Severe to disabling symptoms related to acute condition or exacerbation of severe/persistent disorder	Disabling symptoms related to acute condition or exacerbation of severe/persistent disorder
Risk/ dangerousness	At-risk or limited with minimal need for confinement	Limited, transient dangerousness and minimal risk of confinement	Mild instability with limited dangerousness and low risk for confinement	Moderate instability and/or dangerousness with some risk of confinement	Marked instability and/or dangerousness with high risk of confinement	Significant danger to self/others exists
Commitment to treatment/ follow-through	Ability to form and maintain treatment contract	Ability to form and sustain treatment contract	Ability to sustain treatment contract with intermittent monitoring and support	Limited ability to form extended treatment contract; requires frequent monitoring and support	Inability to form more than initial treatment contract; requires close monitoring and support	Inability to form treatment contract; requires constant monitoring and supervision

TABLE 8–3. Continuum of behavioral health care: patient variables *(continued)*

| | Patient variables | | | | | |
	Primary care	Outpatient	Multimodal outpatient	Intermediate ambulatory	Acute ambulatory	Inpatient/Residential
Social support system	Ability to form and maintain relationships outside treatment	Ability to form and maintain relationships outside treatment	Ability to form and maintain relationships outside treatment	Limited ability to form relationships or seek support	Impaired ability to access or use caregiver, family, or community support	Insufficient resources and/or inability to access or use caretaker, family, or community support

Source. Copyright 1999, Association for Ambulatory Behavioral Healthcare. Used with permission.

of the key differences, but an extensive description of each modality is beyond the scope of this chapter. Readers interested in in-depth reviews of specific interventions should refer to texts such as that edited by Schreter et al. (1997). The case examples included in this chapter, which focus on modalities with which the reader is less likely to be familiar, are given both to orient the reader to these modalities and to demonstrate the flexibility and creativity with which service designs can accomplish the desired treatment functions.

Inpatient/Residential

The inpatient/residential level of care provides the most intensive behavioral health interventions currently available on a 24-hour/day basis. From a functional perspective this level is used for crisis stabilization, acute symptom reduction, and improvement in functional capacity when symptoms or functional impairments are so severe that the patient or others are at imminent risk of harm. Thus, lengths of stay tend to be brief. This level offers the highest degree of safety and security through low patient-to-staff ratios that permit frequent, if not constant, observation and supervision tailored to each patient's level of acuity. Self-injurious and assaultive behaviors, when extreme, can be managed through physical restraint and seclusion. The physical environments of services within this level are designed to minimize opportunities for self-harm and are often locked to prevent elopement.

To enhance safety and to assist patients in improving their level of organization, the milieu in these settings is planned and highly structured. Schedules are commonly posted, and each day is filled with a series of activities that serve to orient, organize, and educate, bringing patients into constructive contact with each other. Individual, group, and family interventions are used as appropriate to meet patient needs. Treatment is medically supervised and psychopharmacological interventions are routinely employed to reduce acuity.

Patients who require this level of care typically fall into one of several categories. Many have acute psychotic disorders that produce severe impairment in reality testing. Individuals with depressive disorders accompanied by psychosis or severe functional impairment may also require such intensive treatment. Suicidality or homicidality, when the patient is unable to contract for safety, may also dictate such a level of intervention.

This level of care can be delivered through numerous service types. Acute inpatient units have traditionally met the identified treatment functions, often in general hospitals or freestanding psychiatric hospitals. These units are generally locked, use psychopharmacological interventions for stabilization, and engage patients in the milieu and therapeutic activities as they stabilize. A variation on traditional inpatient acute care has involved the creation of crisis stabilization beds or units; there are usually a small number of beds, the average length of stay is very short, and the staff is specially trained in crisis intervention. Often these units are located in hospitals or community mental health centers, and their entire thrust is the rapid return of patients to the community. Interventions in this modality may focus on engaging family or community support systems or addressing conflicts between the patient and individuals in these support systems.

Even more innovative has been the provision of 24-hour care in crisis residential programs that offer high levels of structure, supervision, support, and intervention in a more homelike setting (Bourgeois 1994). This modality is illustrated in the following case example.

Crisis Residential Care

G.L. was a 22-year-old single white male who was attending college away from home when friends began to notice significant changes in his behavior. Previously an above-average and socially active student, his attendance at classes became irregular, he withdrew from contact with friends, and he increasingly ignored his personal hygiene. G.L. became distrustful and suspicious of others, was confused in his thinking, and began to engage in bizarre, ritualistic behaviors. His roommate, unable to persuade G.L. to seek outpatient treatment, turned to university staff, who arranged for G.L.'s admission to a crisis residential program.

This program was located in a renovated two-story home situated in a residential area adjacent to the campus. Efforts had been made to reduce the opportunities for self-harm in this setting, but the homelike atmosphere had been maintained. During the 5 days that G.L. was in this program he lived with four other patients who, as a group, were generally in the company of two staff members. He was monitored closely by the staff, evaluated by a program psychiatrist, and started on an antipsychotic medication. The staff oriented him to the program and its schedule, which included a highly structured routine of meals, treatment groups, individual treatment contacts, and therapeutic activities. Although he required considerable direction during his first 2 days, he quickly became increasingly organized and more engaged with others. He was assessed each day, and his medications were adjusted. In consultation with his parents, the staff arranged for his discharge after 5 days to the family home and a nearby day treatment program.

Acute Ambulatory

From a functional perspective, the next level of care offers highly intensive services without providing constant monitoring and supervision. As in the inpatient/residential level, acute ambulatory care shares a focus on crisis stabilization, acute symptom reduction, and alleviation of severe functional impairments that prevent an individual from living in the community without intensive supports. However, patients typically remain in their natural environments for most of the day. This maximizes the supports available in those environments and minimizes disruption of the individual's activities and routine.

Acute ambulatory services are highly structured with scheduled activities and an active therapeutic milieu. Programming is usually offered for 4–6 hours/day, 4–7 days/week. Patient-to-staff ratios are low, affording high levels of staff contact with patients and intensive intervention. The care is medically supervised, and the almost daily contact affords an excellent venue for assessing the effectiveness of medications and making medication adjustments. Backup systems are available 24 hours a day to ensure adequate response to crises that occur while patients are not with program staff.

Individuals for whom this level of care is appropriate typically have severe symptoms or functional impairments that are either of acute onset or an exacerbation of a severe and persistent disorder. The intensity of these treatments is warranted by the level of clinical instability, functional impairment, and potential risk to self or others. Although risk of harm may be significant, it should not be considered imminent for those appropriately admitted to this level of care. The presence of social supports or some ability by the patient to contract for safety may obviate the need for round-the-clock interventions. Although modalities in this level are often referred to as *alternatives* to inpatient care, they are in fact the most appropriate level for individuals with the clinical characteristics described earlier.

Acute ambulatory care includes modalities such as partial hospitalization, outpatient detoxification, and intensive in-home crisis intervention. The first two services are facility or office based and have largely replaced inpatient care for the treatment of acute psychiatric illness and severe addictions. Partial hospitalization programs are known for their family-like environments, offering perhaps the most intensive and supportive therapeutic milieu available. The emphasis on providing structure, interpersonal contact, and pharmacologic interventions is highly organizing for those in acute distress. In addition to serving as an alternative to an inpatient admission, partial hospitalization is frequently used as a brief "step-down" from inpatient care.

Ambulatory detoxification is the functional equivalent of partial hospitalization for those with addictive disorders. It combines a structured regimen of pharmacologic interventions, clinical monitoring, and supportive therapies to accomplish a medically safe and psychologically tolerable withdrawal from substances of abuse. Group interventions are emphasized, and often 12-step self-help programs are incorporated into the programming. Educational and cognitive-behavioral approaches are used to improve problem-solving, decision-making, and relapse-prevention skills. Like partial hospitalization, ambulatory detoxification is often used as an alternative to an inpatient admission but can also serve as a step-down from inpatient care.

Intensive in-home crisis intervention programs demonstrate creativity in addressing the functions of this level of care, but in a completely different format. A team of professionals builds a therapeutic milieu in the community by conducting assessments and interventions in home, work, and school environments. Used most frequently for children or adolescents exhibiting severe functional or behavioral impairment, this approach facilitates assessment of the behavioral contingencies in the child's environment and engagement of family members, teachers, and significant others to alter those contingencies.

Intensive In-Home Crisis Intervention

J.S. is a 12-year-old male who exhibited increasingly self-destructive behavior such as head banging and assaults of both peers and family. A crisis occurred when he refused to attend school one morning, repeatedly hitting his mother as she tried to force him out of bed. The mother called the police, who took J.S. to the local emergency department. Staff members from an in-home crisis program assessed J.S. and met with his mother in the emergency department. They arranged for his discharge home, where team members remained with the family for the first 24 hours until the mother felt safe and J.S. was back in school. Staff escorted J.S. back to school and met with the mother, outpatient therapist, and school personnel. They discussed the precipitants to the current crisis and revised the behavioral management plan. Medications were reassessed and adjusted by the outpatient psychiatrist in consultation with the in-home team, whose members evaluated J.S.'s clinical status daily. Other interventions conducted in the home included modeling of behavioral interventions for the mother, supportive counseling for J.S. and his mother, family meetings involving J.S.'s older siblings, assistance with organizing and completing homework assignments, and therapeutic games. The hours of daily contact with J.S., his family, and teachers were gradually decreased over a period of 4 weeks, at which time his outpatient therapist assumed responsibility for continuing care.

Intermediate Ambulatory

The next level of care, intermediate ambulatory, focuses on the functions of clinical stabilization, symptom reduction, and relapse prevention. Of intermediate intensity, the modalities in this level of care may be used to further stabilize an individual recovering from an acute episode or to decrease symptoms and improve functioning in an individual who has a chronic illness.

Like the two previous levels, intermediate ambulatory care offers a structured and active therapeutic milieu that can be either program or community based. Although a backup system is typically available 24 hours/day to respond to crises, staff contact and programming is limited to 3–4 hours/day, 2–3 days/week. Thus, in contrast to higher levels of care, the burden of responsibility and control is shared more among the staff, the patient, and his or her support system. Medical consultation is routinely available to the patient, although at this level it is less likely that a physician will supervise the care.

Individuals receiving this level of care are quite heterogeneous. This stems from the fact that a patient experiencing a first episode of illness may require this level of care only briefly to achieve stability after hospitalization, whereas a chronically ill individual may require this level of care on a continuing basis to prevent relapse. In either case, there is generally a moderate level of instability or some level of risk to the patient or others that warrants this relatively intensive level of care. This level has been used extensively with individuals who have substance abuse disorders as described below.

The modalities within this level, although functionally related, are in other respects quite diverse. Each, in its own way, provides an intermediate level of structure, monitoring, and support. Day treatment is a facility- or office-based strategy that combines a clinical and a rehabilitative focus. A multidisciplinary staff relies heavily on the treatment milieu and group interventions to assist individuals in learning to manage their symptoms and improve their functioning. Lengths of stay tend to be intermediate, averaging several months or longer. Psychosocial rehabilitation programs are structurally similar to day treatment programs but have a less clinical focus. In these programs the emphasis tends to be on improving the skills necessary to live independently or to obtain employment.

In contrast to day treatment and psychosocial rehabilitation, intensive outpatient programs (IOP) have a treatment milieu that is more loosely structured. During a typical day in an IOP, a patient is likely to have an individual meeting with a member of the staff and to participate in a few groups. The focus of these interventions tends to be both clinical and educational. The patients attending such groups will change frequently because IOPs often are used only briefly to stabilize an individual. A principal application of IOPs has been in the treatment of addictions, both for those who are early in the recovery process attempting to establish sobriety and for the relapsing individual who has been unable to maintain an alcohol- or drug-free lifestyle with routine outpatient care. A substance abuse IOP is described in the following case example.

Intensive Outpatient Treatment

M.A. was a 26-year-old, single white female who was abusing alcohol and cocaine. What had begun as recreational use of substances 2 years earlier was now a major clinical problem. She was deeply in debt because of the money spent on drugs and alcohol, had missed an increasing number of days from work, and was in jeopardy of losing her job because of absenteeism and poor performance. Her supervisor referred her to the employee assistance program, which facilitated her admission to an evening IOP focused on substance abuse. She attended for 3 hours each evening, 3 evenings per week with the goal of achieving abstinence. Urine toxicology screens were conducted frequently to assess her progress toward that goal. The core of the program was a series of groups in which she worked with staff to identify the "primary triggers" that led to substance use and to learn strategies for controlling her use and preventing relapse. M.A. also attended educational groups that covered the effects of alcohol and drugs on the body and 12-step strategies for recovery. With the assistance of program staff, M.A. found an individual sponsor to accompany her to Alcoholics Anonymous meetings on weekends and each weeknight that she did not attend the IOP. As she approached the end of her stay in the program (which lasts approximately 8 weeks) she was connected with an outpatient relapse prevention group and encouraged to draw heavily on the support of 12-step programs and her sponsor.

Most divergent in form from the other modalities in the intermediate ambulatory level is assertive community treatment. This modality is used principally for severe and persistently ill individuals who are prone to relapse and are noncompliant with office-based treatment. Assertive community treatment teams are multidisciplinary in nature and are responsible for directly providing most of the services an individual needs. These services are almost exclusively provided through outreach to home and community settings.

Assertive Community Treatment

G.L., the college student discussed earlier who was first admitted to a crisis residential program, was discharged to a day treatment service of a community mental health center. The goal was to facilitate his stabilization; however, he attended only several days before refusing further treatment. His psychotic symptoms and bizarre behavior increased. His suspiciousness of his family prompted him to leave the safety of his home, and he was soon penniless and homeless. The assertive community treatment team assumed responsibility for his care and began conducting outreach visits to him in the local shelters, soup kitchens, and city streets. Team members made few demands of him but offered food, clothes, and guaranteed access to beds in shelters, which were in short supply. The outreach workers slowly developed a relationship with him, establishing some level of trust. He eventually, although reluctantly, agreed to meet with the team's psychiatrist in one of the shelters and consented to resume medications that the staff then supplied routinely. His willingness to meet with clinical staff and to take medications continued to wax and wane. The extensive outreach efforts of the assertive community treatment team were considered essential to maintain his current, albeit impaired, level of functioning. Future treatment goals included obtaining entitlements and housing for G.L., increasing medication and treatment compliance, and connecting him with social and vocational rehabilitation programs.

Multimodal Outpatient

The modalities in the multimodal outpatient level serve to prevent a decline in functioning and are used when routine outpatient services are insufficient to accomplish that task. The objective may be to prevent a further decline in the functioning of acutely ill individuals or to address the devastating long-term effects that severe and persistent mental illness has on functional capacity. Treatment is of intermediate intensity, with approximately 4–8 hours of contact per week. For acutely ill individuals, the duration of treatment is usually quite brief, perhaps 4–8 weeks; for those with a severe and persistent illness, the length of treatment is intermediate to long term. The modalities in this level provide structure, interpersonal contact, and education through a supportive milieu.

The individuals for whom this level of care is appropriate fall into at least two somewhat distinct groups. The first group includes individuals with acute illnesses who are not recovering or are continuing to decline in functioning while receiving routine outpatient care. The second group includes those with severe illnesses who are moderately impaired by persistent symptoms and social and vocational functional limitations. There is a relative stability, however, to their clinical and functional status that is maintained or enhanced through their participation in these multimodal outpatient treatments. Notably, their ability to engage in treatment and in nontreatment relationships allows them to cope with their illness with the addition of only moderate levels of support.

As in acute and intermediate ambulatory care, the functions of multimodal outpatient treatment can be addressed through modalities that are either office or community based. Multimodal outpatient treatments combine traditional outpatient interventions into a package of services to meet the needs of acutely ill patients. A typical package might combine a twice-weekly individual therapy, a group therapy, and a medication management session.

Multimodal Outpatient Treatment

R.G. was a 22-year-old male who had an anxiety disorder that included panic attacks. Despite routine outpatient treatment, the frequency of his panic attacks was increasing. This resulted in decreasing attendance at his college classes. To prevent further decline in functioning, the university counseling center assembled a multimodal treatment that involved two individual therapy sessions per week and weekly attendance at two groups, one focused on cognitive-behavioral strategies for managing anxiety and the second focused on relaxation training. He also met weekly with a psychiatrist to review his response to the current medication regimen and to adjust the medications accordingly. Although this multimodal intervention did not immediately lead to a reduction in his symptoms and reported distress, he did begin to attend classes more regularly. After 6 weeks, R.G.'s symptoms began to subside. He completed the relaxation training group and reduced his individual therapy sessions to once a week. Medication management sessions were tapered to once monthly. He continued to attend the cognitive-behavioral group for the remainder of the semester, in large part because of the peer support that it offered.

Clubhouse programs provide a community-based multimodal outpatient treatment. Those such as Fountain House in New York City or Thresholds in Chicago tend to offer social, recreational, educational, avocational, and vocational activities that are often consumer run. The peer support offered in these environments is typically high, and patient involvement in such programs is designed to counter the regressive pull of severe and persistent psychotic and depressive illnesses. Patients can build a life structure around such programs, as they usually offer activities, a social network, and meals.

Clubhouses

G.L., the former college student described earlier, received assertive community treatment for 2 years. After being admitted to a supported apartment program and connected with an outpatient psychiatrist at the mental health center, he was introduced to the local clubhouse program. He was slow to engage in clubhouse activities, but eventually joined a computer group and a music group that met weekly. He prided himself on his computer skills, soon began tutoring other clubhouse members, and volunteered to do the computer layout of the monthly clubhouse newsletter. G.L. ate several meals at the clubhouse each week but remained reluctant to get more involved in clubhouse social activities or governance. He refused opportunities to run for a seat on the consumer board that managed clubhouse affairs. He shied away from the frequent parties and dances hosted by the clubhouse but would attend the celebrations of major holidays. His outpatient clinician considered G.L.'s clubhouse participation essential in countering his inclination to isolate from others.

In contrast to office-based and clubhouse interventions, home care is used to provide structure, monitoring, interpersonal contact, and assistance with daily living in the patient's home environment. This approach can be particularly useful with patients who are avoidant of therapeutic settings such as mental health centers and clubhouses. Depending on an individual's needs, paraprofessional staff can be deployed to assist with activities of daily living and to provide social support. They may spend a substantial number of hours with the patient each day. Nurses often make brief visits to administer medications and assess clinical status. This is particularly useful with patients who are medication noncompliant and prone to relapse. Social work and occupational therapy personnel are occasionally deployed to address family issues, social service needs, or functional skill deficits.

Outpatient Level

The function of outpatient treatment is to reduce patients' symptoms and alleviate their distress. Routine contact with a behavioral health professional provides a certain level of monitoring and structure. The treatment milieu is contained both within the outpatient sessions and in the all-important relationship between the patient and therapist. Although some level of structure and safety is provided, the patient in outpatient treatment functions independently, drawing on support from family and significant others.

The contact between a patient and an outpatient therapist ranges between 1 hour and 3 hours per week. The therapist or a covering clinician is on call after hours to respond to crises. Medical consultation is available as needed, although some outpatient care is delivered directly by psychiatrists providing both the therapy and psychopharmacological interventions.

There is tremendous diversity in the forms of outpatient care. At a broad conceptual level, outpatient interventions may focus on one or more of the following: psychopharmacology, psychotherapy, case management, and skill development. The theoretical approach guiding these interventions also varies widely. The most common include biological, psychodynamic, behavioral, cognitive, and existential approaches. Outpatient interventions also vary in their basic format, which may be individual, group, family, or multiple family in nature.

Outpatient Treatment

J.M. is a 46-year-old male who consulted a psychologist regarding difficulties related to his job. Although he was experiencing symptoms of anxiety and depressed mood, J.M. was uninterested in considering a trial of medications. After several outpatient visits, his mood improved and he began to feel more hopeful. The psychotherapeutic work focused initially on helping him understand the nature of his reactions to the job stressors. The work then shifted to helping him develop some additional assertiveness skills, which he began to use in the workplace. After six sessions, the psychologist suggested that they meet again in a month, at which time J.M. reported that both his work situation and his symptoms were much improved.

Primary Care

Research has clearly documented that the majority of Americans experiencing mental health or substance abuse problems do not seek help from a behavioral health professional. Rather, they are more likely to present to a general medical practitioner. This has led to efforts to introduce into primary care settings education, screening, and detection programs as well as behavioral health interventions for "uncomplicated" disorders. The function of this level of care is to facilitate the identification of mental illness and substance abuse and to connect patients with appropriate treatment in either a primary care or a behavioral health setting. By imbedding these interventions in routine medical visits, access to treatment is theoretically maximized and the stigma associated with seeking help is minimized.

This level of care has taken several forms (Pruitt et al. 1998). Specialized training has been offered to primary care staff in the detection of behavioral health disorders, basic treatment of uncomplicated disorders, and the process of referring complicated or severe disorders to behavioral health professionals. Specialized paper-and-pencil or computerized instruments have been developed and implemented in primary care settings to assist medical staff in screening and detecting such disorders. Alternatively, behavioral health staff have been deployed to primary care locations to consult with medical caregivers, conduct screenings and assessments, and provide on-site mental health and substance abuse treatment. By nature, the primary care venue of this level of care offers little structure and requires that the patient function independently, aided by family and community supports.

Primary Care

G.C. was a 34-year-old, single female who lived in the inner city. She was unemployed and uninsured. When she had medical problems she presented at the emergency department or primary care clinic of the local city hospital. G.C. recently presented at the clinic complaining of fatigue, difficulty sleeping, and loss of appetite. On a screening instrument that she completed in the waiting room, she acknowledged experiencing sadness, feelings of worthlessness, weight loss, and early morning awakening. The primary care physician conducted an interview and physical examination and ordered various laboratory tests to rule out a range of physical disorders as the source of the symptoms. He then prescribed a course of antidepressants and subsequently reviewed this treatment decision during rounds, which were attended weekly by a consulting psychiatric clinical nurse specialist. G.C. was seen in the primary care clinic biweekly as her symptoms remitted during a period of 8 weeks. She was given educational materials about depression that outlined early warning signs, and she was encouraged to contact the clinic if the symptoms recurred.

DISCUSSION

At this time no single level of care model dominates the field. There is no compelling theoretical or research evidence that demonstrates the superiority of one approach over others in conceptualizing levels of care or ordering available modalities on various dimensions. Level of care models constitute our attempt as professionals to provide a language for thinking about and communicating regarding the services we offer. Although the existing models have differences, the concepts and language being used are sufficiently similar that communication has been enhanced by these attempts to provide frameworks for understanding the current array of behavioral health treatments.

Equally important, the considerable attention being devoted to defining levels of care and associated placement criteria is fostering increased attention on the importance of having a comprehensive range of treatment options that can meet the rapidly changing needs of individual patients. The traditional focus on assessing whether a patient is appropriate for a program is ever so slowly giving way to an emphasis on selecting an array of services that address a patient's needs with respect to treatment function, intensity, form, and duration.

Conceptual models that help us better understand our treatments do more than help match treatments to patients. Unfortunately, in many geographic areas a comprehensive array of services is not available. Understanding the similarities and differences between levels of care and the modalities within levels helps professionals select adequate substitutes for preferred, but perhaps unavailable, services.

The challenge for professionals in the future is to avoid being bound by existing level of care models while exploring innovative treatments that may address patient needs more creatively and flexibly than currently available treatment modalities. There is a danger that existing level of care models may become highly codified through the standards published by professional groups and the level of care criteria published by managed behavioral health organizations. If providers are forced to organize their services in accordance with these models to obtain treatment authorization and payment, the barriers to innovation will be enormous. As managed care organizations continue to merge, becoming fewer in number and more powerful in terms of the control they exert, they will be less able to accommodate provider innovation.

As highlighted earlier, treatment modalities vary on multiple dimensions, including function, intensity, form, and duration. To some extent, we have only begun to scratch the surface in exploring the possible variations—the unique ways in which specific treatment functions can be accomplished using interventions of different intensity, form, and duration. Innovation may involve combining existing treatments. This occurred when day hospitals were combined with "inns" or residential beds to provide alternatives to inpatient care for those with mental disorders or addictions. Innovation may involve merging differing treatment approaches to better serve the needs of special populations. For example, intensive outpatient mental health programs have been combined with relapse prevention and self-help strategies to create dual diagnosis programs for those with a major mental illness who are simultaneously abusing substances.

Other needs cry out. The search for effective outreach and prevention strategies is still in its infancy. As the population of the United States ages, finding novel approaches to caring for the elderly becomes another pressing agenda.

Our knowledge about disorders and their treatment is increasing. For the moment, the organizations that authorize and pay for mental health and substance abuse treatment have considerable flexibility regarding the services they approve. We must capture the moment, searching for more effective and cost-efficient ways to meet the needs of those we serve.

REFERENCES

American Psychiatric Association: Practice Guidelines. Washington, DC, American Psychiatric Association, 1996

American Society of Addiction Medicine: Patient Placement Criteria for the Treatment of Substance-Related Disorders. Chevy Chase, MD, American Society of Addiction Medicine, 1991

American Society of Addiction Medicine: Patient Placement Criteria for the Treatment of Substance-Related Disorders, 2nd Edition. Chevy Chase, MD, American Society of Addiction Medicine, 1996

Bourgeois P: Crossing Place: a community-based model for acute care. Continuum: Developments in Ambulatory Mental Health Care 1:61–69, 1994

Gray GV, Glazer WM: Psychiatric decision-making in the 90s: the coming era of decision support. Behav Healthc Tomorrow 3:47–54, 1994

Kiser LJ, Lefkovitz PM, Kennedy LL: The continuum of ambulatory mental health services. Behav Healthc Tomorrow 2:14–16, 1993

Kiser LJ, Lefkovitz PM, Kennedy LL, et al: The Continuum of Behavioral Health Care Services. Alexandria, VA, Association for Ambulatory Behavioral Healthcare, 1999

MCC Behavioral Care: Clinical Guidelines for Mental Health and Substance Abuse Treatment. Eden Prairie, MN, MCC Behavioral Care, 1996

McFarland B, Minkoff K, Roman B, et al: Utilization management, in Managed Mental Health Care in the Public Sector: A Survival Manual. Edited by Minkoff K, Pollack D. Amsterdam, Netherlands, Harwood Academic Press, 1997, pp 151–168

Merit Behavioral Care Corporation: Utilization Management Guidelines. Maryland Heights, MO, Merit Behavioral Care Corporation, 1997

Pruitt SD, Kapow JC, Epping-Jordan JE, et al: Moving behavioral medicine to the front line: a model for the integration of behavior and medical sciences in primary care. Professional Psychology: Research and Practice 70:230–236, 1998

Schreter RK, Sharfstein SS, Schreter CA (eds): Managing Care, Not Dollars: The Continuum of Mental Health Services. Washington, DC, American Psychiatric Press, 1997

Srebnik D, Uehara E, Smukler M: Field test of a tool for level-of-care decisions in community mental health systems. Psychiatr Serv 49:91–97, 1998

9

Therapeutic Processes Across the Continuum

Laurel J. Kiser, Ph.D., M.B.A.
Lawrence L. Kennedy, M.D.

Integrated delivery systems (IDSs) join an array of clinical services offering treatment at various levels of intensity. Yet the principle of coordinated care speaks to a broader issue than operating as part of a network. Coordination of care requires movement past the structural/functional aspects of integration to the clinical elements that make integration work. Integration of care requires coordination, coherence, and consistency between previously independent or loosely affiliated services. In this chapter we focus on the therapeutic processes that support integrated delivery, starting with promulgation of systemwide processes of care. Therapeutic processes refer to the philosophies, procedures, practices, and techniques used to create or support recovery and wellness.

The establishment of systemwide therapeutic processes is an important indicator of the degree of integration achieved. How do organizations create these processes? Basic to the establishment of systemwide processes of care is promulgation of a mission and statement of values that support a healthy workplace and treatment environment. Common understanding and acceptance of organizational culture, goals, and expectations as well as an administration and staff committed to success at the organizational level are necessary foundations. It is on this basic framework that systemwide processes of care can be built.

Within IDSs, it is at the systemwide level that principles of care are put into operation through the establishment of consistent philosophies, policies, procedures, and practices across the entire service system. This is not to say that these "four Ps" are applied verbatim within every program at each level of care; an effective IDS must be developed "both within each distinct level of care and across the broader 'array of services'" (Lefkovitz 1995). Interservice planning teams are one mechanism for establishing, communicating, and monitoring consistency. Clinical administrators given responsibility and flexibility move outward from this center to establish therapeutic processes compatible with the overall system.

A critical principle of care for IDSs stipulates that services operate in a coordinated fashion. Coordinated care means that across the service array there is continuity in function and therapeutic process, that patients moving through the system are generally treated with a similar philosophy of care and theoretical formulation. A common understanding of human nature, normal and abnormal development, and psychopathology permeates each service offered, shared by the organizational leadership, program administrators, clinicians, and support staff.

However, movement of patients from one level of care to another indicates a need for treatment differing in intensity, either more or less intense. Thus, the clinical processes offered at each level of care must differ in ways that are substantial and meaningful. Levels of care differentiated by clearly delineated functions require therapeutic processes that support that function and facilitate patient movement through the system. Part 1 of this chapter highlights the coordination of clinical processes across the levels of care, and Part 2, the development of patient ecologies that support treatment throughout the array of services offered.

PART I: CLINICAL PROCESSES ACROSS THE LEVELS OF CARE

As a patient's needs change during an episode of care, so do the clinical processes, practices, and techniques used to address those needs. Each level of care varies according to the function and intensity of treatment offered. Distinct levels of intensity are in many ways defined by applying clinical processes in differing ways across the continuum. In this section, starting with therapeutic alliance, we review a variety of clinical processes (e.g., individual, group, and family psychotherapies; pharmacotherapy; case management) as applied across the continuum of care.

Therapeutic or Working Alliances

Ralph Greenson (1967), a psychoanalyst, has written extensively about the concept of the *working alliance*, also known as the *therapeutic alliance*. Greenson stresses the significance of the patient's ability to step back from the intensity of a "transference" reaction to the analyst and to become a collaborative participant in his or her own treatment. In plain English, the working alliance stresses the patient's contribution to the treatment process and recognizes that the patient cannot be a mere recipient of treatment but must be a partner if treatment is going to be successful.

Compliance with medications provides a good illustration. Often patients do not take medications as prescribed either because they do not trust the doctor or they do not feel they have had sufficient opportunity to express their fears and concerns about the medications. The prescribing psychiatrist must recognize that by working to increase trust and the patient's understanding of the illness, a greater partnership will be formed. The patient can then tell the doctor about symptoms or signs he or she is experiencing that may indicate excessive or insufficient dosage, thus aiding the doctor in prescribing the medication correctly.

Therapeutic or working alliances are necessary components of treatment, whether it includes hospitalization, group therapy, or individual therapy (Allen et al. 1984). As more and more seriously ill patients are treated in multiple settings along the continuum of care, the concept of therapeutic alliance with its invitation to the patient to actively engage as a partner in the treatment process becomes increasingly important and meaningful. As patients move away from the protected 24-hour setting of a hospital unit where they are under constant observation, they are expected to take increasing control of their treatment. Patients' ability to participate in treatment is probably the best and most significant indicator for moving them to a level of care lower than 24-hour hospitalization. It is this unique process of patients participating in treatment and simultaneously observing themselves in their own participation that makes it possible to treat them outside of 24-hour settings.

For example, the patient entering a partial hospital setting will be attending the program only a certain number of hours each day. During program hours patients engage with a number of treaters who have an opportunity to participate with them and to observe their behavior. Professionals are constantly assessing how the patient is responding to treatment. However, what the patient does when away from treatment has a powerful effect on whether a partial hospital program is effective. Does the patient, for instance, engage in self-destructive behaviors such as promiscuous sexual activity, self-induced vomiting, self-cutting, and abuse of drugs? The patient must bring this information to the treaters; only then can they know to what extent the patient is participating in treatment.

Individual Psychotherapy

In traditional practice of both inpatient and of outpatient behavioral health care, the primary responsibility for developing the therapeutic alliance fell to the individual psychotherapist. This individual had the most in-depth and meaningful contact with the patient. Integrated models of service delivery tend to minimize the primacy of the individual therapist's role and to refocus attention on the complementary roles of each professional member of the treatment team.

As the roles of providers have shifted, so has the practice of individual psychotherapy. Figure 9–1 depicts the curative role of individual psychotherapy across the continuum of behavioral health care. At the least intensive and the most intensive levels of care, the curative function of individual psychotherapy is minimized. In the intermediate levels of care, individual psychotherapy is used to help patients not only understand their illness but also develop new insights, coping mechanisms, skills, and behaviors that improve their level of functioning and quality of life.

Many patients have their first exposure to psychotherapy when hospitalized in a crisis. It is at that time they begin to learn the "talking cure." They learn that talking about their difficulties may offer new understanding and clues to future prevention. Individual therapy, as practiced in inpatient and acute crisis intervention programs, involves three to four sessions focusing on assessment of the patient's current symptoms and functioning and immediate reductions in symptom distress. Individual therapy also includes introducing crisis management skills or providing support and "holding" while medications and structure diminish psychotic processes.

At the other end of the continuum in primary care settings, the curative function of individual therapy is also minimized. Primary care physicians are trained to conduct brief screening interviews and prescribe medications. The typical visit with a primary care physician is limited to 10–15 minutes and often includes discussion of physical as well as psychiatric conditions. Behavioral health care professionals working in primary care settings augment these functions by providing problem-oriented individual treatments that are limited in scope and duration.

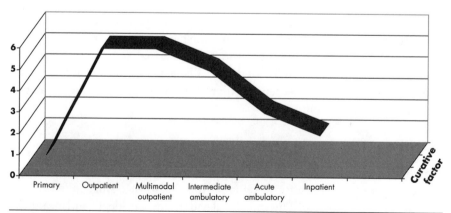

FIGURE 9–1. Curative role of individual psychotherapy.

Traditional forms of individual psychotherapy still play a major role in out-patient care and often in intensive outpatient and intermediate ambulatory behavioral health care services. Individual work at these levels allows a more in-depth exploration of both current and lifelong issues and struggles, strengths and weaknesses, and skills and deficits with a corresponding focus on change to alleviate suffering.

Case Management

In almost any treatment setting it is valuable for the psychiatric patient to have one person who provides the overall planning function. In traditional practice, the individual therapist often assumes this role. As the role of the individual therapist has evolved within IDSs, case management has become a popular way of helping patients plan their treatment and negotiate the system (see Chapter 7).

Case managers help patients maneuver through the complexities of various treatment systems and gain access to the treatments prescribed. Case managers are like patient advocates, helping patients when they encounter difficulty dealing with individuals or systems in a variety of treatment settings. The case manager role is similar to the so-called supportive psychotherapist who helps the patient deal with the realities of everyday struggles rather than intrapsychic or interpersonal problems. The focus is on daily living and helping the patient to use his or her strengths to find the best treatment possible. For example, the patient may find the details of financial arrangements complex and need help with them. The patient may also need direction and assistance in seeking medical help for general medical problems or coordinating general medical and behavioral health care. Alternatively, a patient may need help in negotiating housing arrangements in a community board and care program for psychiatric patients. The case manager is also valuable during periods of crisis, helping the patient seek the level of care needed.

Case managers and psychotherapists need to understand their respective roles with the patient, especially as the patient enters and leaves various treatment modalities. Even though case managers are not specifically psychotherapists, it should be noted that often their relationship with the patient becomes an important and sustaining one for the patient. Hence, a good case manager develops an understanding of the patient and provides encouragement and support in appropriate ways. Case managers need to maintain appropriate boundaries as they help the patient deal with a variety of therapeutic milieus. For example, the case manager needs to have a contract with the patient allowing for the release of information or discussion of the patient's care with other treaters. Without this collaboration, pieces of the treatment may become fragmented or may be excessive or work at cross purposes. In addition, it is important that patients feel they have "okayed" any such communication. The patient is, after all, the central person in his or her own treatment.

Medications

Medications have taken an increasingly important role in the treatment of mental illness, particularly since the early 1950s. The introduction of chlorpromazine for the treatment of psychotic illness, particularly schizophrenia, and the many antipsychotic drugs that have followed, created remarkable change in the locus of treatment of many severely mentally ill patients. In recent years advances in antidepressant drugs have represented another major factor in the increasing use of biologic agents (Pincus et al. 1998). Improvements in medications allow for expanded use of the whole continuum for treatment of serious mental illness.

Across the continuum of care patients assume differing levels of responsibility for medication compliance. Thus, issues related to medication management such as titration, safety, monitoring of side effects, and compliance vary according to level of care. On an inpatient unit, for example, nurses dispense medications with both timing and dosage controlled by medical staff. As patients move to less intense levels of care, they assume greater responsibility for taking their own medications. Promoting an alliance with the patient in terms of taking medication requires much effort. One important means of promoting patient compliance is specific groups in which medications are discussed and education provided.

In addition, in more intensive and restrictive levels of care, the staff is actively engaged in monitoring medication effects—targeted response and side effects. For example, in inpatient settings staff can observe changes in appetite, sleep, energy, and thinking and can track these changes across multiple settings. The physician with sufficient and reliable observation data, not solely dependent on patient report of medication effects, can safely increase dosages more rapidly. In less intensive and restrictive levels of care, such as outpatient, the physician assumes less supervision of medication management because patients at these levels of care are usually more capable of reporting response accurately.

One critical medication management issue within IDSs is to ensure that the appropriate follow-up is done with regard to patients' medication as they move around the array of services offered. When a patient moves between levels of care, accurate and timely information about medications must be transmitted. In addition, when patients shift from higher levels of care, in which multidisciplinary teams encourage cooperation between physicians and other clinicians, into services such as multimodal outpatient or psychosocial clubhouses that necessitate developing collaborative arrangements for patients on medications, enhanced communication channels regarding medications become particularly relevant.

Additionally, coordination of therapy processes and medication management becomes an important issue in integrated systems. In traditional practice it often has been the patient's psychiatrist who performs the role of pharmacotherapist and of psychotherapist. However, in recent years there has been a tendency toward more efficient use of psychiatry and increasing the use of multidisciplinary teams to provide treatment. Within these systems, staff members often provide other active therapies with medications prescribed by the staff psychiatrist or patient's psychiatrist. This requires a collaborative effort and probably works best when the psychiatrist and the nonmedical therapist work in close concert (Prentice-Dunn et al. 1981). Changes in the patient's mood and reactions to various issues that arise in the psychotherapy process can lead to a need for changing medication prescriptions, and vice versa—changes in the medication may require adjustments in the psychotherapy process.

Finally, at the least intensive and restrictive levels of care, in many instances, a primary care physician who is not part of the behavioral health treatment team prescribes a patient's medications. In these cases ensuring sufficient collaboration between the primary care physician and clinicians is essential. This may be done through direct contact or through the medical director in an outpatient clinic setting. Or, in intensive outpatient programs there may be a psychiatric nurse who can make contact with other physicians and gain their support in coordinating a treatment plan for the patient. This practice is particularly relevant in the treatment of geriatric patients for whom it is helpful to have one physician prescribe all of a given patient's medications. In some settings the pharmacist who dispenses the medications may play an important role by helping patients understand their medications, the side effects, and the importance of compliance.

Group Psychotherapy

Various types of group psychotherapy have played a major role in psychiatry since the 1940s and are becoming increasingly popular in systems aware of population-based care issues. A useful aspect of group psychotherapy for many patients is the recognition that talking about symptoms provides relief. Patients notice that others have similar symptoms, and it is helpful for them to hear how other individuals deal with their illnesses. This mutual feedback is an important curative factor for patients. In addition, groups give all patients an opportunity to provide therapeutic assistance to others and to avoid being simply the recipients of therapy. This can be ego strengthening for patients because they experience themselves in a helpful role. However universal the curative aspects of group psychotherapy are, as with other therapeutic processes, group psychotherapy models have to be adapted for each level of care along the continuum.

Specific models of group treatment have been developed for inpatient units based on concepts borrowed from outpatient group psychotherapy (Yalom 1983). Inpatient group psychotherapies are usually limited to small groups of patients, normally 8–12, with the frequency of group sessions related to the length of hospital stay. For example, on a 3- to 5-day crisis hospitalization unit, group psychotherapy sessions may be held four or five times a week. Group psychotherapy in this setting focuses on the immediacy of the patient's situation and on the here and now. It provides an excellent opportunity for processing the arrival of new patients and preparing for discharge of others. New patients may share their anxieties and obtain direct information and assistance from other patients. Patients facing discharge may share their plans and get encouragement and feedback from other members. Yalom (1983) and others (Rice and Rutan 1986) have recognized that there is seldom a consistent membership in these groups, and each session is viewed as a separate group because it may have membership different from any of the previous sessions.

As patients transition to ambulatory levels of care, the emphasis in group psychotherapy is often on movement back into jobs, school, and home (Kennedy 1993). "Change" issues are powerful forces in such groups. Because patients' lives have been disrupted by their illnesses, they are struggling to determine when they are ready to return to their preillness roles as students, spouses, parents, and workers. Patients in the group learn to recognize that some patients are apt to jump into things impulsively without any plan or careful thought given to when they are ready for a change, whereas others delay and undermine their own efforts to move ahead. Group members can be particularly helpful in this regard by pointing out repetitions of old behavior. Many patients learn some of the precipitating factors that led to their illness and work to develop new lifestyles, new living arrangements, and even new jobs and new relationships. The group provides a place where they can try out ideas, where they can use relationships with others in the group and learn in the here and now how they interact with people in ways that may be therapeutic or harmful.

Services that have a therapeutic community as a basic philosophical model for treatment use groups of many types as the primary active therapy (Kennedy 1993). The frequency of group psychotherapy in these services can range from multiple sessions daily to just twice weekly. Such groups emphasize the importance of belonging to a community and the significance of relationships in the patient's life and treatment.

Group psychotherapy is also useful for patients participating in treatment at the outpatient or primary care level and is often the only modality used. Outpatient and primary care programs may be able to design groups for different types of patients. Diagnostic groupings, functional groupings, or age groupings may be important. Yalom (1983) recommended the placement of higher- and lower-functioning patients in separate groups. He believed the task is somewhat different for the two groups. Higher-functioning patients may be able to tolerate a much more active and expressive group psychotherapy process, whereas patients with more limited coping skills need a more supportive approach. A group also may be designed around a specific problem with a focus on skill building and problem resolution.

Group psychotherapy at the primary care level may also be targeted at prevention and wellness and thus integrated into other medical specialty practices. Prevention and wellness groups provide a combination of education, behavior modification, and support for patients who need to make lifestyle changes. Groups at these levels of care can be either short term or long term in focus but typically meet only once or twice weekly for 60–90 minutes.

Combinations of individual and group psychotherapy may be particularly useful for patients needing continuing support and may also be used for gaining insight. Borderline patients may find it particularly useful to be in both individual and group psychotherapy simultaneously (Horwitz 1980). Patients can take what they learn in their individual psychotherapy to the group session and vice versa. It is essential that when patients are in such combined therapies, the therapists develop a contract with each other and the patient to be able to converse collaboratively.

Group psychotherapy can facilitate transitions between levels of care by allowing patients to be introduced to a group in the next level of care and even begin attending sessions before they terminate care at the previous level (Kennedy 1993). That approach gives them a connection with a group of patients and a group therapist that helps them depart from the structure and comfort of their previous treatment. For example, patients moving to an intensive outpatient level of treatment from partial hospital care may include group psychotherapy in their ongoing treatment regimen. Programs can facilitate this move by making it possible for patients to use the same group in both levels of care so they can move away from the day hospital and reenter work while continuing in the group. It is also useful for other patients in the group because they hear about one of their members attempting to "make it."

Psychoeducational Activities

Increasingly, a variety of psychoeducational activities are being used as effective active therapy for the whole spectrum of behavioral health care patients.

Several examples illustrate the variety of psychoeducational approaches:

- Programs for patients who have suffered severe trauma provide a trauma educational program (Allen 1995) in which patients are taught about the psychological effects of trauma, both immediate and long range, and are given direct information on ways to deal with symptoms such as dissociative states.

- Educational groups focusing on medication provide patients with information regarding how their medications work and possible side effects along with an opportunity to discuss their varied experiences with medication (Nand 1991).

- Programs for patients who are chronically mentally ill provide considerable opportunity through psychoeducational activities for patients and their families to learn about chronic mental illness. The National Alliance for the Mentally Ill, an organization of consumers and families, has been effective in providing a wide array of educational materials for families.

- Psychoeducational services and materials are also commonly included in programs for substance abuse, eating disorders (Piran and Kaplan 1990), depression, bipolar disorder (Goldstein and Miklowitz 1994), and patients with Alzheimer's disease and their family members. Gunderson et al. (1997) developed psychoeducational groups for families of borderline patients.

Such psychoeducational activities can be effectively used across the entire continuum of care to educate both consumers and family members or other caregivers. Psychoeducational materials may be presented to patients either in activity group format or through handouts. The design of psychoeducational programming, however, must take into account the consumer's ability to receive and comprehend the information presented. The presentation of psychoeducational materials to a patient hospitalized during an acute exacerbation of symptoms has to be handled quite differently from presentation to a patient attending an outpatient group.

Crisis Management

Crisis intervention is a necessary component of behavioral health care because patients with psychiatric and substance abuse disorders become unstable and experience acute crises resulting from an acute psychotic episode, manic excitement, suicide planning or suicidal gestures, and other out-of-control behaviors. In traditional systems, individuals in crises often end up in the emergency department with triage to inpatient care. Thus, the hospital often is viewed as the setting in which crises are handled. IDSs attempt to eliminate the use of this expensive and often inefficient crisis care.

Within an IDS, many hospitalizations can be averted as other programs become adept at dealing with crisis management. For this reason all programs must have services for crisis management. However, the structure of those services needs to differ according to the level of intensity of the treatment provided and the stability of the target patient population. The following guidelines meet those crisis management needs:

1. All IDSs should have an on-call psychiatrist available 24 hours/day, 365 days/year to deal with medical emergencies.

2. Additional on-call services need to be available. Many IDSs develop crisis teams responsible for providing emergency care to patients across the entire system. Often these teams are associated with a central assessment unit. Crisis teams may provide office-based care or care at various program sites or they may be dispatched to a patient's home for crisis intervention. Crisis teams provide assessment, deescalation, encouragement of problem solving, and enhancement of the patients' and their families' competencies in crisis resolution, support, and triage. Crisis teams also begin psychopharmacology or evaluate and adjust current medications as necessary.

3. Patients in intensive ambulatory services presenting with unstable conditions may experience frequent crises. Some crises will be handled appropriately without a change in programming, whereas others may require heightened structure or intensity. Patients in partial hospitals and other such programs may have crises that need to be handled first by the program itself. Program staff members familiar with the patient's treatment plan and current condition provide the most knowledgeable assistance to patients in crisis.

4. However, crises that arise after program hours can be referred to the crisis team if necessary. If a patient is referred from an intensive ambulatory service for crisis assistance, it is essential that pertinent treatment information be readily available to the crisis team. It is also particularly important to have crisis services immediately available to patients so that they do not have to move to a higher level of care. Examples of such services include ready availability of apartments or some other kind of respite care that provides the patient with immediate help in a crisis and well-developed programs, such as Crossing Place (Bourgeois 1994) in Washington, D.C., that actively treat the patient in crisis in a residential noninstitutional setting.

5. In community-based settings, crisis services need to include assistance for the patient's family, existing support relationships, or caregivers, because

they may have felt abused or mistreated by the patient during the crisis situation.

6. It should be noted that when patients require crisis episodes of hospitalization while participating in a lower level of care, every effort must be made to return them to the lower level of care as soon as possible. In many situations in which these levels of care are part of the same integrated system, patients may be able to start attending ambulatory care activities or psychotherapies while they are still hospitalized. In this way patients do not lose their connection with the staff and patients in the program and can move out much more readily than patients without a built-in support system. Also patients can process the crisis and hospitalization with program staff and hope to acquire additional knowledge about their propensity for relapse and under what conditions it is most apt to occur. This helps patients become more actively engaged in treatment.

Special Treatment Procedures

Of course, crises can occur at any point across the continuum of care as patients attempt to take greater responsibility for themselves. Many services deal with the potential for patient crises by developing and implementing special treatment procedures. Special treatment procedures for dealing with patients displaying aggressive, acting-out behaviors; noncompliance with program rules; and suicidal, homicidal, or runaway ideation are a necessary part of behavioral health care programming (Kiser et al. 1991). Special treatment procedures designed for use in IDSs must adequately address the issue of safety and involve the family, social support network, and community as necessary while maintaining the patient in the least restrictive treatment environment.

Often nonacute behavioral health care programs simply do not offer special treatment procedures, believing such procedures are appropriate only on inpatient units. However, special treatment procedures can be implemented effectively at all levels of care given that they do not violate the program's mandate—that is, they outline procedures that can also be used by families, friends, parents, or guardians in the home environment. For instance, although typical of many inpatient services, manual and chemical restraints are rarely used in ambulatory behavioral health care services. Other interventions, such as crisis deescalation, that allow a patient to regain self-control are implemented.

Suicide Precautions: Ambulatory Levels of Care

An assessment of intention and risk is always the first step in suicide prevention. If manageable risk is determined, various interventions can be implemented within ambulatory and outpatient services. A close observation protocol consisting of 30-minute checks with evaluation of suicide risk at the end of program hours every day can be implemented in partial hospital or intensive outpatient programs. Such a close-observation policy reflects the philosophy of maintaining the patient in the least restrictive setting without providing services beyond the resources of the family or support community. This philosophy is opposed to using the program staff for one-to-one continuous observation to prevent suicidal action when a family is unlikely to have similar resources available. However, patients are typically at highest risk for suicidal ideation after treatment hours and on weekends. This observation is addressed through development of no-harm contracts and after-hours phone contact with suicidal patients. At prearranged times the patient is phoned, usually by the case manager or individual therapist, and support and coping mechanisms are reviewed. Additionally, a plan for continued supervision after program hours is developed using family and community supports, telephone contact, beeper services, and other monitoring techniques.

Family Therapy

As professional responsibility and control for patients diminish across the continuum, involvement and commitment of family and social support networks become essential. Many programs use family therapies; this use is consistent with the fact that family dynamics and conflict frequently contribute to mental health problems and crises. Often patients admitted to inpatient services can be observed to quickly de-escalate once they are removed from these daily stressors. However, when patients are discharged from the hospital without resolution of family problems, symptoms reemerge quickly. The use of family therapies is also consistent with research demonstrating that family involvement is a predictive factor in the successful completion of treatment and follow-up, especially for children and adolescents (Prentice-Dunn et al. 1981).

At all levels of care, family treatment provides an opportunity to focus on family dynamics to facilitate change in the home environment. However, involvement of family and the purpose of family therapy change according to the level of care being provided. For example, when the patients are children and adolescents, a powerful difference between family treatment in ambulatory behavioral health care services, such as partial hospital, and inpatient settings is the emphasis on maintaining parental authority. In partial hospitalization and other ambulatory behavioral health care services, parents are involved in every level of decision making and problem solving (Kiser et al. 1991).

PART II: PATIENT ECOLOGY

All the world's a stage
And all the men and women merely players

Shakespeare, *As You Like It*

Historically the specialized environment in which we provide treatment was labeled the *milieu* and was found primarily in an inpatient unit, residential treatment program, or partial hospital setting—any facility-based setting providing intensive psychiatric services. However, as provision of psychiatric services moves dramatically away from office-based outpatient care or facility-based inpatient treatment toward an integrated, comprehensive service array, the traditional practice of milieu treatment is affected, and applying the concept to any and all of the settings in which patients live, work, or interact becomes critical. Thus, we define *therapeutic ecology* as a cohesive, consistent therapeutic environment created within a program, home, or community through the coordination of people, space, materials, equipment, and activities.

In an IDS, treatment is based on service intensity matched to patient needs (Kiser et al. 1993), with patient needs for a therapeutic ecology or milieu just one of the factors to be considered. The benefits of a therapeutic milieu are necessary in all treatment settings; the structure and objective of this specialized environment change as the patient moves among levels of care. The continuum model of IDS suggests that if a service does not include an active therapeutic milieu on site then the treatment plan prescribes active intervention to extend milieu-based therapeutic benefits to the home, workplace or school, and community as needed. "This approach requires an initial abstract conceptual leap from the way people, space, and things interact in a traditional geographically located inpatient unit or partial hospital setting to a *'virtual'* reality that has a real meaning in the patient's experience" (Spencer, personal communication, 1995).

Understanding the Patient Ecology

"A *milieu* is simply any environment in which a patient or anyone else lives. *Milieu treatment* differs in being a specialized environment which is designed to fulfill the general purposes of preventing 'bad' things from happening and allowing 'good' things to occur" (Gunderson 1978, p. 332). "Too often milieu has been invested with a somewhat mystical aura, as if there were some secret manufacturing process that combined institutional input into a substance which then influenced patient behavior" (Lawton and Cohen 1975, p. 202).

A solid understanding of the relationships between behavior and setting can help demystify the process, and *ecological psychology*, as the study of behavior in context, provides a valuable framework.

According to ecological psychology, understanding behavior requires exploration of interrelationships between a setting and the behaviors occurring within that setting, taking into account both the ecological environment (the objective, real-life settings) and the psychological environment (individuals' perceptions of their environment). It is concerned with the natural phenomenon, termed a *behavior setting*, composed of humans behaving and the space, time, and objects within which the behavior is transacted (Barker 1968).

Imagine walking into a room filled with 25 executive office chairs around a large conference table. In front of the table is a screen and computer projection system. A woman dressed in a suit is sitting at the head of the table with a microphone on the table before her. Do you know what to expect and how to behave? You understand what to expect and how to behave based on the *standing patterns of behavior* that define the common set of behaviors typically observed within a specific setting. The arrangement of space, objects, and people provides cues regarding the behavior expected within the setting. Of importance to the understanding of the patient ecology is the observation that standing patterns of behavior created within a setting are often more powerful determinants of behavior than are the individual personality differences of setting participants.

Ecological psychology outlines numerous characteristics and properties related to behavior settings (Barker 1968; Barker et al. 1978). Anyone working in a therapeutic milieu will recognize these as aspects of the environment that affect behavior and can be manipulated to create change. Setting characteristics include participants, space, time, objects, and patterns of behavior that are naturally established within the boundaries of a setting. Properties of behavior settings include *timing*, *duration*, and *sequence* of events; characteristics of the group of people or *population* participating; and their degree of *penetration* (level of involvement or role) in the setting.

Effective Patient Ecology

Is it possible to describe the characteristics and properties of behavior settings that create an environment conducive to patient well-being? Research on the treatment milieu suggests the following characteristics (Gunderson 1978; Hoge et al. 1988; Lefkovitz 1995): a safe and unambiguous physical and psychological climate; a consistent and cohesive group of participants; continuity and stability of activities; clear, reasonable expectations; active participation by participants; open and honest communication; trusting relationships among participants; and shared decision making.

Within the context of a therapeutic behavior setting, the interrelationships between the environment and the standing patterns of behavior allow "good things to happen" through promotion of five therapeutic factors: safety and containment, structure, support, involvement, and empowerment (Gunderson 1978; Hoge et. al. 1988). Table 9–1 provides an overview of those five factors.

Patient Ecologies and Integrated Delivery Systems

Attention to patient ecologies across the service array requires a focus on the specific functions of each level of care and the needs of the patient population served at each level of care. Acutely ill patients often require a patient ecology focused on the most basic issues of safety and containment. Patients able to function more adaptively and receive treatment in less intensive levels can benefit from a focus on involvement and empowerment. The patient ecology moves from primarily facility based to the patient's real-world environment.

The therapeutic milieu within acute, intensive residential programs must be primarily concerned with maintaining a closed system within the treatment setting, ensuring that the system is highly planned and consistent, maintaining a focus on providing safety and containment, and requiring intensive levels of staff direction and participation. Within nonresidential levels of acute treatment the milieu is maintained within an open system; the system is highly planned and consistent; the system is focused primarily on safety, containment, and structure; and high levels of staff and support system participation are required. In services providing transition or rehabilitative treatment, the patient ecology is planned; is within both the program and the home; is focused primarily on structure, support, and involvement; and requires moderate levels of staff and support system participation. Services that function to prevent relapse or deterioration when outpatient treatment is not sufficient require an ecology that is planned, primarily within the home and community, and focused on involvement and empowerment and that requires low levels of staff and support system participation. At outpatient and primary care levels that function to identify, prevent, and diminish mild to moderate symptoms, services addressing the patient ecology focus on the patient's natural setting, stress involvement and empowerment, and are derived primarily through representation of the therapeutic relationship between sessions.

Therapeutic Milieu and Short-Term Care

Acute inpatient units and partial hospital programs, where many milieu concepts originated, no longer have the luxury of using the traditional therapeutic milieu. Challenges to the traditional milieu are driven primarily by cost-cutting strategies implemented in response to managed behavioral health

TABLE 9–1.	Five therapeutic factors	
Factor	**Aspects**	**Therapeutic benefits**
Safety and containment	Elimination or diminution of potentially dangerous objects and interactions Realistic and clearly delineated rules and limits Close supervision and monitoring Special procedures for handling dangerous or highly disruptive behaviors	Increase risk taking Engage in self-exploration Try new behaviors Learn new skills
Structure	Organizing the time, space, and activity of each patient's day through the management of space Regular schedule of activities Size and composition of groupings Organizational chart with lines of authority	Consistency Daily routine Expectation, development of predictable patterns of behavior Sense of purpose
Support	Staff and peer emotional and psychological reinforcement Tangible supports, such as help with a task or financial assistance	Decrease in stress level and symptoms Opportunity to build reciprocal relationships Enhanced self-esteem
Involvement	Structured opportunities for active collaboration Open communication Shared decision making Companionship Expectation for acceptance	Improve communication, problem-solving, and decision-making skills Strengthen sense of identity Enhance productivity Develop relationships
Empowerment	Dispensing positive reinforcement Providing success experiences Encouraging autonomy	Develop a sense of shared reality and universality Feel more accepting of self and others Express hope and commitment to change

care. Cost-cutting strategies affect the use of dedicated space for specific programs and groups, the assignment of staff to a specific service on a regular basis, decreased lengths of stay, and part-time attendance schedules (Lefkovitz 1995). How do providers maintain the benefits of a therapeutic milieu without a program, a stable group of patients, a regular schedule of attendance, and so forth?

A first step is accepting that the function of treatment in acute inpatient and partial hospital programs is changing and that the milieu must change as well. The therapeutic milieu designed for short-term crisis stabilization must accommodate the realities of a constantly changing patient population characterized by acute, severe symptoms; high risk levels; and instability. These realities create an atmosphere within most intensive treatment settings that is intense, complex, dynamic, and volatile (Lefkovitz 1995) and require a therapeutic milieu focused primarily on establishing safety and containment. Providing this safe and secure environment for a rapidly changing census requires constant staff planning and adjustment, with higher levels of staff direction and engagement in the milieu. Staff members must also alter expectations for patient behavior and participation within the milieu, accepting more limited prospects for change, affective sharing, and relationship development.

Many of the techniques used within a traditional therapeutic milieu (patient government, group management techniques, level systems) are no longer applicable or require substantial modification. However, a variety of new techniques bolsters the therapeutic milieu within short-term, intensive treatment settings. One example is use of treatment plans with a long-term focus that orient the patient early in the planning process to the stages of care and the likely transitions between levels. This approach allows patients to prepare for their participation in the current programmatic milieu as well as future ones. Patients with an understanding of both the goals and the time frame for treatment at a specific level of care can more easily assume appropriate expectations for their behavior and interactions within each setting. Opportunities for transition planning are also provided. For some patients this might involve the use of peer assistance or a "buddy system" designed to allow patients to orient and support new patients as they move through the system of care. For others this might involve attending several groups or activities in the next level of care before any transition. Coordinating treatment elements where appropriate is also encouraged, such as use of one physician to manage medications throughout a patient's episode of care or operation of a systemwide crisis safety net.

In addition to programmatic management of the therapeutic milieu, acute ambulatory treatment settings must develop policies to help patients control their behavior both on the unit and at home or in the community. For example, partial hospital programs can provide treatment for patients with significant suicidal or elopement ideation if they are able to maintain appropriate levels of observation during program hours, have policies for structure after hours, and have the ability to liaison with community resources.

Creating the New Milieu: The Therapeutic Patient Ecology

The traditionally defined therapeutic milieu, although still considered essential to effective treatment, has less applicability in today's delivery system. Modifications to the programmatic milieu are necessary, and new means for creating therapeutic environments are being explored. Programs such as partial hospitalization have long been aware of the need to have an impact on the patient's home, neighborhood, and community to create improvements that generalize beyond program walls. These programs use a variety of theoretical foundations to structure their thinking regarding this extended milieu, such as family systems theory (Minuchin 1974), family rituals (Wolin 1984), social network theory (Biegel et al. 1994; Meeks and Murrell 1994; Wellman 1990), and psychiatric home health care.

Assessment. As in other areas of clinical care, sound ecological interventions require an assessment of the patient's world. Included within the structure of this assessment is the patient's evaluation of desired changes, goals for functional adaptation, and choices regarding his or her own relationships and roles and those of other people in the patient's life (Biegel et al. 1994). Assessment of the patient's natural milieu or environment can be based on a variety of useful approaches, such as assessments of family systems, family ecology, family ritual, social network, or psychiatric home care. Assessment techniques may involve interviews, completion of forms, and/or direct observations. Information can be gained from the individual patient, family members, significant others, friends, neighbors, coworkers, teachers, peers, other clinicians, and so on.

There are few patient ecology assessment instruments for use in clinical settings. One example is a patient ecology instrument designed to measure four relevant domains: conflict, burden, connectivity/isolation/access, and structure/safety/stability. Developed as a decision-support tool, the Patient Ecology Scale (see chapter appendix) provides an indication of the readiness of the patient's natural ecology to support the recovery process as well as the patient's ability to use such support.

A family systems assessment can be accomplished during a standard clinical interview. The clinician and patient discuss family membership, family subsystems, formal and informal relationship dynamics (e.g., power, conflict), and coalitions, all of which can be summarized through a family systems ecomap. Relevant intergenerational issues might be explored through gathering a family genogram or history across multiple generations. The family systems assessment underscores the current life cycle of the family and the family's structural properties such as roles, boundaries, rules, and communication style (State of Maryland 1987). Review from a family perspective of strengths and weaknesses and perception of the problem provides additional pertinent information for planning interventions in the home.

Another family assessment focuses on family ritual integrity. Family ritual integrity encompasses perceptions, behaviors, family processes, and parental practices with respect to deliberate planning, ritualization, meaning making and spirituality, daily routines, role clarity, and people resources. It can be measured through a semistructured interview covering the following topics: religious background and activities, storytelling in the family, deliberateness in planning for the future of the family and the results of that planning thus far, people resources during times of family need, and detailed descriptions of two special occasions and daily routines (Bennett et al., unpublished).

A family ecology assessment provides information about the family fit and interaction with community resources. This assessment focuses on the background, existing patterns of interaction, and perceptions of family members regarding these resources. A family ecology evaluation addresses effective resource linkages that can be built on, conflicted resource linkages that require intervention, tenuous/burdened linkages that need support, and absent linkages that must be constructed (State of Maryland 1987). Methods of assessing family ecology include direct questions to family members, observation of the family during crisis, and creation of a family ecomap showing relationships between the family and important social, community, and professional resources.

Various techniques and assessment instruments are available for measuring different aspects related to individual support systems. A social network inventory provides an indication of family and kinship ties; informal network supports such as church, social clubs, and neighbors; formal support networks such as coworkers and self-help groups; and relationships with professional caregivers. Standardized inventory instruments include the Network of Relationships Inventory (Furman and Buhrmeister 1985) and The Questionnaire of Social Network and Social Support (SONET) (Amann 1991). Another technique used to gather such information is a social network map, similar to the family ecomap. Patients sketch out maps of their social support systems using concentric circles to indicate closeness (Carson and Arnold 1996). Structured interview formats such as the Interview Measure of Social Relationships (Brugha et al. 1993) provide similar information.

Much of the work on evaluating patient living environments stems from the field of psychiatric home care. Assessment in this field provides a comprehensive picture of the home environment, physical needs of the patient, functional adaptation, and a risk profile specifically identifying physical and psychological safety issues and danger zones. Activities of daily living and maintenance of functioning are major aspects of home care, and instruments such as the Activities of Daily Living Scale (Duke University 1975) aid assessment of this critical domain.

Intervention Techniques. Following this comprehensive assessment, targeted interventions designed for implementation in the patient's natural environment are incorporated into the treatment plan. As in the programmatic milieu, it is necessary to ensure that safety needs are quickly addressed. Thus, it is important to write a crisis plan with all patients as they enter or move to ambulatory levels of care. Crisis plans identify potential areas of vulnerability and outline a course of action to be followed in the event of a crisis. A no-harm contract is usually implicit in the design and acceptance of the plan. Crisis plans are to an ambulatory therapeutic ecology what special treatment procedures are to the programmatic milieu. They provide a written statement of the policies and procedures to ensure safety of the patient.

Crisis planning is a multifaceted process, developed in a stepwise fashion:

Step 1: The crisis plan describes the naturalistic safety net available to the patient using the patient's own problem-solving abilities and support system. This might involve establishing deescalation plans and/or distress signals, having the patient observed by family members/supports, or removing potentially dangerous objects. Providing home safes for storage of medications or weapons is sometimes warranted.

Step 2: The crisis plan specifies a range of peer/self-help emergency support systems available. The Alcoholics Anonymous model of sponsorship is an excellent example.

Step 3: The plan outlines access to professional emergency services. This part of the plan explicitly details the availability and use of emergency rooms, call systems, check-ins, and electronic monitoring as needed.

Once safety is established within the natural ecology, therapeutic assignments become relevant. These assignments cover a broad range of prescribed interventions designed to promote change in the patient's natural environment. Time management interventions, structured activities, and weekend planning are described as examples.

Time management interventions are often beneficial for helping patients spend less and less of their day in the treatment milieu. Simple concepts such as agreeing on a time to get up and dressed in the morning and a time to go to bed at night can help structure the day. Additional organization can be created with the use of other time management strategies such as making appointments, finding and scheduling activities or chores both within and outside the home, doing volunteer work, and so on. Some patients find the use of electronic schedulers with alarms helpful for maintaining their daily schedule of activities.

Prescribing selected activities can also increase a patient's sense of purpose, pleasure, and quality of life. For instance, child and adolescent patients often benefit from involvement in sports, music, or club activities. It is always important to match the patient's current level of functioning, interests, and abilities with the activities chosen. Contact with the clinician or case manager and the participants or leaders of the activity can be both beneficial and limiting and should be carefully considered.

Weekend treatment plans provide a simple way of extending treatment goals into the patient's real-world environment. The concept of weekend treatment planning is not limited to weekends but can be applied to any block of time between therapy sessions. This is especially relevant for patients who move quickly from inpatient to less intensive programming. As less and less time is spent in treatment settings, it is helpful for patients to set goals and develop strategies for generalizing treatment to routine daily functioning. Components of weekend planning include assessment of risks and vulnerabilities, planning and problem-solving, goals for practice or skill building, assignments, and monitoring. Monitoring the success of weekend treatment planning can range from "check-ins" scheduled periodically during nontreatment hours or use of electronic monitoring devices to a patient journal or self-report of compliance.

Family therapy and other interventions designed to alter family relationships are often helpful. Therapy sessions can be held in the office setting or in the home. Family conflict and reciprocity are two important areas for attention. Resolving family conflict may involve education, role-play, and practice of conflict resolution techniques. Increased reciprocity and decreased burden may be achieved through therapeutic assignments in which patients practice ways of giving something back to their families, such as volunteering to complete a household chore.

A variety of intervention strategies target family rituals. First and foremost, families (including all family members) are encouraged to participate in deliberate planning as to family goals, expectations, quality of relationships, rituals, routines, roles, and people resources. Second, families are helped to plan and carry out important family rituals and to maintain healthful daily routines. They practice a range of activities from "bigger" rituals and routines such as holiday meals and dinner times to more "mundane" routines such as observing regular bedtimes for children and developing leisure time hobbies. Third, they concentrate on developing well-understood and acceptable roles when it comes to carrying out the duties that need to be done in the family on a regular basis or during special occasions. Finally, families explore their relationships with people outside the nuclear family whom they can call on if they need assistance. Thus, interventions around family rituals focus on much of what is lost as families confront the mental illness of a family member: development and maintenance of daily routines, planning and carrying out family events despite disruptions, and celebration of individual and family successes.

In addition to therapeutic assignments and work with families, ecological intervention strategies target social support systems. Findings regarding the social support systems of individuals with severe and persistent mental illnesses suggest that functional adaptation and maintenance of recovery may be related to positive social supports and vice versa. It seems clear that social support systems are negatively affected by chronic illness and tend to diminish in size, complexity, and energy as the illness progresses (Biegel et al. 1994; Meeks and Murrell 1994). Strategies to prevent network deterioration or strengthen network functioning may reduce relapse rates and the need for intensive, restrictive interventions such as inpatient or residential care.

Interventions designed to alter social networks stem originally from intensive case management with individuals with serious and persistent mental illnesses. Two approaches are described in the literature: strengthening natural support networks and creating prescribed support networks. Natural support networks typically comprise family, friends, and other community relationships. Altering natural support networks can involve a variety of intervention approaches: building new network ties, maintaining and strengthening existing ties, enhancing family ties, and/or diminishing or disconnecting maladaptive network ties (Biegel et al. 1994). Prescribed support systems typically involve community-based organizational leaders or members; patient-derived support networks such as mentors, sponsors, or self-help groups; and professional networks composed of doctors, nurses, clinicians, case managers, clergy, teachers, and counselors. Prescription of professional or formal support networks can be used to offset deficits in an individual's natural support system.

Finally, establishing an effective patient ecology often requires intervention targeting the workplace or school. One method for planning these in vivo interventions makes use of the person-environment fit model by focusing on changes both within the individual and within the setting. Many adults derive much of their identity and sense of purpose from their work. When mental illness affects this aspect of their lives, workplace interventions may become necessary and can range from placement in a sheltered workshop, liaison with vocational rehabilitation services, and job skills training and counseling to on-the-job interventions. Workplace interventions are most successful in collaboration with the employer's employee assistance program. Strategies for intervention on the job might include temporary or permanent job assistance, restructuring, or rescheduling and any change in job duties, responsibilities, and/or schedules required to meet the needs of the patient to remain on the job and to be productive. Job mentoring, which involves the assistance of a coworker or supervisor, is another option. This coworker, who is informed about the patient's illness and understands the job-related concerns, helps the patient by modeling appropriate job skills and behaviors, cueing the patient regarding inappropriate or dysfunctional actions, and so on.

Just as the workplace serves as an important environment in the lives of many adults, school becomes the focus of attention for many children and adolescents. School-based interventions focused on the individual may involve teaching new skills, either academic or social; tutoring; and behavioral contracts or assignment of a behavioral aide to enhance school-related functioning. School-based interventions can also focus on altering the child's school milieu to create behavior change. The variety of interventions possible for altering the school milieu in aid of a child with severe attention-deficit/hyperactivity disorder include changing the child's schedule to mix classes requiring greater levels of attention and inactivity, such as literature or math, with those requiring more interaction and movement, such as physical education; placing the child in a smaller classroom with fewer distractions; and/or allowing the child to take more frequent short breaks during class time. Other school-based interventions can target the development of special and supportive relationships between students and teachers, counselors, coaches, or other school personnel. The establishment of such special relationships can be prescribed or structured initially but, it is hoped, will become part of the child's naturalistic support network.

Finally, work- or school-based interventions may involve assessing goodness of fit. Not all employees do well in every job setting nor do all students do equally well in every school setting. Sometimes recommendation of a new job or school becomes an important therapeutic intervention. Take for example the case of a depressed, withdrawn adolescent attending a large high school. Studies have shown that large schools tend to provide less pressure for involvement, with fewer opportunities for active participation, leadership, and responsibility (Barker et al. 1978). Placement in a small school with increased environmental pressure for participation may improve functioning and chances for successful engagement.

Table 9–2 provides a compendium of techniques designed as ecological interventions in programmatic and naturalistic settings.

CONCLUSIONS

One of the myths regarding behavioral health care is that an individual therapist can provide individual therapy in any treatment setting with the same

TABLE 9–2.   Ecological interventions

Therapeutic factors	Programmatic milieu	Naturalistic settings
Safety and containment	Positive peer culture Clear rules and limits Special treatment procedures Staff supervision of milieu	Crisis plans On-call systems/mobile teams No harm contracts In-home services Home safes Bracelets/computer check-ins
Structure	Organizing time, space, and objects Floor plan Size and composition of groups Organizational chart Daily routine and schedule of activities	Organizing the time, space, and activity Behavioral contracts Drug screens Paymaster Computer organizers
Support	Positive peer culture Group support activities Staff availability Guided problem solving	Peer support networks Homemakers Paired to Care/Big Brother programs Church/volunteer Work assistance program
Validation	Active collaboration by patients Attendance and activity schedules Open communication Shared decision making Patient government Patient responsibilities for maintaining milieu	Success experiences in activities of daily living Establishing real-life expectations Volunteer work Self-esteem scavenger hunt
Involvement	Positive atmosphere Success experiences Reward systems Reasonable expectations	Family routines and rituals Job training Volunteer work Mainstreaming in school/activities Shadowing Patients' involvement in their own recovery

results—that is, a clinician with experience on an inpatient unit can treat patients equally well in a partial hospital program. The fallacy involved in this way of thinking is that the process of individual, group, or milieu work is static with regard to level of care. Clearly, appropriate therapeutic processes must also match patient needs with the differing functions of services offered at different levels of care. As clinicians become more adept at treating patients throughout an episode of care using multiple levels of care, our sophistication in adapting clinical processes will undoubtedly improve.

REFERENCES

Allen JG: Coping with Trauma: A Guide to Self-Understanding. Washington, DC, American Psychiatric Press, 1995

Allen JG, Newson G, Coyne L, et al: Scales to assess a therapeutic alliance from a psychoanalytic perspective. Bull Menninger Clin 48:383–400, 1984

Amann G: Social network and social support deficits in depressed patients: a result of distorted perception? Eur Arch Psychiatry Clin Neurosci 241: 49–56, 1991

Barker RG: Ecological Psychology: Concepts and Methods for Studying the Environment of Human Behavior. Stanford, CA, Stanford University Press, 1968

Barker RG, Barker LS, Fawl CL, et al: Habitats, Environments, and Human Behavior: Studies in Ecological Psychology and Eco-Behavioral Science from the Midwest Psychological Field Station, 1947–1972. San Francisco, CA, Jossey-Bass, 1978

Biegel DE, Tracy EM, Corvo KN: Strengthening social networks: intervention strategies for mental health case managers. Health and Social Work 19: 206–216, 1994

Bourgeois P: Crossing Place: a community-based model for acute care. Continuum: Developments in Ambulatory Mental Health Care 1:61–69, 1994

Brugha TS, Wing JK, Brewin CR, et al: The relationship of social network deficits with deficits in social functioning in long-term psychiatric disorders. Social Psychiatry and Psychiatric Epidemiology 28:218–224, 1993

Carson VB, Arnold EN: The journey through home mental health care, in Mental Health Nursing: The Nurse-Patient Journey. Edited by Carson VB, Arnold EN. Philadelphia, PA, WB Saunders, 1996, pp 1151–1169

Duke University Medical Center: Activities of daily living, items 56–69, in Older Americans Resources and Services Instrument (OARS). Durham, NC, Duke University Center for the Study of Aging and Human Development, 1975

Furman W, Buhrmester D: Children's perceptions of the personal relationships in their social networks. Dev Psychol 21:1016–1024, 1985

Goldstein MJ, Miklowitz DJ: Family intervention for persons with bipolar disorder, in Family Interventions in Mental Illness: New Directions for Mental Health Services. San Francisco, CA, Jossey-Bass, 1994, p 62

Greenson R: The Technique and Practice of Psychoanalysis. New York, INT University Press, 1967

Gunderson JG: Defining the therapeutic process in psychiatric milieus. Psychiatry 41:327–334, 1978

Gunderson JG, Berkowitz C, Ruiz-Sancho A: Families of borderline patients: a psycho-educational approach. Bull Menninger Clin 61:4, 446–457, 1997

Hoge MA, Farrell SP, Munchel ME, et al: Therapeutic factors in partial hospitalization. Psychiatry 51:199–209, 1988

Horwitz L: Group psychotherapy for borderline and narcissistic patients. Bull Menninger Clin 44:181–200, 1980

Kennedy LL: Groups in day hospital, in Group Therapy in Clinical Practice. Edited by Alonso A, Swiller HI. Washington, DC, American Psychiatric Press, 1993, pp 137–154

Kiser LJ, Heston JD, Millsap PA, et al: Treatment protocols in child and adolescent day treatment. Hospital and Community Psychiatry 42:597–600, 1991

Kiser LJ, Lefkovitz PM, Kennedy LL: The continuum of ambulatory mental health services. Behav Healthc Tomorrow 2:14–16, 1993

Lawton MP, Cohen J: Organizational studies of mental hospitals, in Handbook of Evaluation Research, Vol 2. Edited by Guttentag M, Struening EL. Beverly Hills, CA, Sage Publications, 1975, pp 201–238

Lefkovitz PM: The continuum of care in a general hospital setting. Gen Hosp Psychiatry 17:260–267, 1995

Meeks S, Murrell SA: Service providers in the social networks of clients with severe mental illness. Schizophr Bull 20:399–406, 1994

Minuchin A: Families and Family Therapy. Cambridge, MA, Harvard University Press, 1974

Nand SS, Bailey L: Medication group in a day hospital. Int J Partial Hosp 7:77–83, 1991

Pincus HA, Tanielian TL, Marcus SC: Prescribing trends in psychotropic medications: primary care, psychiatry, and other medical specialties. JAMA 279:526–531, 1998

Piran N, Kaplan AS: A Day Hospital Group Treatment Program for Anorexia Nervosa and Bulimia Nervosa. New York, Brunner/Mazel, 1990

Prentice-Dunn S, Wilson DR, Lyman RD: Client factors related to outcome in a residential and day treatment program for children. J Clin Child Psychol 10:188–191, 1981

Rice CA, Rutan JS: Inpatient Group Psychotherapy; A Psychodynamic Perspective. New York, MacMillan, 1986

State of Maryland: Intensive Family Services: A Family Preservation Service Delivery Manual. Maryland Department of Human Resources, Social Services Administration, 1987

Wellman B: The Place of Kinfolk in Personal Community Networks (research paper). Toronto, Canada, Centre for Urban and Community Studies, 1990

Wolin SJ, Bennett LA: Family rituals. Fam Proc 23:401–410, 1984

Yalom IB: Inpatient Group Psychotherapy. New York, Basic Books, 1983

Appendix

Patient Ecology Scale

Patient Ecology Scale

Rate each of the items below using the scale from Never to Always

In the past month, how often have you:	Never	Rarely	Sometimes	Often	Always
1. Told people that you were OK when you were not					
2. Felt afraid to trust others					
3. Had friends who came to you for help or emotional support					
4. Preferred being alone and spent as little time as possible with other people					
5. Felt like you did not belong anywhere					
6. Felt like family and friends enjoyed being with you					
7. Felt alone					
8. Felt like you did not have any peers					
9. Belonged to one or more groups in your community, like clubs, that you had fun with					
10. Had people to count on to be there for you when you needed them					
11. Been comfortable with your daily routine					
12. Had your days filled with many things to do					
13. Had your day-to-day activities follow a set routine					
14. Feared for your safety					
15. Been harmed by someone					
16. Felt like your life seemed to be in order					
17. Felt like your life was out of control					

Patient Ecology Scale *(continued)*

In the past month, how often has your guardian, family, or friends:	Never	Rarely	Sometimes	Often	Always
18. Felt that your needs were too much to deal with					
19. Thought that you always took and never gave anything					
20. Did not want to see you because you always need something					
21. Felt they had to take care of you, like cooking, cleaning, driving					
22. Changed plans (vacation, work, going out) because of you					
23. Felt trapped by having to take care of you					
24. Watched you and tried to stop you from doing things to hurt yourself or others					
25. Had money problems because they took care of you					
26. Worried too much about your problems					
27. Felt burdened by you when you shared your problems					

In the past month, how often have you:	Never	Rarely	Sometimes	Often	Always
28. Had trouble controlling your temper					
29. Been rude to others					
30. Gotten into an argument when people disagreed with you					
31. Insulted or sworn at someone					
32. Threatened to hit or throw something					
33. Slapped another person					
34. Tried to get along with people but ended up mad					
35. Thrown, hit, or kicked something					
36. Stomped out of a room or house					
37. Gotten angry over nothing					
38. Disagreed with someone and told them so					

10

Staffing Across the Continuum of Care

Paul M. Lefkovitz, Ph.D.
David E. Ness, M.D.

Integrated service delivery presents new opportunities for personnel in their roles, their identities, and the ways in which they relate to one another. A shared vision for service delivery that minimizes barriers and makes the patient the *raison d'être* for the system has profound implications for staff. The values and processes that underlie service delivery integration encourage new and synergistic perspectives for mobilizing staff resources. To appreciate these new perspectives, we first explore the more established views of personnel and their roles.

In traditional systems of care staffing paradigms are often based on the team model that is defined by a specific program or professional discipline. Without question, the team model emphasizes some very important values and characteristics. With teams that are defined by program or department there is often an emphasis on continuity, consistency, and stability of operations. Where professional discipline is the defining variable, competencies and professional standards assume an important focus. These are all undoubtedly positive attributes that contribute to quality patient care. The team model also encourages a strong degree of identification with the program or the department. Loyalties are often intense, and there is a shared vision and set of values. Often, the team develops a consensus about external challenges or even adversaries. In the context of that common bond, morale may be strong.

At the same time, program and discipline-specific staffing models may represent barriers to service delivery integration. As introduced in Chapter 3, conflicting objectives among programs and/or disciplines may lead to fragmentation, inefficiency, and competition among caregivers. Teams often function as autonomous entities with little regard for the patient's journey through the system of care. For example, within a number of systems, staff from various levels of care actively "market" within the organization for patients in competition with one another. Such energy represents a duplication of efforts that can be avoided through an agreed-on process for equitable and appropriate placement of patients within the system. Turf may also be aggressively protected, leading to lack of cooperation and efforts to undermine others on the staff. Staff members have even been known to make derogatory comments to patients about other programs that they see as competitors within the system.

Service delivery integration offers some perspectives that can minimize these natural hazards that exist in any organization. In Chapter 2 the concept of *integrative mechanisms* was introduced. We discuss several integrating mechanisms in this chapter as they relate to personnel resources. One of the most potent of these involves redefining the team.

REDEFINING THE TEAM

It is important to understand the dynamics surrounding the team, whether the team is defined as a program, a department, a hospital, or a service line. The team defines loyalties, shared values, vision, passions, allies, adversaries, and identity for its constituent members. These team-based ties can be quite powerful and can motivate committed effort. Yet teams can also be quite exclusive and inherently competitive in nature. Teams can build fortifications around their boundaries to protect what lies within. These are frequently known as *silos of operation*. Silos of operation severely compromise patient care and organizational efficiency.

For example, a few years ago in one very traditional state hospital setting, the psychology and psychiatry departments found themselves competing actively for stature and financial resources. One new staff member commented that much of the time spent in department meetings was devoted to political strategizing. His efforts to refocus discussion on issues of quality of care were met with negative reactions and resistance from other department members.

In another example a hospital-based partial hospitalization program found itself competing for patients with the hospital's home care program. Home care staff loyal to their modality routinely made disdainful comments to referral sources about the partial hospitalization program. A bitter rivalry ensued, with the result being that the staff of those two programs could not work effectively together. Transfers between the two programs were rare. In that system patients were deprived of the full continuum of care.

In these two instances the needs of the teams were placed ahead of the objectives of the broader organization and the patients they were entrusted to serve. Redefining the team can minimize this pitfall. In an integrated system, teams may be organized around patient populations and their unique needs rather than around programs, levels of care, or professional disciplines. The organizational structure that best supports this notion is the service line model or one of its variants. That does not mean that program-based teams and professional departments should not exist. Such structures are necessary and helpful, but they alone should not drive the way personnel shape their professional roles. For example, if the partial hospitalization and home care personnel described above could have viewed their roles as supporting a geriatric continuum of care in a complementary manner, they might have been able to open up the necessary dialogue for mutual cooperation.

There is great power in redefining a team. Team loyalties and rivalries can be established and shifted rather quickly and dramatically. Consider a group of young persons assembled to play a game of basketball in school. As the group is divided into two teams, it takes just moments for loyalties to develop; as they begin to play, members can be observed rooting for one another, encouraging one another, and glaring at the opposition. Let's assume the game ends and the teacher draws different sides; two entirely new teams emerge. Within minutes, each new team is passionately rooting for individuals who, just before, had been adversaries.

In a health delivery system old rivalries among levels of care or departments can quickly drop when the team is redefined around a common denominator. Often these are service lines defined by population, such as youth, chemical dependency, or those with serious mental illness. Primary staff identification quickly migrates to the identified population served, and personnel begin to view their work in the context of the broader needs of their targeted clinical constituents. Care becomes more patient focused, and the boundaries between levels of care become less sharply defined. Personnel become much more willing to work together on the patient's behalf because the patient defines the team's reason for being. An excellent example of this process was in the hospital-based chemical dependency setting described in Chapter 2.

It should be noted that any divisions established within a system might become silos of operation. For example, youth services may actively compete for resources with geriatric services. However, although that is true, those silos would have little impact on an individual patient's movement through the system. Therefore, although all silos are detrimental and should be avoided, those that cut across levels of care are the most damaging to patient care and to service delivery integration.

CONTINUUM-BASED STAFFING

The continuum-based staffing model (Lefkovitz 1995, 1996) was proposed as a response to rapidly changing conditions in behavioral health care. Declining lengths of stay in all levels of care, increasing demands for cost effectiveness, and the expanding continuum of services all argue for new staffing models. A continuum-based staffing model addresses those challenges by viewing the episode of care as extending across the entire continuum rather than within a single program.

Continuum-based staffing introduces the concept of extending personnel across program boundaries. Staff members maintain a primary program assignment, perhaps accounting for 70% or 80% of their productive hours, but devote their remaining time working in another level of care. Depending on the support for the concept, the process may involve one person per program or several volunteers; participants may be added over time. Exchanges of staff should ideally be budget neutral so that each program maintains its staffing needs and budgetary targets.

The benefits of this simple concept may be seen at multiple levels. For the organization, continuum-based staffing produces a more fluid and seamless delivery system. This model facilitates cross-training, which equips personnel with a broader array of competencies and skills. The system also benefits from a workforce that is more diversely trained and can more easily accommodate possible redeployment needs in the future. Also the flow of personnel among levels of care reduces boundaries and competitiveness between programs.

For the program itself, the benefits of a stable core staff are present and yet the model opens up a diversity of new skills and approaches from other teams. In fact, specialized skills and talents can intentionally be sought out. Additionally, programs are likely to see improved communication with other programs as familiarity among staff members increases.

For the patients, there is increased familiarity with staff as they transition through levels of care. This familiarity is likely to enhance their comfort level. Patients also benefit from improved quality of care as a result of working with a team that consists of staff who are more familiar with their needs. All of these factors enhance the seamlessness of movement through the system.

Finally, for the staff, a major benefit is the opportunity to work with patients over a broader spectrum of the continuum and witness more significant clinical improvement. With declining lengths of stay in all levels of care, staff members are increasingly disappointed with the amount of improvement they see in their patients. Involvement in a broader range of services will allow staff to recognize that significant change still takes place but that progress is simply spread over more points along the continuum. This can have a very positive impact on the morale of the staff. Another benefit that continuum-based staffing offers for staff is the broader set of skills they acquire, which may enhance their job opportunities within or outside the system. Table 10–1 summarizes the benefits of continuum-based staffing.

This model is employed in selected areas of the first author's (P.M.L.) hospital-based setting with promising success thus far. Particularly in the chemical dependency services continuum, personnel are quite mobile in their movement among various levels of care. The resultant esprit de corps is high, and the blending of skills, approaches, and enthusiasm across the continuum presents distinct benefits for the patients and programs as well.

NEW ROLES FOR STAFF

Service delivery integration needs its own champions to help ensure its success. Although all leaders in an integrated system require new perspectives and skills, opportunities for new roles also emerge. One way to approach this need is to establish a role for a *continuum specialist* (Lefkovitz 1996). A continuum specialist is a professional who serves as a *facilitator* for a designated continuum of care. This individual should not function as another layer of management or merely an extension of the designated leader. Rather, the continuum specialist supports and advocates the clinical, administrative, and financial considerations that facilitate service delivery integration in all of its facets. Without the establishment of a unique role for such advocacy, it may very well not exist within the organization.

TABLE 10–1. Benefits of continuum-based staffing

To the organization	Enhances fluid patient movement
	Results in more diversely trained workforce
	Reduces barriers among programs
To the program	Preserves stable core of staff
	Makes new skills available to the team
	Improves communications with other programs
To the patient	Enhances ease of movement through system
	Increases familiarity and comfort with personnel in "new" levels of care
	Creates better-informed staff
To the staff	Permits involvement with patients over broader spectrum of continuum
	Brings about exposure to greater patient progress
	Improves morale
	Enhances acquisition of broader skills, in support of mobility and promotion

---

Specific duties of the continuum specialist might include identifying gaps in the continuum of care, initiating program development efforts, mediating philosophical and procedural disputes among programs, leading performance improvement activities, establishing clinical pathways or case management processes, problem solving patient flow issues, facilitating regulatory compliance, and representing the continuum to the broader community. Ideally, the continuum specialist would operate very proactively, identifying opportunities for greater service delivery integration. The specialist would also serve as a consultant, responding to requests for assistance from management and line staff. The continuum specialist should also become a trusted advisor to leadership in helping maintain efficient operations, improve quality, and shape the vision for the future.

In the role as facilitator, the continuum specialist needs to have expert process skills. It is especially important for the individual to maintain therapeutic distance in addressing problems within the organization. The ability to maintain neutrality in resolving disputes and improving performance is key in helping the organization move ahead in promoting greater service delivery integration.

It is helpful if the continuum specialist role can be combined with a part-time clinical role, allowing the specialist to rotate every few months through different parts of the system. In that way the continuum specialist could experience firsthand the barriers that exist within the system and the opportunities for greater integration that present themselves. Such a unique perspective is not likely to emerge from any other traditional role within the organization. Also, rotating clinical assignments would allow the continuum specialist to be viewed as being knowledgeable about all modalities of clinical care, thereby enhancing credibility.

The continuum specialist role should be occupied by a respected, senior-level clinician with experience in multiple levels of care. A high degree of familiarity with mediation skills and group process techniques is important. The person will need to be viewed as a teacher and mentor. The individual should also have a strong grasp of systems-oriented thinking. The continuum specialist will need to successfully champion the notion that the "whole is greater than the sum of its parts" to be effective in this unique role.

In the first author's (P.M.L.) hospital, four continuum specialist positions were established, one for each service line: adults, youth, senior adults, and chemical dependency. These roles contributed significantly to service delivery integration as the organization transitioned from a traditional level-of-care model to a service line structure.

Continuum integration brings other opportunities for new roles as well, such as competency-based personnel assignments. This view asserts that functional competencies are more critical to effectiveness and efficiency than are traditional disciplinary roles. Opportunities are therefore opened up for personnel with established competencies to be matched to work assignments that require their particular skills. Obviously, there are certain legal and regulatory limits associated with this model, but it does make available some interesting and creative possibilities. Certainly, a much more flexible and resilient workforce would result. Also, nontraditional staff assignments may bring new vantage points in service delivery evaluation and implementation.

MULTIDISCIPLINARY TEAM

The multidisciplinary team has been an established fixture of behavioral health care for many years. "In many behavioral health care organizations, the concept of teamwork is inherent in the philosophy of care. Much care in behavioral health settings is delivered using an interdisciplinary team" (Joint Commission on Accreditation of Healthcare Organizations 1996, p. 12). In the integrated system, however, the multidisciplinary team takes on new importance and meaning. Multidisciplinary teams were the first formalized effort in behavioral health care to bring about service delivery integration. Prior to their establishment, various departments essentially worked in isolation from one another. The arrival of the multidisciplinary team signaled a change in thinking that recognized the value of synthesis of thought and coordination of efforts.

In the integrated setting, multidisciplinary teams help facilitate many of the ingredients for successful service delivery integration. Such teams support a shared language and a consistent conceptual framework. They also provide for cohesion and trust, all of which are necessary for system integration. As delivery systems become more complex in their integrative efforts, the challenges to the multidisciplinary team will grow. These teams will increasingly cross level-of-care and other boundaries. Yet the ideals of producing one shared clinical vision that serves the patient in bringing about consistent and cohesive treatment will always remain part of the tradition and culture of the multidisciplinary team.

CHANGING ROLES FOR PROFESSIONAL DISCIPLINES

Service delivery integration has implications for the professional disciplines that operate in behavioral health settings. The specific impacts vary from discipline to discipline in light of their unique traditions, histories, and roles. This section explores service delivery integration in the context of some of the traditional disciplines found in behavioral health settings. The array of professions covered is not intended to be exhaustive but more illustrative of the interplay between traditional professional roles and the new dynamics of service delivery integration.

Psychiatrist

In an integrated system of care, decision making is necessarily more dispersed than centralized and care is coordinated rather than directed. In such a system the role of the psychiatrist involves working with multiple leadership structures rather than being the ultimate caregiving authority, as was the case in the past. The psychiatrist's authority needs to be exercised with a full awareness of the system's context. As Anderson (1998) asserted, however, "The importance of the role of physicians in clinical integration cannot be overemphasized" (p. 55). In the multifaceted role of leader and clinician, the physician plays a pivotal role in influencing the course of service delivery integration.

Roles and Functions Within an Integrated Environment

Assessing and Assigning Appropriate Levels of Care.   When helping to make level of care decisions, psychiatrists need to use their combined medical knowledge, psychological understanding, and appreciation of the system's dynamics. They should incorporate the input of other caregivers, which brings a variety of data about the patient, and include any relevant medical considerations (for example, the need to monitor medication side effects). Because other caregivers will have to live with the psychiatrist's decision, the doctor needs to be sensitive to the balance between medically desirable measures and therapeutically feasible ones. An example would be the decision not to prescribe medication that might be sedating or calming.

Providing Continuity Across Different Levels of Care.   Psychiatrists traditionally have been based in program "slots" (e.g., inpatient, partial hospital). However, patient care stands to benefit greatly from having the same psychiatrist (as well as other clinicians) available to follow along with the patient's transition from one level of care to another. The psychiatrist who treated a patient during an acute episode on the hospital unit knows more about the patient's medical and mental condition than a newly assigned outpatient doctor can possibly learn by merely reading the discharge summary. Furthermore, when the experience has been positive for the patient and family, the inpatient psychiatrist will have earned their trust, and this can be highly beneficial for the completion of treatment.

Tasks that are relevant to providing continuity include activities such as communicating with staff from each program about key items in the patient's history and psychiatric care. The psychiatrist also needs to remain available to the patient and staff in case of emergency, so there is medical support to facilitate changes in level of care.

Training and Skills Needed for Integration

Locus of Training. Traditional psychiatric residency training begins in the hospital and progresses to the outpatient clinic. This type of training allows the resident early exposure to the most severe cases and conditions. It also provides a safety net made up of the nursing staff and the attending psychiatrist to support residents as they acquire clinical decision-making skills. As is the case with severe medical illnesses, there is a confidence-building advantage to having the trainee experience the most pathologic situations first.

A more naturalistic setting could be argued for, however, one in which the trainee is exposed to outpatient clinical decision-making tasks with less of an institutional safety net. In the outpatient levels of care, it is crucial to assess risk, functional capacity, environmental influence, treatment alliance, and other factors that affect the feasibility and safety of treatment. The old Massachusetts Mental Health Center Day Hospitalization and Inn Program, which was a model of its kind (Gudeman et al. 1985), provided Harvard PGY-II psychiatric residents with their initial training in the partial hospital. Such experiences give the psychiatrist-in-training a feel for the clinical complexity (as well as the anxiety) of decision making with an acute but outpatient population.

Nature of the Supervision: Working Within the Integrated System. So that psychiatrists can be prepared for an integrated setting, more emphasis should be placed on the development of skills that facilitate teamwork, communication, management of computerized data, assessment of needed levels of care, and other tasks as outlined above. Many of these might fall under the heading of *administrative psychiatry*. A key item relates to the handling of the physician's authority. Traditional models have had all authority flowing downward from the physician to other members of the treatment team. Although that has changed greatly, there is a legitimate role for the physician's use of authority, particularly where this may give necessary focus to treatment with both medical and psychosocial issues. It is crucial that the psychiatrist-in-training acquire the ability to balance authority with team collaboration.

Psychologist

Psychologists bring unique perspectives and skills into an integrated system of care. At the same time, their traditional roles present interesting challenges in adapting to the special needs of service delivery integration.

Roles and Functions Within an Integrated Environment

Involvement Across the Continuum. In many respects the roles that psychologists often play in health care systems are quite compatible with integrated delivery models. Often psychologists function as members of a treatment team in organized settings. They often work collaboratively with other professionals in support of the best interests of the patient. Psychologists working within the context of this model may have few difficulties adjusting to the strategies of continuum integration.

Psychologists also frequently provide specialized consultative and clinical services across the continuum. This is particularly true of psychological assessment. In addition, many psychologists engage in clinical research or performance improvement activities throughout the system of care. Involvement with a diversity of programs provides many psychologists with comfort and perspective across the treatment spectrum.

Psychologists also function in a variety of therapeutic roles across the continuum of care. They are generally well prepared by virtue of their training for a broad range of clinical responsibilities, for example, traditional individual psychotherapy, brief therapy, cognitive behavior therapy, group therapy, and family therapy. Psychologists are also active in supervising the work of others in those domains of activity.

New Opportunities. New opportunities for psychologists are likely to emerge from the movement toward integration of the continuum. Their empirical and conceptual-oriented background can assist in developing paradigms for clinical benchmarks, care pathways, and other attempts to standardize best practices across levels of care. Also, many psychologists may find themselves in positions of leadership across the continuum, as has been the case in the managed care industry.

New opportunities may also come from evolving boundaries around the profession of psychology. The movement toward prescriptive authority could have significant impact on the use of psychologists across the continuum.

Advancing Psychology as a Profession. In years past, psychology typically was organized as a distinct department within the health care system. In many instances this organizational structure helped set the stage for spirited interdisciplinary rivalries between psychology and other disciplines, most frequently psychiatry. In recent years it has been more common to integrate psychologists with other professionals into clinical teams or service-related departments.

Yet debate regarding the issue of professional autonomy continues among those committed to advancing psychology as a profession. At the University of Missouri Health Sciences Center, the organizational placement of psychologists within the system recently became the object of some controversy. Psychologists had been integrated throughout the system in various departments, such as rehabilitation and neurology. A proposal was made to create a distinct psychology department, which would have required psychologists to relinquish their existing appointments. The originator of the proposal asserted, "The power of the profession is diluted because we are spread across departments" (Rabasca 1998, p. 19). A competing proposal for a separate psychology department would have allowed psychologists to retain their primary appointments while pursuing secondary appointments in the psychology department, citing "requiring psychologists to leave their current departments and join the new department would create unnecessary competition" (Rabasca 1998, p. 19). These are daunting issues for systems to grapple with inasmuch as the pursuit of professional identity can sometimes conflict with the ideals of service delivery integration.

Training and Key Skills Needed for Integration

The training of psychologists tends to emphasize conceptual models and systems thinking. Organizational and industrial psychologists, in fact, view the system as the principal focus of attention. This orientation helps prepare psychologists for the strategies that might be adopted in an integrated system of care. Their background should assist in understanding the importance of uniform, well-developed conceptual platforms and clinical processes for care delivery.

However, in an integrated setting, psychology's emphasis on a conceptual model may also present some challenges. Psychology, probably more than any other discipline, encourages students to adopt a consistent, cohesive, and concretized theoretical model for understanding psychopathology and psychotherapeutic intervention. Whether the model is psychodynamic, behavioral, or multimodal, psychologists learn the value of a consistent conceptual foundation with which to make clinical decisions. This is an invaluable tool for solo practitioners who must rely on their own judgment. A clear model can also facilitate clinical consistency throughout a system of care. At times, however, a firm reliance on a conceptual model can also set the stage for conflicts with those of different persuasions and, in the extreme, it can lead to conceptual orthodoxy (see Chapter 3). To bridge such gaps, psychologists and others must seek common denominators to ensure that communications and planning are collaborative.

Psychology has worked diligently to achieve its status as a respected independent profession and, as a result, has made many vital contributions to behavioral health. The vision for psychology, among many of its leaders, no doubt encompasses further evolution of its vistas. Within an integrated delivery context, the challenge will be for the profession to continue to realize its potential while supporting a sense of collaboration with others within the system.

Psychiatric Nurse

Integrated delivery models may have a dramatic impact on the profession of nursing (Shortell et al. 1996). The expansion of the behavioral health continuum and the relentless movement in the locus of care toward less intensive treatment alternatives are likely to bring about changes in the roles and functions of nursing professionals.

Roles and Functions Within an Integrated Environment

With the pressure to reduce the frequency and expense of patient visits, it falls increasingly to nurses to provide the psychiatrist and others with information about response to treatment. Where the setting is closed and the data are easily retrievable, such as an inpatient psychiatric unit with daily rounds, this task is much simpler than in situations in which assessment requires gathering the observations of family members or program clinicians who are working in different places.

Because the contact between clinicians and patients in the integrated environment may be more diffused than it is in a single program, there is a greater risk that medical problems may be missed. Therefore, medical problems must fall directly under the spotlight of the search for psychiatric symptoms. This is even more of a priority among populations that traditionally receive less thorough medical care, for example, patients on welfare. It is often the nurse who detects these problems and brings them to the psychiatrist's attention.

Checking for medication side effects is another problem that applies universally to nursing. It is mentioned here because of its added importance in the integrated environment where there is more of a risk that things may get "lost in the shuffle." Undetected medication side effects, or medical problems, play a part in integrated treatment in the sense that if undetected or not addressed, they may throw the patient back into a more intensive level of service.

Case Management. Nurses frequently occupy the important role of case managers in integrated settings (Herrick et al. 1991). Some observers recommend that clinical nurse specialists with master's degrees act as case managers for acute care patients whose course of treatment falls outside established parameters (Henry 1998). Robertson (1998) characterizes nurses as the "backbone" of any successful case management system, and goes on to say, "Acting as care managers for their patients…nurses assume a proactive, outcome-focused approach, enhancing their autonomy and accountability" (p. 159).

Educating Patients and Families About Medication. Although patient and family education falls within the psychiatrist's bailiwick, the burden of the job often falls on nurses. Nurses are often the clinicians most accessible to the family and best positioned to educate the family about medicine. Education is a critical factor in reducing recidivism, and it is needed at all levels of care in an integrated system. It can be done individually or, with much therapeutic potential, in group settings.

Psychotherapy. Essential aspects of the nurse's role are psychotherapeutic. Too often we identify *therapy* as only being that which occurs for 50 minutes behind the closed doors of a therapist's office in a dialogue about personal issues. All patient contact, however, presents the potential for an interaction that promotes healing. This is particularly true of educational meetings. However, it also applies to contact that concerns medical issues. A good example would be the preparatory work done with a patient who has been avoidant about obtaining gynecologic care but who needs evaluation. In addressing such situations, the nurse often takes the lead. It is crucial to use knowledge of the healthy and unhealthy uses of denial, the patient's characteristic ways of dealing with anxiety, psychodynamic factors, and cognitive items. These are the same items that are important in psychotherapy.

Beyond these more traditional functions, nurses (particularly nurse practitioners) are doing more formal psychotherapy across the continuum of care. This is a function likely to continue to grow in the integrated settings of the future.

Home-Based Psychiatric Nursing Care. Nurses are providing leadership and clinical direction in the movement toward more home-based care. This important expansion of the continuum offers a unique and valuable role for nurses within an integrated setting. Home-based care is one type of service that can truly serve as a preventive measure and can reduce hospitalization. The home visit can identify problems before they become acute and can support the physician's management of some appropriately selected problems by telephone, without the need for costly and inconvenient patient visits to a facility. The job is not easy, however, because it requires a high level of independent judgment and assessment skills. The reward is a richer view of patients' real environments and a reaching out to patients on their own terms.

Advanced Practice Nursing. Nurses are exploring new frontiers of service delivery as advanced practice nurses in many settings. Particularly in those states that have given prescriptive authority to qualified nurses, new roles and functions are emerging. These developments are well in synch with the ideals of service delivery integration in which there is a blending of roles and functions. In integrated systems, these opportunities are likely to become increasingly important.

Training and Key Skills Needed for Integration

Nurses must undergo training throughout the full range of psychiatric treatment settings to obtain proper preparation for an integrated continuum. Supervision needs to focus on skills that are not routinely part of the nurse's repertoire, such as how to evaluate readiness for transition to another level of care. Another key item would be training in the difficult area of home psychiatric nursing visits. Given that the nurse is a key liaison for medical and psychopharmacologic issues across different programs, the person's training should include learning to understand and negotiate the systems issues that arise, such as coordinating the management of medications between program and home (or supportive living situation), facilitating medical visits, ensuring active communications among the different caregivers, and coordinating care when home visits are used.

Social Worker

The social worker performs myriad roles in an integrated behavioral health system. The broad skills that social workers possess find application in many facets of the integrated setting, including assessment, counseling/therapy, case management, family and environmental involvement, education, and advocacy. Social workers generally are encountered in all levels of care throughout the continuum.

Roles and Functions Within an Integrated Environment

Assessment and Coordination of Care.   The social worker often plays an important role in assessing appropriate level of care. Working with other team members, social workers often draw on their traditional expertise in exploring environmental factors. For example, assessment of family dynamics might reveal not only a lack of support but even actively destructive conditions that could undermine efforts at treatment. The social worker's interviews with key individuals in the patient's life are crucial to learning about these dynamics, assigning levels of care, evaluating readiness for a less intensive level of care, and determining the treatment plan.

In addition to performing assessment functions, the social worker is a key clinician in coordinating movement along the continuum. Central to this task is the ability to conceptualize and plan for an entire episode of care. The social worker is also the person to evaluate how transitions are progressing, and whether the new level of care remains safe and effective.

Conducting Individual, Group, and Family Therapy.   Although different organizations will assign therapy tasks to members of different disciplines, frequently it is the social worker who will conduct individual and group therapies, and usually it is the social worker who will conduct family counseling sessions. Because one goal of treatment in an integrated environment is to move the patient from a more acute to a less acute level of care, therapy should support this movement.

As treatment progresses to less intensive levels, the social worker may help the patient and family focus on developing coping and adaptive skills, on managing stressful situations, and on identifying destructive patterns in the home environment that might lead to relapse or at least to treatment noncompliance. As more complete recovery from the acute episode occurs, therapy may address adaptive skills at a more complex level. It is always productive to educate the patient and family about the nature of the disorder and to try to identify ways of reducing the likelihood of future difficulties.

In an integrated system the social worker may serve as the primary link among the different levels of care the patient will experience. This underscores the advantage of being able to focus the therapy partly on the issues of transition and being able to gain an intimate sense of what the transitional issues are for each patient.

The social worker is also likely to draw on well-developed skills in family systems theory to render home-based services. These skills may be applicable to children within the family context, the infirm, the elderly, or others who are homebound by virtue of their psychiatric condition. Ongoing monitoring and assessment, therapy, and case management are important services rendered within the home setting. The social worker is a natural choice for the delivery of such services.

Training and Key Skills Needed for Integration

Systems-oriented thinking represents a traditional area of strength in social work education. An orientation to systems dynamics (e.g., families, institutions, workplace, the community) builds skills and insights that are crucial to the integrated treatment environment. These skills help to provide an appreciation of the big picture in an integrated delivery setting. They also help the social worker to successfully maneuver within the work environment itself.

Social work education also stresses the importance of the patient's environment and support system. This focus lends itself well to service delivery integration where there needs to be a blending of available resources as the patient moves through the continuum of care.

Social workers are also oriented, by virtue of their training, to be comfortable functioning within a treatment team. A team-oriented spirit tends to be inculcated early on in social work education. Driven by the sense of community that helps define the profession of social work, attitudes and values are passed along that help social workers function well as members of a collaborative work group. These same qualities help to minimize the barriers to service delivery integration discussed earlier, such as turfism and conceptual orthodoxy. Thus, social workers seem to be well prepared for roles of leadership and support in an environment attempting to embrace integrated service delivery.

Activity and Expressive Therapists

Activity and expressive therapists of various specialties are also represented on the behavioral health team. Art therapists, music therapists, dance therapists, recreational therapists, occupational therapists, activity therapists, and others bring special talents and perspectives to the mental health enterprise.

Roles and Functions Within an Integrated Environment

Milieu Development and Therapy.   Typically, activity and expressive therapists function as part of an interdisciplinary team in inpatient, residential, and partial hospitalization settings. The structured interaction they bring to these settings adds greatly to the cohesion and spirit of the therapeutic milieu. They are less often found in outpatient settings, largely as a result of reimbursement practices and the fact that their traditional roots are linked to therapeutic communities.

Their unique contributions to the development of the milieu flow directly from the nature of their work. Each of the activity and expressive therapies provides a special vehicle to connect with patients that is not available in the context of cognitive, psychoeducational, and other more traditional talking therapies. Some refer to this phenomenon as "getting in under the patient's radar." Therapeutic activities, properly presented, are innocuous and inviting and tend not to raise patients' defenses. Yet these therapies access patients' feelings and memories in a way that can be very powerful. Therefore, activity and expressive therapies bring contributions to the milieu that enrich it with more affective life, stronger interpersonal bonds, and opportunities for new skill acquisition.

Assessment.   Activity and expressive therapists, particularly recreational and occupational therapists, often have a role in patient assessment. This is an opportunity to evaluate the patient's leisure, work, and other skills as they contribute to day-to-day functioning. The assessment should address unique dimensions that are not dealt with in assessments completed by other members of the team. However, there is always a risk of duplicating the efforts of others and exposing patients to unnecessary, repetitive tasks. Such inefficiencies can result from lack of coordination, a desire to fit in with other members of the team, or turfism ("our assessments are better than theirs"). Interdisciplinary review of documentation forms should help prevent turfism.

Role as a Member of the Team.   Activity and expressive therapists are vital members of the treatment team. In a truly integrated setting their roles are interwoven with those of other professionals. However, in practice, some activity and expressive therapists feel they are not accorded due recognition as full members of the team. This may be evident in failure of other professionals to read their assessments and notes. It may also be evident in limited opportunities for input in the development and modification of treatment plans. As systems embrace the values of service delivery integration, the contributions of these professionals will increasingly find their way to a level playing field with those of others.

Historical Trends.   Activity and expressive therapists have played a pioneering role in the evolution of the continuum of care. As partial hospitalization developed in the 1970s, these therapists were prominent in staffing and leading new programs. With the emphasis on the therapeutic milieu in partial hospitalization, it was only natural that they would be tapped to add their unique skills to the mix.

Since that time, activity and expressive therapists have enjoyed a fair degree of mobility within the continuum of care. There tends to be liberal movement within the delivery system, and in many settings these therapists are assigned to various units outside a centralized department. Therefore, they gain a good deal of familiarity and comfort with different levels of milieu-based care. This is a form of continuum-based staffing, as discussed earlier in this chapter, that can benefit both patients and staff.

Reimbursement trends within the industry have tended to adversely affect the activity and expressive therapies. Inpatient charges are now typically bundled, resulting in an inability to charge for activity and expressive therapies. At the same time, credentialing requirements among third-party payors have made it difficult or impossible for these professionals to extend their services into the outpatient realm. Unfortunately, therefore, staffing levels have declined over the years.

Future Opportunities.   Although these fields are experiencing declining use in traditional parts of the continuum, new opportunities are emerging. Some see an increasing role for activity and expressive therapies in home-based care, working with individuals and families. Also, where financial risk is borne by the provider, credentialing may be less of a factor and staff deployment can be based on functional skills rather than on "approved" disciplines. Finally, creativity has been the impetus of new applications for activity and expressive therapies. For example, music therapy shows promise as an effective agent in the palliative care of those who are dying.

Training and Key Skills Needed for Integration

Activity and expressive therapists are particularly well prepared to deal with patients in groups. Such skills will always make these professionals particularly well suited for milieu-based settings. However, the training of activity and expressive therapists should not be limited to inpatient environments. Professional schools should emphasize diverse levels of care to support cross-training and mobility within the system.

With declining lengths of stay in all levels of care, key skills for activity and expressive therapists will include relationship-building techniques. To achieve therapeutic gains, it is necessary to bring about therapeutic trust in the leader and the group more quickly. Also, brief solution-focused models of therapy should augment traditional approaches to keep pace with current needs across the continuum.

SUMMARY

The structure and dynamics of integrated service delivery affect the roles of personnel in myriad ways. As we have illustrated in this chapter, integrated delivery bestows many new opportunities while introducing interesting challenges. These dynamics cascade over the various mental health disciplines in different ways as they interact with their unique traditions, roles, and attitudes. Service delivery integration cannot be pursued successfully without careful consideration of these complex and fascinating factors.

REFERENCES

Anderson BJ: Values and value, in Clinical Integration: Strategies and Practices for Organized Delivery Systems. Edited by Tonges MC. San Francisco, CA, Jossey-Bass, 1998, pp 39–58

Gudeman JE, Dicket B, Hellman S, et al: From inpatient to inn status: a new residential model. Psychiatr Clin North Am 8:461–469, 1985

Henry SA: Administrative integration through product and service line structure, in Clinical Integration: Strategies and Practices for Organized Delivery Systems. Edited by Tonges MC. San Francisco, CA, Jossey-Bass, 1998, pp 83–108

Herrick CA, Goodykoontz L, Herrick RH, et al: Planning a continuum of care in child psychiatric nursing: a collaborative effort. J Clin Psychiatr Nurs 4:41–48, 1991

Joint Commission on Accreditation of Healthcare Organizations: A Guide to Performance Improvement in Behavioral Health Organizations. Oakbrook Terrace, IL, Joint Commission on Accreditation of Healthcare Organizations, 1996, p 12

Lefkovitz PM: The continuum of care in a general hospital setting. Gen Hosp Psychiatry 17:260–267, 1995

Lefkovitz PM: Managing staff across the continuum of care. Open Minds May:4–5, 1996

Rabasca L: Structuring departments for greater impact. APA Monitor 29:19, 1998

Robertson S: Clinical maps and care maps: a system-level care management strategy, in Clinical Integration: Strategies and Practices for Organized Delivery Systems. Edited by Tonges MC. San Francisco, CA, Jossey-Bass, 1998, pp 151–178

Shortell SM, Gillies RR, Anderson DA, et al: Remaking Health Care in America. San Francisco, CA, Jossey-Bass, 1996

11

Documentation Management

Joan Betzold, M.Ed., A.B.Q.A.U.R.P., A.B.R.M.

Practitioners have long seen documentation of care as a necessary evil, something that takes them away from the activity they do well and enjoy most—direct care. It is a tremendous challenge to convince practitioners that the documentation they provide is an integral part of care and that the quality of it directly influences the care provided (Betzold 1994b).

Many practitioners have been taught the axiom "if it isn't documented, it didn't happen." This, then, becomes the principle guiding documentation and its quality. Documentation is and always has been so much more; documentation is basic communication. Communication between providers is of paramount importance, particularly when they do not physically see each other, as in different shifts or in a continuum of services with different sites and programs (Betzold 1994a).

However, documentation in today's environment goes even further than basic communication. Documentation creates an organizational memory that serves to support the organization and its employees in any future litigation or in licensure and accreditation surveys (Betzold 1995b). Additionally, today's documentation of care has to accurately reflect the care given to justify reimbursement to a payor (Betzold 1995a). These requirements add additional pressure to an already busy practitioner. Frequently organizations fail to transmit the importance of or requirements for documentation to their employees and contractors until there is a serious legal, reimbursement, accreditation, or licensure problem. At that point, it is an expensive and time-consuming process to overhaul and reteach staff (Betzold 1996).

Other pressures have affected documentation. Notably, in the past decade behavioral health care providers have been adding services to their primary products in an effort to diversify, capture revenue that would have gone to others, or offer services that would not have been rendered at all. This has created tremendous challenges for documentation because the recipient of services is treated by the organization for a longer time and may receive various levels of care, sometimes receiving multiple services simultaneously. As with most things, medical record processes grow out of need in response to changing circumstances. It is therefore likely that an organization that has grown over the years is faced with medical records processes that are redundant, inefficient, ineffective, labor intensive, and that can even hamper or interrupt care. That is where the concept of the seamless or continuous medical record can prove useful (Betzold 1999a, 1999b)

As a recipient of services moves through the different levels of care in a provider organization or network, one continuous record documents all treatment without interruption. This concept seems quite logical and full of common sense, but putting it into operation is daunting. The basic problem is that the record mirrors the care provided, and that care often is not seamless or continuous.

Seamless Record

Creating a seamless record is a process that takes place over a long period and, once it is achieved, has to be constantly safeguarded, evaluated, and upgraded. From the outset, a number of challenges need to be recognized: 1) organizational buy-in; 2) access into the system; 3) communication between levels of care; 4) transferring within the system; 5) exiting from the system; 6) forms, policies, and procedures; 7) billing on a seamless record; and 8) computerized patient record.

Organizational Buy-In

The leadership of the organization or integrated delivery system (IDS) must take the lead and insist on care being integrated in reality as well as reflected in the integrated record. Anything less will adversely affect the outcome of care. Within general medical systems the organization or network must adopt a basic philosophy that care of the patient requires input of both the physical and the behavioral components of treatment. This means that all practitioners become part of the treatment team and are represented in the assessment of the patient and the development of the problem list and treatment plan. An integrated record flows simply from such a philosophy.

Access to the System

Access to the system of care is of paramount importance to the efficiency of care, satisfaction of the care recipient and other customers, proper documentation, and the resulting appropriate reimbursement. Regardless of whether the system is a single organization or a multiorganization system, access into the system is frequently the first major hurdle in developing a seamless record.

There are many ways to approach access to care; the one that makes the most sense in terms of documentation is a central access system. Unfortunately, many organizations interpret *central access* to mean a single point of entry. What *central access* really means is one *way*, not one *place*, to enter treatment. Therefore, an organization contemplating a seamless record first reviews its screening and admission process not only from the standpoint of documentation but also from the standpoint of the recipient of service. Frequently this examination reveals an admission process that is inefficient, riddled with redundancy, and a test of endurance for the recipient of service.

Central access processes need to be as consistent as possible, regardless of the location, diagnosis, level of care needed, or how the potential recipient of service begins the interaction with the provider organization. The assessment process and resultant documentation need to clearly demonstrate how, when, by whom, and why a decision to admit a recipient to a particular level of care was made. This process needs to be as uniform as possible across the continuum and within a network. Emergencies would be the only exception to the standard process.

A biopsychosocial assessment is the first step in the documentation process for a continuous medical record. This assessment is a screening and assessment tool designed to gather data and evaluate them with ever-increasing intensity. Each section addresses issues that assist caregivers in clinical decision making: whether to refer out of the system or treat within the system and what level of care and what specific services the potential recipient of service needs. Particular components assessed are based on variables such as the level of care, population served, laws, reimbursement requirements, and accreditation standards. Good technical practices as well as accreditation standards, reimbursement requirements, and licensure requirements would indicate that the components outlined in Table 11–1 are included in the assessment (Betzold 1997c).

Information on each component is gathered and then evaluated. Each component tells a critical part of the recipient's story and adds to the overall assessment and the demonstration of need. The cumulative product of the biopsychosocial assessment is the evaluative or integrated summary. This is the practitioner's summary, integrating the aforementioned assessments; it includes the practitioner's opinions regarding strengths, weaknesses, support systems, reliability of information, special needs, justification of the level of care, anticipated length of stay, and recommendations for consultations. This assessment should promote the best use of system resources and should incor-

TABLE 11–1. Components of a biopsychosocial assessment

Identifying information (e.g., name, address)
Financial/insurance information
Present illness/medications
Current physical status/allergies
Disabilities
History and physical examination
Nutrition
Sleep
HIV risk assessment
History, including
    Medical/psychiatric/counseling history
    Marital/committed relationship history
    Abuse history
    Educational history
    Legal history
    Sociocultural history
    Alcohol/drug history
    Sexual history
    Vocational/employment history
    Spiritual history
    Military history
    Recreation/leisure history
    Family health history
    Family psychiatric history
Risk assessment, including suicide history, violent/homicide potential assessment
Mental status examination
Integrative summary

porate any processes required by third-party payors and accreditation bodies (Betzold 1996b).

If *central access* means one *way*, then the biopsychosocial assessment has to serve multiple populations so that it is not necessary for each population to have a separate assessment. However, additional areas of evaluation should be added for special populations. For example, children and adolescents require a developmental history and immunization history. In addition, the assessment for children and adolescents would focus more on school issues, whereas the assessment for the adult would focus on vocational issues. When working with the mentally retarded population, a developmental history is necessary as well as a specific section devoted to information on onset, test scores, communication, self-care skills, and current or past agencies providing services.

Communication Tools

Communication of care is paramount for the success of an integrated continuum, and the record is the primary means of communication. The first step is designing a documentation process that does what it is supposed to do—that is, communicate effectively. Two tools significantly aid this process: a list of problems and a treatment plan (Betzold 1996d).

Problem List

From the instant a recipient of care interacts with the provider, a list of problems needs to be generated. The integrated or evaluative summary should detail the problems on the problem list with initial treatment recommendations. The problem list is simply an organizing tool—a critical one—that ensures that none of the problems identified in the evaluation process or in the early portion of treatment is lost.

Problems are captured and prioritized on the problem list to be targeted later in the treatment plan. This list should identify every problem or need for the recipient of care and outline decisions made by the treatment team as to whether a problem will be addressed immediately, deferred to another level of care, or not treated at all. The details of these decisions should be in the progress notes. Any problems deferred require an explanation in the note as to why.

The problem list is a living document. As problems continue to be identified, they are added; as they are resolved, they are identified as such. This becomes the first major tool for communication between levels of care (Betzold 1996d).

Treatment Plan

From the integrated/evaluative summary and the problem list comes the treatment plan. This plan is the map of care; the patient has only one treatment plan during an episode of care. The plan has input from all the different providers at each level of care. It contains specific goals and objectives written in behavioral terms that address each problem identified as a priority for treatment. Each objective includes a corresponding modality, its frequency, and the names of those who will provide it. The treatment plan clarifies which objectives are transfer criteria (it is hoped to a lower level of care) and which are discharge criteria. The treatment plan also provides justification for the current level of care and transfers to higher levels of care (Betzold 1996d, 1996e).

Transferring Within the System

The next hurdle for documentation occurs when a transfer of care is necessary. The biggest challenge is to convince every aspect of the organization that the seamless medical record is possible and that there is no need to start over with new documents or, even worse, to close the chart when a recipient of service changes level of care. Frequently, the business end of the organization has the idea that charts must be closed when a transfer occurs. It is fundamental that all aspects of the organization agree about what a transfer is and what a discharge is. Two types of transfers occur within an integrated delivery system—one within the system between levels of care and one short-term transition to a care facility outside the system with immediate return to treatment within the system.

When a transfer is documented, the goal is to have the chart continue along with the recipient. This requires a number of events to take place. The receiving level of care needs to know about the transfer and needs to be briefed on all aspects of the current care, including the reason for the transfer. The need for the transfer should be well documented in the treatment plan and progress notes so that there is no reason to re-evaluate the individual at the new level of care. A summary of care (see Table 11–2) should be transferred along with recommendations for what is yet to be done in treatment. Then the organization needs to have a process by which the documentation—problem list, treatment plans, and progress notes—are continued by the receiving level of care.

A major challenge to the concept of transfer occurs when a recipient of care leaves the organization or network and it is known that the recipient will be back. An example of this might be a recipient of services who transfers to an acute care hospital to give birth and then returns in a few days to continue in the organization's women's program. If the organization or network chooses to discharge such patients, and the recipient of care returns to the system, then an assessment must be performed again, admission paperwork redone, treatment plans reinitiated, and other documents re-created. The process of care documentation will have to start all over, and the organization will incur the expense of closing the chart. This process is very costly in terms of resources for the organization. In addition, this process may interrupt care with another assessment and create a situation in which the treatment provided at the previous level is not built on but rather lost.

The answer is to create or use a product such as case management. In this way the organization can legitimately provide necessary and useful liaison services and have a place to document and bill for them. When the patient transfers to the hospital, the case shifts to case management with a transfer summary, progress note, and changes in the treatment plan. Then when the recipient of care returns to the treatment program, the case is transferred back to the appropriate level of care, again with the proper documentation.

Exiting From the System

Discharge from an IDS is straightforward, but it is different from discharge from a single program and presents some unique challenges. A discharge

TABLE 11–2. Components of a transfer and discharge summary

Transfer summary	Discharge summary
Identifying information	Identifying information
Type of transfer	Reason for referral to the system
Reason for transfer	Assessment findings and problem list, including admitting diagnosis
Status of problems, both old and new	
Medications or other special treatment procedures	Course of treatment, including levels of care, modalities, providers' names
Specific objectives for transfer	Progress in treatment
Contacts made to assist transfer	Final assessment, including diagnosis at discharge, prognosis, referrals, and recommendations for care outside the system

occurs when a recipient of service leaves the organization or network. When the word *discharge* is used, it puts many wheels into motion that often cannot be stopped or ignored. A discharge requires that a discharge summary be written and the chart closed within specified time frames dependent on laws, accreditation standards, good technical practice, level of care, and reimbursement requirements (Betzold 1997a).

The chart should be closed using a standard process. Gathering data from all sites to complete this chart should not be an issue if there is a continuous record. One major obstacle is getting practitioners to understand that the last level of care before discharge is responsible for writing the discharge summary. This summary needs to include a review of all care given during this episode, regardless of how many levels of care or separate programs were involved (see Table 11–2). Many practitioners do not want to review care from other levels in the discharge summary because they feel they are going to be held responsible for all treatment received throughout the episode of care. Practitioners need only refer to the transfer summaries and detail what happened at each level of care based on that information. They may even wish to highlight caregivers' names associated with the different levels of care. Another concern is that there not be multiple copies, or "shadow records."

A challenge to the concept of discharge occurs, for example, in the case of an outpatient recipient of care who does not show up for a long period but the provider knows the person is likely to resurface in the future. Specific policies and procedures need to be developed that will address such situations. Whenever patients miss appointments, they should receive a call or a letter notifying them that the practitioner is aware of their absence and that they need to make another appointment. This action needs to be documented in the record and appropriate copies made. When the patient has not been heard from in a specified period, then another letter or documented call needs to be made. If nothing is heard from the recipient or the person continues to miss appointments, the chart should be closed. The number of calls and the length of time between contacts should be detailed in policies and procedures; however, contact should be made within 1 month from the time recipients were last seen. Risk management issues are enormous for keeping charts open for longer periods. These policies and procedures should be made as uniform as possible between levels of care in a continuum or a network.

Billing

A seamless or continuous record presents many organizational challenges. A major challenge is to ensure that the business side of the organization supports the clinical side and feels that it is part of the care that is given. Patients may have very good treatment experiences but find the billing office so difficult to deal with that they will never come back and will forever say negative things about the organization.

It is important that complete and thorough information be given in a timely manner to the business component so that it can bill accurately and properly. Business office employees need to be included in meetings in which information is disseminated and decisions are made about what information is gathered, by whom, and when. In other words, the business component must be included when the continuous record is designed or the process will not work effectively.

Some billing departments may want to bill at the end of a stay, but this is not possible in a continuum because the stay in the organization may be extended to various levels of care. Billings along the way, by day, week, month, or level of care, are more appropriate. It is typical to find some of the business departments of organizations resistant to such a concept.

Forms, Policies, and Procedures

Forms, policies, and procedures are the backbone of a seamless system, and standardized forms are a must. It is imperative that an IDS have a basic medical record that has as many uniform forms as possible. Specialty forms need to be limited. As an example, an organization that provides care to a child and adolescent population as well as a mentally retarded/developmentally disabled population should be able to use the same developmental history for both populations. Labeled only as a developmental history (out of respect for the adult mentally retarded/developmentally disabled population), it could be completed by a parent or a guardian for either population. There is no need for two forms.

Once the basic seamless record model is achieved, it must be diligently guarded and protected. Often practitioners and managers develop forms themselves. Frequently forms are created that are unnecessary and are never evaluated for duplication within the system. There must be a forum in which these ideas are evaluated and reviewed against the entire record. It is critical that each new form be looked at in regard to how it would be used by the entire organization or network, how necessary it is, and what parts could enhance a current process or replace other processes more effectively. Often forms can be eliminated and the information just put in the progress notes (Betzold 1997b, 1997c). Forms need to be evaluated and the total number of forms reduced by combining and deleting redundancy. This process not only streamlines the documentation, it also frees staff time and saves money for paper, copying, and so on. In the event that forms change, are added to, or are eliminated as a result, formal approval, training, and implementation processes should be in place. It is critical to control the form approval process to protect the seamless process.

Staff Competencies as Affected by a Seamless Record

A seamless record adds many additional staff competency requirements because it is critical that staff understand the documentation process and have a familiarity with the forms from all parts of the continuum. In an IDS, staff will interact with all the different levels of care and must understand any forms and processes that are unique to levels of care other than their own. They must also understand the policies and procedures and time lines behind those forms.

Staff at all levels of care must be able to comprehend the purposes of other levels of care, their approaches and philosophies. They must be able to follow and interface with the treatment plans of other levels of care and prepare their own documentation in ways that will be compatible with subsequent caregivers at different levels of care. Staff must clearly know the purpose, philosophies, rules, and policies of their own level of care and be able to clearly and professionally articulate them in treatment team meetings with members of other levels of care. They must remember that they represent their level of care at that meeting and must be seen as capable, organized, cooperative, informed, team players, ethical, and recipient-of-care oriented.

Computerized Patient Record

Many organizations look to the development or purchase of a computerized patient record (CPR) as the solution to all of their problems concerning the delivery of seamless care. Computerized medical records cannot solve an organization's documentation problems or create seamless care or create a seamless medical record. An organization or network *cannot* delegate leadership and planning to an information management system. A CPR cannot think, organize, allocate resources, streamline, eliminate redundancy, evaluate, or make decisions. The organization or network needs to do a number of things before *any* purchases are made.

First, the organization needs to recognize that the perfect product for every system does not exist. No system has ever been designed that will meet the unique needs of every organization or network. Second, the purchase of a CPR involves the input of many people, all of whom have different expectations, needs, and agendas related to the automation of data. Third, the organization or network must understand what it is really trying to do, that is, build a record to document seamless care within an organization or network (Betzold 1996c).

Planning is the first and most important thing for success in selecting a CPR. The CPR plan needs to be part of the IDS's strategic plan. As part of the planning process, it is important to answer some basic questions about the current medical record:

- What data are currently automated?
- What hardware is currently in the system?
- What software is now being used?
- What pieces are compatible? What pieces are networked?
- How computer literate are the staff?
- What functions should be automated?
- What are the needs within the IDS and outside the IDS?
- How much money is available?
- Are there time constraints?

As part of the planning process, the IDS needs to put together written guidelines to evaluate possible software purchases. When establishing these guidelines an organization must consider

- The stability of the product
- The stability of the vendor
- The service record of the vendor
- What is needed to do the job, and what is unnecessary
- Value
- Finding a vendor who will collaborate with the organization on development projects and share the risks and rewards
- The life of the product—today's cutting-edge technology may be obsolete tomorrow
- Identifying a few good vendors, staying with them, and having them work together

- What staff members think and need
- What the IDS *needs*, what it *wants*, and what it *must have*
- The specific internal and external requirements needed to have the organization "talk" internally as well as to outside agents
- The market and understand the trends, threats, and other factors that influence what is needed to compete
- Refining the criteria as the organization becomes a more sophisticated consumer

The next step in the planning process is to evaluate the current medical record process. Some critical questions must be examined in this area. If the current process is not working well, the introduction of a CPR could prove disastrous. The following questions need to be addressed:

- Do the staff understand the fundamental principles of documentation?
- Are the needed clinical/medical and administrative data being captured?
- Are the current records compliant with appropriate state and federal laws?
- Do the current records meet applicable accreditation standards?
- Are managed care requirements being met with the current records?
- Are there reimbursement issues with the current records?
- Is the current process effective and efficient?
- Is the process seamless?

After all those questions have been thoroughly investigated and reviewed, a detailed plan needs to be developed. After the evaluation of the current system is done, possible improvements would be incorporated into the plan. This is also the time to eliminate forms and processes as needed to ensure as little redundancy as possible. Systems under consideration for purchase would be further evaluated, including interviews of current and past customers and on-site visits to current users. The plan would include exactly what hardware and software would be needed. It would address computer literacy and any necessary employee training. In addition the plan would identify when the goals would be achieved, who would be responsible, and how much money would be allocated.

It used to be that a plan of this nature was adequate for up to 5 years. Unfortunately with the incredible rate of change in health care technology, a plan such as this is probably not useful for more than 6 months to 1 year. Any organization undertaking this process needs to recognize that fact and be willing to see that the investment in hardware and software will probably diminish quickly in value. It is estimated that the average life of a computer is 4 years. Thus, this plan would be approved by the leadership and put into action with updates at least quarterly.

Organizations need to be aware of the many pitfalls in purchasing a CPR. The decision must be based on what is best for the organization or network and the recipients of care—not on someone's desire to build a private empire or employees' fear of computers. Employees, contractors, and sales representatives may have hidden agendas. Sales representatives may embellish a product's capabilities in order to sell it; thus it is crucial to be aware of unnecessary "bells and whistles" as well as the required add-ons and upgrades needed to do the job. Organization staff may be resistant to the change; therefore, the training plan should be adequate and properly carried out by knowledgeable instructors. These issues need to be addressed during the planning process or the organization may find itself with a system no one can or will use.

In light of these pitfalls, it is good advice to have a nonbiased expert do all or part of the evaluations for you, or at the very least, have the expert review your evaluation and your plan before you purchase anything. Technology can be a useful and powerful tool. You can solve problems, but you can also create new ones. Once an organization becomes computer driven, other issues rise to the surface, such as the security of records, disaster planning, and confidentiality.

CONCLUSION

Creating a seamless or continuous medical record is a task that faces health care organizations head-on in today's ever-demanding, increasingly complex, and constantly changing environment. Single-provider organizations and the networks they form have to be able to do more with less. There is no allowance for waste, inefficiency, redundancy, staff underperformance, multiple and conflicting agendas, or for any other factor that has a negative impact on the smooth delivery of care. Organizations that want to survive and thrive in this environment will have to look at their operations, including the medical record component, and realize that there is a better way. The business of providing good care and good value requires that organizations use their resources to their best advantage and convince payors that they provide the best care for the best price and that a seamless or continuous medical record is a vital and fundamental component of that success.

REFERENCES

Betzold J: Clinical supervision: changing roles for a changing industry. Professional Counselor Aug:45–47, 1994a

Betzold J: Documentation. Professional Counselor Oct:16, 1994b

Betzold J: In retroactive denial. Professional Counselor Dec:20, 1995a

Betzold J: Programming: documentation keys to success under managed care. Professional Counselor April:22, 1995b

Betzold J: The critical connection between documentation, reimbursement and survival. Paradigm Spring:10–18, 1996a

Betzold J: Documentation evaluation/Integrated summary. PSC Healthcare Consultant May/June:3, 1996b

Betzold J: Electronic medical records. PSC Healthcare Consultant Sept/Oct:5, 1996c

Betzold J: Master treatment plan, part I. PSC Healthcare Consultant Sept/Oct:3, 1996d

Betzold J: Master treatment plan, part II. PSC Healthcare Consultant Nov/Dec:3, 1996e

Betzold J: Discharge summary. PSC Healthcare Consultant July/Aug:3, 1997a

Betzold J: Integrated progress notes. PSC Healthcare Consultant Jan/Feb:3, 1997b

Betzold J: Integrated progress notes. PSC Healthcare Consultant Mar/Apr:3, 1997c

Betzold J: "Seamless" comes before "integration," part I. PSC Healthcare Consultant Mar/Apr:16, 1999a

Betzold J: "Seamless" comes before "integration," part II. PSC Healthcare Consultant May/June:10, 1999b

12

Reimbursement

Rates and Rate Structures

Mark Tidgewell, C.P.A.

Ⅰn this chapter I present an overview of reimbursement mechanisms and their effects on integration of care and system development. The following topics are covered: the cost of care, rate structures, risk-based contracting, capitation management, performance incentives, and relationships with payors.

COST OF CARE

Cost to the Purchaser (Employer or Health Plan)

Successful integrated systems of care, like other business enterprises, understand the view of their customers and respond with products that deliver value as defined by their customers. Most purchasers, whether they are governmental programs, health benefit plans, or employers, place considerable emphasis on the price of the service. Although there has been an increased focus on quality of care and access to service in recent years, the fundamental issue of cost remains critical to the purchaser. Successful integrated systems are able to deliver both acceptable quality and competitive price in the local market.

Integrated systems of care may limit their offerings to clinical services or they may provide administrative services and assume risk (subject to state regulation). If the system provides only clinical services, pricing will usually be at market rates for similar services in the region. If additional services are offered, the system may be compensated for administrative services and risk assumption. The market will determine the rates to be paid. For example, if a purchaser is willing to pay $4.00 per member per month (pmpm) for behavioral health services to a health plan or carve-out vendor, the $4.00 pmpm would be the total revenue the integrated delivery system (IDS) received. That revenue must be sufficient to meet the financial requirements of the system, including the cost of care, administrative costs, working capital, and the contribution to equity or reserves.

Nearly all large employers cover behavioral health services, but not to the same extent they cover other medical care. In fact, insurance plans often impose greater restrictions on behavioral health benefits than they do on general medical care. Benefits are restricted through limits on days or visits, total dollars spent on care, or cost-sharing requirements. According to the National Alliance for the Mentally Ill, spending on behavioral health declined by more than 54% during the 1988–1998 period, from $154 per covered life in 1988 to a mere $69 per person in 1998 (National Alliance for the Mentally Ill press release, 1998).

Service demand, however, remains high. The National Institute of Mental Health estimates that as many as 40 million Americans may have some form of mental illness. Bipolar disorder, or manic depression, affects about 2 million people every year, and schizophrenia affects another 2.5 million (National Institute of Mental Health 1998).

How much is all this behavioral ill health costing? The National Institute of Mental Health (1998) says severe mental illness pulls about $70 billion a year from the economy. Depression, the most common behavioral dysfunction, adds another $40 billion. Absenteeism, low productivity, and short- and long-term disability account for as much as 55% of the annual depression bill—about $22 billion. Although employers may acknowledge these estimates for the economy as a whole, most have not clearly quantified the cost/benefit impact on their individual businesses. Accordingly, employers and the health plans from which they purchase products continue to be focused primarily on cost for acceptable benefits and quality.

Employers are most likely to cover traditional forms of behavioral health services. A survey conducted by Mercy/Foster Higgins, an employee benefits consulting firm in New York composed almost entirely of large employers with about 4 million employees, showed that the annual cost of behavioral health benefits in 1997—the most recent behavioral health figures available—averaged $230 per employee in indemnity plans, $170 in preferred provider organizations (PPOs), $165 in point-of-service plans, and $150 in health maintenance organizations (HMOs). In freestanding mental health (carve-out) plans, behavioral health costs averaged $185 per employee (Mercer/Foster Higgins 1999).

Two items are worth noting in regard to this study. First, the costs are per employee per year, rather than the more common managed care approach of using per covered person (member) per month. For example, the rate of $150 per employee per year for those covered in HMOs would translate to $5.43 pmpm assuming a ratio of 2.3 covered persons to each employee. Second, the costs are considerably above the current market for behavioral health benefits offered by HMOs in many markets. It is not uncommon today for carve-out programs to receive capitation for commercial populations in the range of $2.50 to $3.50 in many regions of the country.

For mental health services, nearly all the Mercer/Foster Higgins (1999) survey respondents covered inpatient psychiatric care and outpatient psychotherapy, but they varied in their coverage of other modes of treatment. About two-thirds covered intensive nonresidential treatment, such as partial hospitalization, and about one-third covered nonhospital residential care. For substance abuse services, most covered inpatient and outpatient detoxification treatment and outpatient therapy. About two-thirds covered intensive nonresidential treatment and case management and referral services. About one-third covered nonhospital residential substance abuse care, whereas less than one-fifth covered methadone maintenance. These figures show that although little variation exists for traditional forms of care, notable differences exist for others. Generally, carve-out plans are most likely to cover the listed services, followed by point-of-service plans; HMOs are generally the least likely to cover a given service.

Employers often restrict behavioral health benefits by placing more limits on their use or imposing greater cost sharing than they do for other health care services. In most plans, these restrictions are the same for both mental health and substance abuse services. Limits are placed on annual or lifetime benefit payments and/or the use of deductibles, copayments, or coinsurance for services. In 1995 employers most commonly used limits on the maximum dollar amount per lifetime and the maximum number of days per year for psychiatric inpatient care. The major exception is in HMO plans, which used limits on annual number of days more than did other types of plans.

IDSs must develop an understanding of the purchasers' current costs and acceptable level of quality in order to develop a marketable product or service. These values will vary significantly from region to region and from benefit plan to benefit plan.

Cost of Providing Services

The largest single expense an IDS will have is the cost of providing clinical services. Depending on the nature of the arrangement between the IDS and its providers, payment may be made using fee-for-service, case rates (a form of capitation), subcapitation, or some mix that varies by service.

Regardless of the methodology chosen by the IDS, the rates must be based on market conditions in the region. Professional fees can vary widely by region and by discipline, as illustrated in Table 12–1 (Fee, Practice and Managed Care Survey 1998).

Other Costs and Financial Requirements

Assuming the IDS is more than a discounted fee-for-service arrangement, the system will also have other costs and financial requirements. These include the cost of utilization management, quality assurance, provider network management, claims (encounter) processing, reporting, customer service, and related services.

In addition to the costs of clinical services and administration, an IDS will have other financial requirements that must be met. These include working capital, an accumulation of equity and reserves needed to support the level of risk assumed by the IDS, and other requirements such as repayment of development expenses. Often it is not feasible for the IDS to generate a sufficient flow of funds to meet these other financial requirements during start-up periods or during a significant expansion. Accordingly, the integrated system will often use a sponsoring organization to meet these requirements over the short term. However, it is essential that the integrated system meet these obligations on its own over the long term. The system, therefore, must generate sufficient gains and positive cash flow to cover these amounts and any related repayment obligations.

TABLE 12–1. Managed care fees for individual therapy and group sessions

Individual therapy			
Discipline	**Mean, $**	**Median, $**	**Mode, $**
Marriage and family therapists	64.83	60	60
Professional counselors	66.24	65	n/a
Psychiatrists	93.39	89	70
Psychologists	81.02	80	70
Social workers	68.66	65	60
Group sessions			
Discipline	**Mean, $**	**Median, $**	**Mode, $**
Marriage and family therapists	41	35	25
Professional counselors	42	44	50
Psychiatrists	41	35	35
Psychologists	45	40	40
Social workers	41	40	35

Source. Data from Chavez and Barry 1998

RATE STRUCTURES

IDSs can be effective in assuming risk for the cost of clinical services delivered under a managed care contract. The services may be delivered by a core group of providers, facilities, and professionals that may enter into risk-sharing or risk-assumption arrangements with the IDS. However, most IDSs find it necessary to contract with additional providers on a discounted fee-for-service basis to achieve the breadth of services and access required for serving the covered population. Other rate structures that involve sharing financial risk with providers will be discussed later.

The ability of a provider to accept a discounted financial arrangement is key. Providers may not be able to remain financially viable if they cannot be guaranteed sufficient patient volume, are not organized as groups, cannot deploy less expensive master's-level practitioners to provide services, or practice in extremely competitive markets.

Fee-for-Service

Although there are a wide array of contractual relationships between managed behavioral health organizations (MBHOs) or IDSs and their care providers, the most prominent payment mechanism is discounted fee-for-service (Munson et al. 1997).

Fee-for-service arrangements are characterized by payment for individual services at an established price or within an established price range. With a minimum of utilization controls, this arrangement is otherwise known as indemnity coverage and is what is usually thought of as traditional insurance. Under indemnity insurance, providers can increase revenue by increasing the number of patients treated or units of service rendered. Without restrictions, there is some risk of overtreatment. Financial gain and patient demand for specific services are only two of an array of factors that increase the risk of overtreatment.

All-inclusive per diems are a common form of payment for facility services. Although they are not technically discounted fee-for-service, they function much like discounted fee-for-service arrangements for behavioral health services because the provider assumes little risk beyond the impact of the discount.

Fee-for-Service With Withholds

Fee-for-service with a withhold is another way to align treatment incentives between an IDS and providers. In essence, an IDS contracts with providers to withhold a percentage of a payment until aggregate utilization for members treated by a panel of providers is determined for a given time period. Rather than attempting to control utilization on a member-by-member basis, the MBHO motivates providers by making payment of the withhold contingent on some measure(s) of utilization, potentially in conjunction with other measures of financial performance. A variation of this is to reward providers based on their performance relative to other providers in the network (Broskowski 1997). Thus, although a similar percentage of each provider's payment is withheld, the sum is divided unequally among them.

The best performers receive a greater portion of the withhold than do lower performers. This type of arrangement can raise fears of undertreatment, particularly because few IDSs and MBHOs have adequate outcome assessment mechanisms in place to define *best performance* by criteria that effectively demonstrate patient improvement.

Case Rates

Case rates have become increasingly popular in recent years. A case rate is a fixed fee per patient, per treatment episode, possibly based on the assignment of the patient to a given type of treatment or level of care. The case rate approach to payment was developed as a way of sharing financial risk with providers. The case rate is calculated by estimating the expected average expenditures for service users for a single level or multiple levels of care for a specific time. For example, a case rate may cover outpatient services only, or all services from inpatient through outpatient. The time interval, sometimes called the *risk window*, covered by a case rate may be short, for instance, this admission plus 10 days or longer, or this service plus the next 12 months.

The case rate provider assumes no risk for the underlying rate of patients per 1,000 requiring treatment in the population. The provider is at risk, however, for the frequency and intensity of service needs per treatment case, and the underlying cost of the services provided. In other words, the case rate carries with it the risk (and potential reward) of fixed fees or global fees. In exchange for provider risk assumption, both the provider and the IDS/MBHO benefit from a less costly and intrusive care management process (Chavez and Barry 1998). Extensive concurrent utilization management is eliminated, and treatment is provided at the discretion of the provider. Case rates are essentially capitation arrangements for individual cases.

Case rates serve to align financial incentives between provider and management entity. In accepting a case rate payment mechanism, a provider agrees to cover all necessary treatment for an established "episode"—12 months, for example. The provider must balance current treatment utilization with an eye on the longer term. Initially some providers may have difficulty adjusting to a case rate system because there is a tendency to view any case with a cost in excess of the case rate as a loss. In fact, there would be a loss only when the average cost of all cases exceeded the case rate. Provider education and monitoring are critical to the success of a case rate system. Managed care entities often find that stop-loss and appeal mechanisms are important to provide the financial security that providers seek, because they can ensure providers have some recourse when statistical averages are not met.

Administration of case rates can present significant challenges to an IDS or MBHO that has responsibility for processing of claims/encounters and the administration of a benefit plan. Behavioral health benefits, even in the public sector, often contain discriminatory limitations for the number of covered days, sessions, visits, and so forth. Administrators may be required to administer benefits under a case rate system using fee-for-service rule sets for benefit tracking or reporting and case rate rules for payment. This requires sophisticated and flexible information systems (Broskowski 1997).

RISK-BASED CONTRACTING

Table 12–2 shows the continuum of financial risk-sharing arrangements for managed care contracts—including a global budget, capitation payment, case rate payment, and fee-for-service payment. These arrangements allocate the four major components of financial risk (i.e., risk due to variation in the rate of enrollment, in the cost of producing services, in the volume and types of units used, and in service users per 1,000 enrollees) in very different ways between the purchaser of managed behavioral health care services and a managed care organization (MCO) (Chavez and Barry 1998).

When choosing a risk transfer payment system, purchasers of managed behavioral health services must determine how many distinct subpopulations, and thus distinct rates, to develop. Some purchasers have chosen a single rate blended for all enrollees; others have used several different rate categories. When more than one rate category is used, they can be based on many different types of variables. In many situations the purchaser may also want to divide the total population of eligible persons and services into two or more different risk-sharing arrangements (e.g., adults with serious and persistent mental illness, children with serious emotional disorder, chronically addicted individuals). Indeed, using multiple categories of rates can result in more appropriate matching of payment to estimated costs of service provision and, ideally, can be used to mitigate incentives for the MCO to undertreat those with highest needs.

Global (or Fixed) Budget

A payment arrangement that transfers full financial risk for the components of financial risk mentioned earlier from the purchaser of managed care to an

TABLE 12–2. Risk transfer payment models

Payment model	Variations	Comments
Global budget (payment for total population)	No excluded services Limited excluded services	Under a global budget arrangement, the MCO is at full risk for all four components of financial risk: 1) variation in the rate of membership and enrollment, 2) variation in the cost of producing services, 3) variation in the volume and types of units used, and 4) variation in service users per 1,000 enrollees.
Capitation payment (payment per enrollee)	Full capitation No risk/reward corridor Risk reward corridor Partial capitation No risk/reward corridor Risk reward corridor	Full capitation payment arrangements involve payment to an MCO of a predetermined fixed fee per capita to provide all necessary services for a defined population of enrollees. The MCO is at financial risk for variation in the cost of producing services, as well as for variation in the volume and types of services and variation in users per 1,000 enrollees. It is not at risk for variations in rate of enrollment. Partial capitation refers to situations in which one part of the population is capitated and the other is not.
Case rate payment (payment per user of services)	Period of time Episode of care	Under case rate payment arrangements that involve payment to the MCO (or provider*) of a fixed "case rate" per user to provide a defined set of services as needed to a specified group of users, the MCO is at financial risk for both variation in the cost of producing services and for variation in the volume and type of services required by the individual.
Fee-for-service payment (payment per unit of service)	Services bundled Discounted Not discounted Services not bundled Usual and customary charges Billed charges	Under fee-for-service arrangements, the MCO is not at financial risk for any of the four types of risk. The purchaser assumes all the risk. An MCO paid through a global budget, capitation, or case rate may pay providers using a form of fee-for-service. In this case, the MCO is at risk.

Note. MCO=managed care organization.

*Case rates are used most often to pay service providers, either when they are functioning as an MCO or when they are subcontracting to an MCO.

Source. Substance Abuse and Mental Health Services Administration 1998.

MCO (or from an MCO to a network provider) is a global (or fixed) budget. Under this model, the purchaser of managed care pays a fixed dollar amount to the MCO, both to administer the managed care program and to provide all services for which the MCO is responsible. No matter how high the costs of providing care to enrollees are, or how many additional enrollees join or leave the plan in a given year, the MCO is paid the agreed-on global budget payment.

A global budget arrangement allows the purchaser of managed behavioral health care to predict with certainty the level of expenditures on mental health and/or substance abuse services in a given year. Global budgets are often used when the number of eligibles is unknown, and they are usually based on the previous year's costs, less a predetermined percentage for savings. They are more especially likely to be used when the purchaser is a state or county substance abuse and mental health authority (Latham 1996).

A global budget creates very strong incentives for an MCO to control costs and improve the efficiency of its service delivery and administrative practices, especially if the MCO is to retain all savings as profit or as new operating capital. However, the very strong incentives to the MCO to achieve savings can encourage the entity to provide less than the therapeutically appropriate level of care or to reduce overall access to care, particularly when enrollment is greater than expected.

A fixed budget places the MCO at the highest level of financial risk. If managed care enrollment is higher than expected and/or claims costs greatly exceed the amount in the global budget, the financial viability of the managed care initiative may be put in jeopardy. For an MCO with low financial reserves, the result could be very serious financial difficulties or insolvency. The risk of insolvency is particularly great for small regional MCOs or providers whose budget is dependent on the managed care contract. The loss of such a contract could lead to serious financial troubles. Several states have seen their community mental health centers suffer such a misfortune when they have acted as underfunded MCOs.

Because an MCO may assume a relatively high degree of financial risk under a global budget arrangement, the MCO is likely to seek higher payment rates from the purchaser for assuming that risk. Thus a global budget arrangement may actually result in higher overall costs for the purchaser, especially if the purchaser has insufficient data to accurately estimate need, utilization, and costs. Because of the potentially higher costs of a fixed-budget arrangement, some purchasers have chosen to use a global budget arrangement for selected services or populations only and to use other payment strategies to pay for other types of services or groups of recipients (Latham 1996).

The greatest legal concern in a global budget arrangement is ensuring that the MCO can safely assume the risks associated with it. In determining the rates that are to be paid to the MCO, the purchaser should consider including provisions in the contract to allow for renegotiation of the rates in the event the amount reimbursed proves to be unrealistically low or high. Allowing some renegotiation options may permit a managed care program to remain a viable option for the purchaser if the MCO is on the verge of bankruptcy, is pushing risk too far down to the provider pool, or is taking too much profit from the system.

Capitated Systems

Under a fully capitated, full-risk arrangement, the purchaser pays the MCO a monthly per capita rate to cover all costs associated with providing behavioral health care services to a population of enrollees. The per capita rate for each enrollee is fixed, regardless of whether an enrollee uses any services. It may be set by the purchaser in advance or determined in the context of a competitive bidding process. The MCO assumes all financial risk for variation in the cost of producing services but assumes no risk for variation in enrollment. The latter risk is assumed by the purchaser, who pays an additional per capita payment for each additional enrollee or pays less in aggregate if enrollment reverses.

Fully capitated payment arrangements are like a fixed-budget arrangement in that they provide a strong incentive to control costs and improve efficiency. Although full capitation can create strong short-term financial incentives to unduly restrict enrollee access and use of services, it also can provide equally strong incentives for the MCO to provide high-quality services and to secure effective linkages with other types of service providers to support positive outcomes. The strength of the contract access monitoring and quality monitoring mechanisms and the effective use of incentives and sanctions will in large part determine the way in which a full capitation payment system affects the success of the managed care initiative.

CAPITATION MANAGEMENT

Capitation is a fixed payment, usually calculated on a pmpm basis, for the delivery of a defined range of health care services to a defined population (Broskowski 1997). The fee paid to the provider or IDS is calculated based on the number of members enrolled with the provider during a given time period. A provider may be an individual, a group, a treatment facility, or an IDS. Financial risk is assumed by the provider, and the provider's gain is contingent on expending less money on caring for the capitated population than is received in capitation fees. Overtreatment, as with captitated MCOs, equates to financial loss because additional money for services is not forthcoming. Given the inability to predict utilization accurately across time or populations, it is in the provider's interest to be guaranteed sufficient member volume. The promise of volume allows providers to accept the risk of members who are high users of services because their use will be balanced by low users. This is one reason HMOs employ restricted networks of providers. By doing so, they can establish a fixed pmpm payment, and guarantee providers a certain member volume.

Managing the performance of an IDS under a capitated arrangement is critical to its success. The capitation is usually based on a set of assumptions that includes covered members (lives) and level of care statistics such as access rates, average length of treatment, unit costs, and the computation of a pmpm cost for each group of services. IDS management processes that support capitation differ from traditional provider management processes in a number of ways. The following are some of the key differences:

- Capitation models are usually based on population-based utilization assumptions rather than on the individual patient.

- Some services are supplied directly by the IDS and are easy to track; others are supplied by network providers that file claims. The introduction of claims payment and insurance accounting concepts, such as reserving for unbilled but incurred services, can pose a significant challenge to an IDS. The management must have the skills to manage through analysis of estimates and trends.

- Sophisticated claims processing and information systems are required. These systems are very different in design from facility or provider information systems.

- The provider's financial objective is to maximize revenue and utilization. The IDS's financial objective is to manage the cost of care within limits of a capitation or budget.

Traditional Capitation Models

The following are traditional capitation models:

- *Primary care capitation*: Payment for furnishing services is the pmpm amount.

- *Professional services capitation:* The provider organization receives a pmpm amount for services provided by both primary care and specialty physicians, including office visits, specialty consultations, and surgery. Typically, some tertiary and quaternary services are excluded from this payment and are paid instead on a fee-for-service basis.

- *Global, or full-risk, capitation:* The provider organization receives a pmpm amount for all health care services, including inpatient care and other facility charges, such as ambulatory surgery. Often these arrangements are structured on a percentage-of-premium basis, with the payor retaining a portion of the premium for administration, marketing, and specified services not at risk, such as transplant surgery and out-of-area care. These arrangements can become complex when risk is shared among multiple provider organizations or when providers accept risk for services they do not provide internally.

Disadvantages of Traditional Capitation Models

Despite their widespread use, the three models of capitation described above pose some disadvantages for health care organizations:

- *Administrative costs.* Capitated provider groups normally must increase their administrative activities, such as payor reporting, claims adjudication, data analysis, and funds-flow administration, to manage their capitation arrangements. Such responsibilities can place an expensive burden on providers. Often payors consider these functions to be a normal cost of doing business for which providers are responsible and, thus, usually do not offer providers additional payment to cover these costs. It is not unusual, for example, for capitated organizations to spend 10% of their revenue on administration, on top of the 15%–20% retained by health plans.

- *Inappropriate levels of provider risk.* In markets in which excess premium levels exist relative to utilization, it is financially appropriate for physicians to assume risk. When premium levels are relatively high, providers often are willing to assume risk in hopes of gaining "arbitrage" earnings, which represent the difference between the capitation payment and expenses incurred. In many markets, however, use levels have bottomed out, premium levels are declining, and arbitrage earnings have all but disappeared. Providers in such markets are not likely to benefit from accepting risk and may, in fact, incur losses.

- *Inappropriate provider incentives.* Traditional risk models sometimes have produced results contrary to the intentions of managed care. For example, many independent practice associations that have capitated their specialists have noticed a dramatic increase in referrals from primary care physicians to specialists, a phenomenon often referred to as *dumping*. This increase in referrals has been linked to the absence of marginal costs incurred by primary care physicians in making these referrals. Such situations frequently cause relationships between primary care physicians and specialists to deteriorate.

- *Increasingly negative image of managed care.* The media have recently focused considerable attention on public frustration with managed care and HMOs. Moreover, this coverage has not been balanced with coverage of excess utilization problems associated with fee-for-service payment. As a result, patients are increasingly questioning whether physicians are being paid to deny care. Legislation restricting capitation is already being implemented in some states and may be expected to be introduced in other states soon. In Oregon last year, for example, a ballot referendum outlawing capitation was narrowly defeated by voters.

Capitation rates are rarely adjusted for the risk profile of a provider's panel of members. As a result of practice location or specialty, providers may attract a member mix that has a utilization pattern that is significantly different from the normative pattern used to establish the capitation rate. One benefit of capitation is the freedom the provider has to treat patients creatively. Services not covered under fee-for-service arrangements can be employed, including indirect treatments (e.g., telepsychiatry) or substituting partial hospitalization or residential care services, where appropriate, for more expensive inpatient care.

In contrast to fee-for-service, capitation arrangements can motivate providers to overly restrict use. The nature of some creative revenue-enhancing treatments remains dubious. Such treatments often have no substantial empirical validation and their treatment efficacy may be questionable. Capitation arrangements have numerous derivations, including partial or subcapitation arrangements similar to the shared risk agreements between payors and MBHOs. Another form of capitation is the case rate payment mechanism.

Capitation rates can be very fairly set, provided everyone is working with adequate data. With capitation, both parties—MCOs and providers—should have access to at least 2 years, and preferably 3 years, of each other's utilization data. Needless to say, access to data is especially important to those getting involved with Medicaid managed care because those populations are very complex. It should be remembered, too, that there is not as much flexibility with capitation as there is with case rate; capitation is fixed by contract, whereas case rates—at least as we have administered them—can be changed from time to time as needed in collaboration with providers.

Many MCOs should be able to offer very precise utilization data that can be relied on in setting reasonable capitation rates. For providers who are less comfortable with the process, the MCO can also work in shared risk arrangements, such as utilization targets and accompanying bonuses and takeaways. All of this can be negotiated on the basis of reasonably good data.

Behavioral care subcapitation by medical/surgical groups and HMOs is often very complicated. Benefits designs are frequently poor, many medical groups and HMOs do not particularly value behavioral care, and there is skepticism about the medical offset effect of behavioral health care.

Many employers have contracted for mental or behavioral health services separately from other types of health care to control cost and quality. The contractors are MCOs specializing in the treatment of mental health problems. Capitation rates are paid for a defined set of benefits, which may include substance abuse services. Extraordinary savings have been reported by companies such as Xerox, IBM, and Conoco.

Spurred by the private sector's remarkable savings, many states include some or all mental health services in their Medicaid managed care programs. Several states have even used Medicaid's flight to managed care to trigger the consolidation of the public sector's purchasing of mental health services on a statewide or regional basis. The changeover is intended to save money and improve access and continuity of care.

PERFORMANCE INCENTIVES

To promote continuous quality improvement, the payor may link a portion of the capitation rate to the MCO's achievement of certain performance objectives. The portion is specified in the contract, along with the indicators that will be used to assess performance. All or some of the withheld amount is paid to the MCO, depending on its success ratio.

Performance indicators may address any quantifiable aspect of access, quality, and continuity. Some indicators may be basic—hospital admission rates and lengths of stay, readmission rates for the same mental health problems, length of time for an ambulatory visit following discharge for an affective disorder, and waiting time for mental health and chemical dependency treatment. Other indicators may require rigorous data collection efforts and complex data processing, such as the percentage of members seeing the same professional during a set time interval and the percentage of adolescents screened and counseled for alcohol and tobacco use.

MCOs need sophisticated information systems to authorize benefits, monitor utilization, coordinate care, pay claims, and document performance. Without adequate information, neither care nor financial risk can be managed properly.

Contracts for mentally healthy patients may have tighter use mechanisms than do contracts for chronic behavioral patients, who tend to be public-sector patients. The looser controls that may exist under public case management programs often stem at least partly from a deliberate effort to minimize hurdles to treatment. Looser controls, however, mean higher costs and capitation rates.

RELATIONSHIPS WITH PAYORS

Maintaining an open and positive relationship with the payor is critical to the long-term survival of the IDS. An open and honest exchange of information and frequent communication are needed. All too often, providers become suspicious of payors' motives and become less open with the payor regarding financial performance, quality of care issues, and member service issues. The following are some steps that an IDS should consider in developing and maintaining a positive relationship with the payor:

- Market-based pricing should be maintained. If the IDS finds that its pricing is higher than that of the current market, it should consider taking the initiative to offer the customer a lower price.

- Reporting deadlines must be met. When the IDS fails to meet the deadlines, significant stress between the IDS and the payor can result, and in some cases penalties may be imposed.

- Details of use and cost need to be shared openly (subject of course to patient confidentiality). Failure to be open regarding actual use and cost of services may erode the positive relationship between an IDS and payor, resulting in strained negotiations during contract renewal.

- There should be frequent meetings between the IDS and the payor.

- The IDS should work closely and effectively with the payor's information systems staff. Most IDSs conduct data exchanges with their customers' information systems. Positive working relations with the management information system staff are critical.

- Finally, all complaints should be followed up quickly and resolved, and the payor should know about the resolution.

REFERENCES

Broskowski AB: The Role of Risk-Sharing Arrangements. Baltimore, MD, Annie E. Casey Foundation, 1997

Chavez N, Barry CT: Contracting for Managed Substance Abuse and Mental Health Services. Rockville, MD, Substance Abuse and Mental Health Administration, Center for Substance Abuse Treatment, 1998

Fee, Practice and Managed Care Survey. Juno Beach, FL, Psychotherapy Finances, 1998

Latham SR: Regulation of managed care incentive payments to physicians. American Journal of Law Medicine 22:399–432, 1996

Mercer/Foster Higgins: National Survey of Employer-Sponsored Health Plans 1999. New York, Mercer/Foster Higgins, 1999

Munson BD, Cave DG, Heumann KA: New Payments and Incentives in Contract Capitation. Bronxville, NY, Managed Care Interface, 1997

National Institute of Mental Health: Parity in Financing Mental Health Services: Managed Care Effects on Cost, Access and Quality. Arlington, VA, National Institute of Mental Health, 1998

13

Reimbursement

Assuming Risk

Susan L. Ettner, Ph.D.

Achieving the goal of integrated behavioral health care depends on the economic incentives operating at all levels of the health care system. Through their choice of contractual arrangements, purchasers of health care (e.g., employers and government payors) can affect the incentives of health plans to enroll certain groups of patients or offer certain services. In turn, insurers determine the incentives facing health care providers and patients by deciding on covered benefits, patient cost-sharing requirements, and provider reimbursement methodology. These financial mechanisms can affect which services are purchased by patients and delivered by health care providers. In this chapter I give examples of some of the incentives affecting the behavior of health plans, providers, and patients and describe their implications for the delivery of integrated care.

HEALTH PLAN INCENTIVES: RISK-BASED CONTRACTING

It has become increasingly common for purchasers of health care, such as employers or public insurance programs (Medicare and Medicaid), to contract with capitated health plans such as health maintenance organizations (HMOs) and other types of managed care organizations (MCOs). As with the premiums paid to traditional indemnity insurers, capitated health plans receive a fixed payment for each covered life. Thus in the absence of risk-sharing arrangements with the purchaser, plans bear the full risk of the utilization of the covered population and have a strong incentive to contain costs. Unlike indemnity insurers, however, which have little or no control over the service use of beneficiaries, capitated health plans integrate the financing and delivery of care and thus are able to directly influence the costs of care.

Risk-based contracting may also operate at the level of individual health care providers. For example, MCOs often capitate the physician groups with which they contract, with the group generally receiving a fixed amount for each additional patient. In turn, the groups may salary member physicians, subcapitate them, or pay them on a fee-for-service basis. Even in cases in which the physician is not fully capitated, it has become increasingly common for part of the physician's salary to be put at risk. For example, 5% of the physician's annual income may be withheld, with some or all of the amount returned at the end of the year, depending on the physician's practice style during the year. Payment may depend on factors such as the number of referrals made to specialists or off-formulary drugs prescribed. Thus physicians also have a financial incentive to limit the services delivered to the patient.

In what follows I describe some of the methods used by purchasers to reimburse health plans for enrolling patients (or used by health plans to reimburse physician groups) and how these methods affect the incentives of the health plans to enroll certain groups of patients and deliver high-quality, cost-effective care. In the concluding paragraphs in this section of the chapter I discuss the implications of these methodologies for the provision of behavioral health care along a continuum.

Full or "Pure" Capitation

In the context of risk-based contracting with health plans, *capitation* is the payment of a fixed amount of money per enrollee that does not depend on the actual cost of services rendered. The incentives associated with capitation payments arise because the party at risk for the cost of the services used by the patient (the health plan) simultaneously has control over the use of those services. The result is that capitation payment provides strong incentives for cost containment, along with incentives to deliver suboptimal quality and quantity of care.

Although capitation payments do not depend on the actual costs of the enrolled population, they may (and generally should) be adjusted to reflect the expected costs of enrollees. The appropriate capitation rate for a health plan (or physician group) depends not only on the plan's cost structure but also on the clinical, geographic, and sociodemographic characteristics of the enrollee population, the services covered under the contract, and the patient cost-sharing requirements. All of these factors will affect the use of services by enrollees. Methods used to risk-adjust capitation payments are described in a later section.

An additional point to note about the initial implementation of a capitated payment system is that providers may respond to being capitated by cutting back on the services they deliver. If the capitation rate is set on the basis of utilization patterns within a fee-for-service system, it may overcompensate providers for the costs of care provided within a managed care setting, even if patient populations are comparable.

"Soft" Capitation

Purchasers contracting with an MCO may choose to bear some of the risk. Retaining part of the risk for the health care use of enrollees makes sense when the purchaser is large relative to the capitated plan or has some other reason for being less risk averse. In soft capitation arrangements, the purchaser sets a target amount for expenditures, T, and defines risk corridors. Cost sharing between the purchaser and the MCO will differ, depending on whether the actual expenditures fall below, within, or above the risk corridor. For example, suppose that the target amount is $100 per enrollee and the risk corridor is defined to be plus or minus 10% of this amount, that is, between $90 and $110. Cost sharing within the risk corridor is assumed to be 50%, that is, the MCO keeps only half the profits made by reducing costs below the target amount and incurs only half the losses resulting from actual costs surpassing the target amount. Cost sharing outside the risk corridor is assumed to be 100%; any profits or losses resulting from actual expenditures falling outside the risk corridor are retained entirely by the purchaser.

In this example, if the MCO has actual expenditures of $100, it receives $100. If actual expenditures are $94, the MCO retains only half the profits, that is, it gets $97. If actual expenditures are $108, the MCO incurs only half the losses, that is, it gets $104. If actual expenditures are $80, the MCO receives $85 (actual expenditures plus 50% of the difference between the target and actual expenditures that falls in the "at-risk" portion of the payment schedule). If actual expenditures are $120, the MCO receives $115 (actual expenditures minus 50% of the difference between the actual and target expenditures that falls in the at-risk portion of the payment schedule). Thus, the most per capita profit the MCO can ever receive is $5 per enrollee; conversely, the maximum loss is capped at $5 per enrollee.

A more complicated payment schedule could define multiple risk corridors, each with different risk-sharing rates. Hence, a wide variety of contractual arrangements is possible with soft capitation, depending on the definition of the risk corridors and the risk-sharing proportions specified. Asymmetrical risk sharing is also possible. The purchaser could require that the MCO incur three-quarters of the losses if actual expenditures are between 110% and 120% of the target amount, yet stipulate that the MCO retain none of the profits if actual expenditures fall below 90% of the target amount.

Risk-sharing arrangements give MCOs fewer incentives for cost containment. However, they have other advantages that may make soft capitation contracts worthwhile from the point of view of the purchaser. Because the MCO retains only part of the profits from reducing costs below the target, incentives to underprovide services, skimp on quality, or (in the case of multiple MCOs) compete to enroll low-cost patients are attenuated. Conversely, because the MCO is responsible for only part of the losses in case costs are higher than anticipated, vendors may be more willing to bid for the contract or to submit low bids, particularly in cases in which there is much uncertainty regarding the cost of caring for the beneficiary population.

Mixed Payment Systems

Mixed payment systems typically involve reimbursing health plans or providers partially on a capitated basis and partially on the basis of the population's actual health care costs. The portion of the total payment that is capitated may or may not be risk adjusted, and the portion based on actual costs may use prior-year or concurrent costs. In a stable system the incentives associated with using prior-year versus concurrent costs would not be that different, as long as the health plans understood that their current service use would influence the capitation rate they would receive during the following year. Mixed payment systems can be particularly useful when health plans have private information about the health status of patients that is not readily available for purposes of risk-adjusting payments.

In some cases the purchaser may choose to bear all the risk. For example, an employer may self-insure, yet still contract with an MCO to perform functions such as utilization review. Contracts in which the MCO does not bear any risk are known as *administrative services only* contracts.

RISK ADJUSTMENT OF CAPITATION PAYMENTS

Risk adjustment is the process of accounting for differing patient characteristics when making comparisons across populations. One common application of risk adjustment is in setting capitation payments to competing health plans; for example, a typical risk adjustment methodology might adjust the capitation rate paid to a health plan for the enrollee's age, gender, geographic location, and health status, most commonly measured using diagnoses obtained from medical claims.

In the absence of risk adjustment, all health plans would be paid the same amount, equal to the average cost of caring for all enrollees. Capitated health plans attracting high-cost patients, such as patients who are mentally ill, will be paid less than the actual costs of their enrollees, and plans attracting low-cost patients, such as those in good psychiatric health, will be paid more than actual costs. An inequitable solution will result, in which plans enrolling healthy patients will earn profits, whereas those enrolling the mentally ill population will suffer losses. Worse yet, plans will have incentives to try to avoid severely ill patients ("dumping") and enroll healthy ones ("cream-skimming") because the capitation rate is independent of the expected cost of the patient.

Risk adjustment systems adjust the amount paid to health plans for enrolling a patient with given characteristics for the expected costs of that patient. By "leveling the playing field" in this manner, incentives for cream-skimming and dumping individual patients can be attenuated and overall payments to health plans made more equitable; plans treating sicker, more costly patients will receive higher payments than those treating healthier, less costly patients.

Risk adjustment may be prospective—that is, capitation payments may be based on the characteristics of the population during the previous year—or it may be concurrent—that is, payments are based on the current characteristics of the population. Capitation payment using concurrent risk adjustment is closer to a cost-based or "mixed" reimbursement system because patients receive diagnoses only when they seek treatment for the condition. Because capitation payments can be adjusted upward only when services are used, concurrent risk adjustment provides fewer incentives for cost containment but also fewer incentives to skimp on quality and/or quantity.

Risk Adjustment: A Basic Example

Suppose that we had data on the health status, age, and health care costs of a particular beneficiary population. Our goal is to determine how much to pay competing health plans for each beneficiary the plan enrolls. The simplest method, shown in Table 13–1, is to calculate average expenditures within subgroups of the population defined by the values of the classification variables (health status and age). These averages give us the relative payments for a beneficiary of each type.

TABLE 13–1. Average health care expenditures for subgroups defined by age and health status

	Under age 18	Age 18 and older
Healthy patients	$100	$300
Mentally ill patients	$200	$600

In Table 13–1, I define subgroups of patients based on their status and age group (under age 18 versus 18 and older). In this simplified example, healthy patients under 18 have on average $100 in health care costs, mentally ill patients under 18 have $200, healthy patients age 18 and older have $300, and mentally ill patients age 18 and over have $600. If the budget remains the same over time, then these are the respective amounts that should be paid to health plans for enrollees in each of these categories.

Even if the budget changes, these numbers can still be used to set relative payment rates. Relative to a healthy patient under 18, health plans should be paid two times as much for a mentally ill patient under 18, three times as much for a healthy patient age 18 and older, and six times as much for a mentally ill patient age 18 and older. The payment for healthy patients under 18, X, is obtained by solving this formula:

Total budget = (X)(number of healthy patients under 18) + (3)(X)(number of healthy patients age 18 and older) + (2)(X)(number of mentally ill patients under 18) + (6)(X)(number of mentally ill patients age 18 and older)

Thus,

X = Total budget / [(number of healthy patients under 18) + (3)(number of healthy patients age 18 and over) + (2)(number of mentally ill patients under 18) + (6)(number of mentally ill patients age 18 and over)]

Relative differences in expected expenditures may also be estimated using multiple regression techniques. Regression adjustment is particularly useful when the risk classification factors are continuous rather than categorical, or have large numbers of response categories (e.g., age).

This example illustrates how risk adjustment reduces incentives for health plans to selectively enroll patients. Suppose that there are equal numbers of healthy patients under 18, healthy patients age 18 and older, mentally ill patients under 18, and mentally ill patients age 18 and older. In this case, the average cost of care would be $300. In the absence of risk adjustment, capitated health plans would be paid $300 for each person they enrolled, regardless of the person's age and health status. On average, for every child enrolled, the health plan would make a profit, whereas for every adult enrolled, it would suffer a loss. If the health plans were aware of the relative costliness of adults versus children, they would try to attract children and discourage adults from enrolling. Similarly, within each age group, health plans would profit more by enrolling healthy patients than mentally ill patients. In a real-life setting, access problems for particularly costly populations (in this example, adult mentally ill patients) might result. In contrast, risk adjustment avoids giving plans incentives to selectively enroll lower-cost patients because it allows the health plan to be paid the expected cost of each patient, regardless of that patient's characteristics.

CONSIDERATIONS IN CHOOSING A RISK ADJUSTMENT METHODOLOGY

In general, three criteria should be used to select a methodology for risk adjusting capitation payments: 1) predictive ability of the risk adjustment model, 2) "gameability" of the system, and 3) ease of implementation.

First, a good risk adjustment system should be able to explain a high proportion of the systematic differences in costs across patients. If it does not, then the capitation payment will tend to be too low for sick patients and unnecessarily high for healthy patients, again leading to incentives for creamskimming and dumping. When the risk adjustment methodology is relatively ineffectual at tailoring the capitation payment to the actual costs of the patient, as is often the case with simple adjustments such as age-gender, the added value of risk adjustment may not be worth the effort required to implement it. It is important to make a distinction here between the ability to predict the costs of the entire population and the ability to predict the costs of an individual patient. Although predictive ability at the aggregate level will lead to "fair" capitation payments, only predictive ability at the individual patient level will eliminate incentives for the health plan to avoid sick patients and court healthy ones.

Second, good risk adjustment systems are not "gameable," that is, they do not give incentives for providers or plans to change their behavior in such a way as to increase payments without providing higher-quality care. The simplest example of gaming is a situation in which providers or health plans change the way they code diagnoses and procedures so that they will receive higher payments although they are providing the same set of services to the same patients. In general, risk adjustment systems based on diagnoses rather than procedures are preferable, because they may be less gameable and do not distort the choice of treatment by providers.

Third, good risk adjustment systems are relatively easy to implement. The most important consideration here is the availability of data. Often a trade-off exists between the predictive ability of a risk adjustment model and the types and number of data required to achieve this level of performance. For example, although the use of self-assessed health status and other patient-reported health measures may add considerably to the explanatory power of a risk adjustment model, the expense of regularly collecting such data might be prohibitive. Similarly, a methodology relying on a single year of prior data is likely to be far easier to implement than one relying on multiple years, particularly if discontinuous enrollment poses an obstacle to obtaining sufficient historical data on all beneficiaries. Thus a risk adjustment methodology based on multiple years of data would only be adopted if historic diagnoses were important in explaining variation in costs.

One final consideration in choosing a risk adjustment system is that the weights should be estimated based on data from the health plan being capitated, or at least from a similar plan. Otherwise both the overall capitation level and the relative weights will be inaccurate. For example, suppose that a commercial risk adjustment system is developed using Medicaid data for relatively healthy young women and children. The overall cost levels may be lower than would be the case for a health plan serving an older, sicker population, or a health plan offering more generous insurance benefits. This problem, however, can be solved by adjusting the overall payment level. A more insidious problem is that the relative weights may be incorrect. For example, depression may add to the expected costs of an otherwise healthy young woman, but it might add even more to the costs of treating an elderly widow with cancer. If the increase in payment for enrolling a patient with depression is based on data from the former patient but is applied to the latter patient, the plan will be underpaid for its efforts.

Similarly, depression will increase costs by substantially more in plans offering generous mental health and substance abuse benefits than in a plan with limited benefits. In the extreme case, if a risk adjustment methodology was developed using data from health plans that did not cover mental health and substance abuse services, there might not be any meaningful adjustment to payments for patients with behavioral health problems. Yet if that system were applied to health plans that did offer those services, the health plans would be underpaid for enrolling patients with psychiatric conditions unless there was a medical cost offset.

DESCRIPTION OF COMMERCIAL RISK ADJUSTMENT METHODOLOGIES

The two best-known commercial risk adjustment methodologies are the Adjusted Clinical Groups (ACGs) and Diagnostic Cost Groups (DCGs).

Adjusted Clinical Groups

ACGs were developed by Weiner et al. (1991). In the original version (3.03), the process of assigning a person to a particular ACG involves four stages of classification and uses only outpatient diagnoses received during face-to-face encounters, defined by whether or not the visit is associated with procedure codes requiring patient/provider interaction. First, each qualifying ICD-9 diagnosis code is assigned to 1 of 34 Adjusted Diagnostic Groups, based primarily on the level of persistence or recurrence associated with the diagnosis. The Adjusted Diagnostic Groups are then collapsed into 12 broader categories. On the basis of the constellation of collapsed categories into which the patient's diagnoses fall, the patient is placed into 1 of 25 major ambulatory categories, of which 1 is psychosocial/psychophysiologic. Finally, on the basis of age, gender, and major ambulatory category, people are classified into 1 of 51 mutually exclusive ACGs. A variant of this model uses Adjusted Diagnostic Groups based on all inpatient and outpatient diagnoses and controls separately for age and gender.

Diagnostic Cost Groups

DCGs were developed as an alternative method for paying Medicare HMOs (Ash et al. 1989; Ellis et al. 1996). The Health Care Financing Administration began using Principal Inpatient Diagnostic Cost Groups (PIP-DCGs) to set capitation rates for Medicare risk contractors in January 2000, as specified by the Balanced Budget Act of 1997 (Federal Register 1997; Greenwald et al. 1998).

In general, DCG-type models use diagnoses that involve little discretion on the part of the provider to classify individuals according to expected relative costs. The two best-known versions are the PIP-DCGs and the Hierarchical Condition Categories (HCCs). The PIP-DCG system uses age, gender, and principal inpatient diagnoses to classify enrollees according to their single most important health condition. Each patient is assigned to 1 of 143 diagnostic groups, based on whichever of the patient's principal inpatient diagnoses has the highest future costs.

In contrast, HCCs are based on all inpatient and outpatient diagnoses, in addition to age and gender. Each of the diagnoses received by the beneficiary during the year is first assigned to 1 of 543 diagnostic groups. These are further grouped into 118 *condition categories* on the basis of costliness and clinical relation, which are then ranked within hierarchies from least to most severe or costly. For persons who have more than one condition within each hierarchy, only the most severe manifestation of the medical problem is retained. A regression analysis is then used to assign cost weights to each HCC. The predicted payment for each person is the sum of the incremental costs from each of the categories into which the person's diagnoses fall. Thus, unlike the PIPDCG system, payment for an individual with multiple health problems is adjusted separately for unrelated conditions. However, only a single adjustment is made for related conditions.

Risk-Based Contracting and the
Behavioral Health Care Continuum

In general, risk-based payment is likely to promote integration of care and the use of a full continuum of services better than a fee-for-service system would. That is because with risk-based payment, health plans receive a single payment covering all services and are then free to deliver whichever bundle of services is most cost effective for an individual patient. With fee-for-service systems, prices are set by the payor, and unless they reflect the true relative costs of delivering the services to each patient, the incentives to provide one type of service versus another will be distorted. For example, if providers are paid $80 for each hour-long psychotherapy session and $50 for each half-hour-long psychotropic drug management session, they have a financial incentive to use drug rather than talk therapy to treat the patient. If providers are instead paid a fixed amount per hour to treat the patient, they can decide the best use of their time for this purpose. This point can be seen even more clearly with examples in which certain benefits are not covered at all in a fee-for-service system; capitating health plans and/or providers allows them the flexibility to provide a range of services and still receive reimbursement.

It should be recognized, however, that some of the methodologies used to risk-adjust the capitation payments might still embody adverse incentives affecting the setting of care or type of services provided along the continuum of care. For example, if risk adjustment is based on inpatient diagnoses only, for example, as with the PIP-DCGs, health plans will find it more lucrative in some cases to hospitalize enrollees who otherwise might have been treated in outpatient settings. Some risk adjustment methodologies base payments on the type of services received; for example, some of the diagnosis-related groups used in Medicare's prospective payment system are in fact based on procedure rather than diagnosis codes. A problem with procedure-based risk adjustment is that it may change therapeutic practices. Suppose, for example, that a payor wished to reimburse more for severe than moderate depression and sought to use electroconvulsive therapy as a marker for severe and refractory depression. It seems likely that the use of electroconvulsive therapy would increase in response.

HEALTH PLAN INCENTIVES:
BEHAVIORAL HEALTH CARE CARVE-OUTS

The focus in this book is on integration across a continuum of behavioral health care. Yet because a large proportion of patients with psychiatric disorders are identified and treated in the primary care sector, a major issue in integrated care is the degree to which the financing of behavioral health and medical care are separated. It has become increasingly common for behavioral health care services to be *carved out*, that is, for purchasers of health care to engage in separate risk contracts for medical and behavioral health care. Oss et al. (1997) estimated that the proportion of insured citizens in the United States whose behavioral health benefits were managed by some type of specialty program increased from 44% in 1992 to 75% in 1997. In particular, risk-based network programs increased from 16% of the population in 1993 to 22% in 1997. Under a risk-based carve-out arrangement, the vendor receives a capitated payment per covered life in return for financing all services within a given category, in this case mental health/substance abuse services. A separate MCO is responsible for the medical services used by the same enrollees.

Strong arguments can be made in favor of separate financing of behavioral health care to limit incentives for health plans to dump patients with psychiatric disorders and to guarantee a target amount of funding for mental health and substance abuse services. Nonetheless, separate financing streams for medical and behavioral health care do have implications for the delivery side as well, in terms of incentives for cost shifting and potential loss of continuity. A health plan "integrated" in the sense that it receives a single capitation payment to cover the costs of both medical and behavioral health care will have incentives to ensure that the patient is treated by a coordinated, cost-efficient team of providers.

If the financial risk for services delivered in the primary care versus specialty sectors is borne by separate MCOs, neither will take into account the impact that its utilization management has on the costs of the other. Higher costs to the overall health care system can result. For example, a behavioral health care carve-out vendor would not consider possible medical cost offsets resulting from improved psychiatric care. Conversely, a medical plan would prefer to refer patients with mild psychiatric problems to the mental health specialty sector, even if the costs of specialty care (borne by the carve-out vendor) would be greater than having psychotropic drug management integrated into the patient's primary care.

In terms of promoting an integrated continuum, one attractive option for purchasers may be the use of "administrative services only" contracts with behavioral health care carve-out vendors. Such contracts are quite common in behavioral health and are frequently used by integrated health plans that choose to subcontract with a behavioral health care carve-out vendor. "Administrative services only" contracts permit the benefits of specialized care management and utilization review that can be provided by carve-outs, but a single party still bears the financial risk for both medical and behavioral health care.

Provider Incentives: "Bundled" Reimbursement

An important determinant of the degree to which care is integrated is whether separate reimbursement versus bundled payment is used for services provided across a continuum of care. As an example, an ongoing debate in Medicare reimbursement is whether acute inpatient care and postacute services should be reimbursed separately or together. Separate reimbursement encourages cost shifting, with patients being discharged earlier from the hospital but using more intensive services following discharge; bundled reimbursement, which puts hospitals at risk for both types of service use, provides incentives for hospitals to choose the most cost-effective mix of acute and postacute services.

A comparable situation in behavioral health would be one in which hospitals were paid a single amount to care for an acutely ill patient, regardless of the extent to which the care was composed of inpatient treatment versus other services such as partial hospitalization. Separate reimbursement of each type of service can lead to the provision of suboptimal combinations of services, especially if prospective reimbursement is used for one type of service but not another. For example, it would not be desirable to pay psychiatric hospitals a fixed amount per discharge while their outpatient clinics are paid separately on a fee-for-service basis.

Thus, in considering how to structure reimbursement to encourage delivery of appropriate services along a continuum, it is important to take into account providers' incentives to shift costs. Although cost shifting is not such a concern when provider reimbursement is on a cost or fee-for-service basis, whenever possible, providers paid on a capitated basis should be put at risk for the full range of services that might be appropriate for patients.

Patient Incentives:
Covered Benefits and Cost Sharing

The financial incentives patients face can also have an important impact on the integration of care. As the RAND Health Insurance Experiment (Newhouse 1993) and other studies have shown, patients respond to increased costs of care by cutting back on service use. Price responsiveness tends to be even stronger for mental health services than it is for medical care. Thus cost-sharing requirements and the benefits covered by the insurance plan have the potential for distorting the patient's treatment choices. For example, Medicare imposes a 190-day lifetime limit on reimbursement of psychiatric hospital care; no such limit exists for general hospitals. It seems likely, therefore, that Medicare beneficiaries who are close to, or exceed, the lifetime limit for psychiatric hospital coverage will instead choose to be treated at a general hospital. Another example is that Medicare requires a 50% copayment from beneficiaries receiving outpatient psychotherapy services, but only a 20% copayment for management of psychotropic medications. Among beneficiaries who do not have very strong preferences for one over the other, the change in the relative price of the two therapies induced by the differential cost-sharing requirements may influence therapeutic choices in favor of pharmacotherapy (although Medicare's failure to cover prescription drugs is likely to have the opposite effect).

In the context of the integrated behavioral health care continuum, an example is a circumstance in which inpatient care was reimbursed, but day programs were not. In this case, some patients might prefer to be admitted to the hospital, even if day care would be a more appropriate treatment option for them. Often limits are applied differentially, with different dollar caps on the reimbursement of inpatient versus outpatient care. Even within an outpatient setting, a 10-visit limit on psychotherapy services in conjunction with unlimited coverage of medication management visits to primary care physicians may shift the setting of mental health counseling away from the specialty sector into the general medical sector.

Thus, as with provider reimbursement, insurance coverage ideally should be structured so as to eliminate incentives for the patient to choose one set of services over another perhaps more clinically appropriate set simply on the basis of financial considerations. One possible means for achieving that goal would be for a particular type and severity of psychiatric disorder to trigger the payment of a lump sum that could be used by the patient to fund whichever combination of services is most appropriate for his or her treatment needs. Although empirically difficult to implement, this approach does have the advantage of allowing maximum flexibility for the patient's treatment plan and avoiding the distortion of treatment choices. This type of *indemnity* payment is currently being tested for long-term-care services as part of a Health Care Financing Administration–funded demonstration project for Medicaid patients. Innovative financing mechanisms to promote integration across a continuum of care should be further explored in the context of behavioral health.

References

Ash A, Porell F, Gruenberg E, et al: Adjusting Medicare capitation payments using prior hospitalization data. Health Care Financ Rev 10:17–29, 1989

Ellis R, Pope G, Iezzoni J, et al: Diagnosis-based risk adjustment for Medicare capitation payments. Health Care Financ Rev 17:101–128, 1996

Federal Register, Doc. 98-24085 (Vol 62). Washington DC, Office of the Federal Register, National Archives and Record Service, 1997

Greenwald L, Esposito A, Ingber M, et al: Risk adjustment for the Medicare program: lessons learned from research and demonstrations. Inquiry 35:193–209, 1998

Newhouse J: Free for All? Lessons from the RAND Health Insurance Experiment. Cambridge, MA, Harvard University Press, 1993

Oss M, Drissel A, Clary J: Managed Behavioral Health Market Share in the United States, 1997–1998. Gettysburg, PA, Open Minds, 1997

Weiner J, Starfield B, Steinwachs D, et al: Development and application of a population-oriented measure of ambulatory care case-mix. Med Care 29:452–472, 1991

14

Current Research on Mental Health Systems Integration

Mark S. Salzer, Ph.D.
Edna Kamis-Gould, Ph.D.
Trevor Hadley, Ph.D.

Systems integration emerged in the 1960s in response to the expansion of mental health and social services programs and the perception that it potentially offers increased efficiency and effectiveness (Agranoff 1991) compared with a duplicative, fragmented, and generally haphazard array of services. Far from a simple concept, systems integration is thought to have multiple forms that vary substantially on at least two dimensions: the intensity of interagency relationships (loose to highly organized) and the formality of governance (informal to formal policies) (Konrad 1996). Konrad (1996) described five levels of integration: 1) information sharing and communication (shared information on regular or irregular basis), 2) cooperation and coordination (reciprocal referrals, joint staffing), 3) collaboration (formal collaboration with shared goals), 4) consolidation (umbrella organization with single leadership, possibly shared central administration, divisions remain but with high degree of cooperation), and 5) integration (single authority, operates collectively, activities fully blended).

Interest has waxed and waned over the years, but in the 1990s systems integration received a considerable amount of theoretical and empirical attention, especially in the area of mental health service delivery. The assumption is that systems integration will positively affect the array of services (i.e., diversity) and access to these services, improve service delivery patterns (e.g., fewer hospital services and more rehabilitation services), and decrease fragmentation thought to limit service effectiveness. Individual-level clinical outcomes are thought to be enhanced through two routes. First, clinical outcomes may be enhanced by the availability of an array of services that meet the current needs of the consumer. A key assumption of this model is that clinicians and case managers can assign consumers to the most appropriate level of care and appropriate transitions when their conditions change. A better match between the consumer and delivered services is thought to result in better clinical outcomes. Second, changes in the service delivery process should improve clinical outcomes. For example, coordination of services should produce enhanced continuity of care, decreased dropout rates, use of less restrictive services, more individualized service plans, and more timely services. All these system improvements are assumed to improve individual clinical outcomes.

Although there is interest in systems integration and a belief that it has important effects on systems and consumers, there have been relatively few rigorous studies in the adult and child mental health areas. Nonetheless, we synthesize the initial research findings on systems integration in the delivery of mental health services and find that they shed some light on the enormous potential that systems integration has to enhance systems and alter service use patterns and service processes. Specifically, systems integration has demonstrably affected some very important areas, such as improved identification of need, access to services, the development of a continuum of services, decreased use of expensive inpatient services, enhanced service coordination and continuity of care, and consumer satisfaction. However, initial results suggest the need to be cautious about how the benefits associated with enhanced systems trickle down to individual service recipients through improved individual-level clinical outcomes, such as quality of life and symptom change. These results should inspire further refinement of systems integration theory, expectations, and research approaches as well as highlight future directions for mental health services research.

CONCEPTUAL FRAMEWORK FOR EVALUATING SYSTEMS INTEGRATION EFFORTS

Before reviewing current research, it is important to consider a framework for discussing outcomes that are routinely assessed in systems integration research. This framework is useful for gaining an appreciation of the types of areas in which systems integration has an impact as well as those areas in which an impact has not been found. Systems integration interventions are expected to have an impact in four general areas: systems, service involvement, service processes, and individual-level clinical outcomes. A fuller explication of how systems integration is expected to affect each of these areas can be found in earlier chapters, and we mention the reasoning only briefly here as well as caveats in the interpretation of results in each area.

System Level

System-level variables are those that specifically reflect the operation of the service system. These include variables such as service delivery efficiency (e.g., nonredundancy of services), continuum of care, and service linkages. Changes in these areas should usually be thought of as activities associated with implementing systems integration. These variables are reflective of successful implementation rather than *outcomes* in the traditional sense of the term (see Rossi 1997 for a discussion of endogeneity), and use of variables such as outcome measures is to be avoided.

Service Involvement

Service involvement refers to resource use or service contact within the mental health system and within a specific service type (e.g., hospitalization) and the associated costs. One example is access to mental health care. It is hypothesized that systems integration efforts will increase the availability of mental health treatment (i.e., service slots) and use of service slots across the mental health system. Increased access and placement in housing is another example of service involvement changes that are expected to be associated with systems integration interventions for those who are homeless (see later discussion of ACCESS). Systems integration interventions are also intended to increase resource availability and options and enhance the appropriate allocation of the least restrictive services available. One routine expectation is that systems integration will result in decreased inpatient hospital use (and expectations for decreased costs) and more appropriate service mix and intensity. Additional examples of service utilization changes in other systems affected by systems integration include increased school attendance in the education system, decreased incarceration or arrests in the criminal justice system, and decreased out-of-home placements in the social welfare system.

An important goal of systems integration is to enable changes in resource use so that more efficient and appropriate service patterns are delivered. However, the interpretation of, for example, reductions in hospital length of stay, hospital admissions, out-of-home-placements, or incarceration rates should be done with caution. In particular, attributing decreases in these areas to reduced distress, enhanced individual or family functioning, or improved behavior in the systems integration population is probably not valid. Resource use in all social service sectors depends to a certain extent on subjective decision making that is influenced by service system philosophy. For example, one of the philosophies associated with systems integration in the children's area is an emphasis on keeping children in their homes. This philosophical change alone may account for decreases in out-of-home placements and hospitalization rates regardless of changes in the child's behavior (e.g., Rubin 1992). A similar argument can be made about discretion in the criminal justice system, such as police discretion in making arrests (Bittner 1967; Green 1997) and making decisions regarding parole and sentencing.

Service Process

Systems integration efforts are proposed to enhance the services delivered to the population. In current systems integration research, improvement in service processes is examined by analyzing quality of care indicators, such as timeliness (i.e., how long the person waits to obtain treatment), continuity of care (length of time between hospital discharge and initiation of outpatient treatment or length of time in treatment), and consumer satisfaction with services. Quality of care indicators such as those mentioned above are excellent for evaluating the efficiency of systems integration, but they have yet to be sufficiently linked with individual client outcomes (Salzer et al. 1997) and may not be useful to assess the effectiveness of service processes. Similarly, consumer satisfaction measures are an excellent way to obtain consumer perspectives on service processes. However, using satisfaction measures to evaluate the clinical effectiveness of systems integration remains open to question. A review of the literature in this area indicates that there is ample evidence to suggest that no empirical relationship exists between satisfaction and change in clinical outcome (Lambert et al. 1998). As is discussed later, evaluation of the use of effective service approaches (e.g., effective inpatient, case management, or psychotherapy treatment models) remains rare in systems integration research.

Clinical Outcome

Improving individual-level clinical outcomes of the service system is one of the primary goals of systems integration. Donabedian (1980) provided a definition of *outcome* that we find useful: "a change in the patient's current and future health status [symptoms and functioning] that can be attributed to antecedent health care" (p. 82). Wells and Brook (1989) outlined a number of important outcome domains of interest in mental health besides symptoms, functioning, and quality of life, such as severity of a mental health problem, occurrence of a new medical or mental health problem, subsequent use of medical and mental health services, course of disorder, social disposition and placement, development of coping abilities, and level of distress experienced by family members.

The major issue associated with examining outcomes of systems integration involves the use of comparison or control groups to assist in ruling out threats to internal validity (e.g., history, maturation, regression to the mean). Systems integration studies are increasingly using designs involving control or comparison groups, which is one indicator of increased sophistication and rigor in systems integration research. These issues are discussed in more detail later.

Systems Integration in Adult Mental Health Services Research

The expansion of community-based mental health services for adults with severe mental illnesses away from large inpatient hospitals is viewed almost universally as a positive step in the delivery of mental health services. Strong community-based services enhance the successful community tenure of persons discharged from long-term mental health facilities. However, historical continued funding and expansion of social services resulted in increased fragmentation, duplicity of services, and decreased coordination (Hadley 1996). Moreover, the development of catchment areas further separated agencies, and in some cases catchment areas were established with little attention paid to their affiliation with public mental hospitals (see Goldman et al. 1994 for a discussion of these issues). The resulting need for increased systems integration for adult services seems clear. Results from a few studies in adult services are beginning to highlight areas in which change was brought about by systems integration.

The Rochester Capitation Experiment involved fixed payments to a lead agency to provide one of two service levels to persons with a history of long-term state hospital care (Reed and Babigian 1994). The first care level required the lead agency to provide comprehensive services, including medical care and residential services. The second level required the lead service agency to provide all ambulatory mental health care, including psychiatric medications, but not medical or residential services. The theory underlying this intervention was that services coordinated through a single agency paid a fixed rate would enhance systems integration. More than 700 people were enrolled in this demonstration program between 1987 and 1993. Many positive system-level changes were reported for this experiment, such as enhanced continuity of care and enhanced continuum of services, including rehabilitation services. Positive findings for service involvement were also evident, such as aggressive outreach to combat dropout from treatment and the transfer of care of persons in state hospitals to the community. However, as Reed and Babigian (1994) noted, similar changes were occurring in mental health systems throughout the country, and without appropriate comparison groups, it was difficult to draw firm conclusions about the causes of perceived system improvements.

Another study examined the relationship between network integration and effectiveness in four mental health systems (Tucson, Arizona; Albuquerque, New Mexico; Providence, Rhode Island; and Akron, Ohio) (Provan and Milward 1995). This correlational study defined *integration* in two ways: 1) interconnectedness among provider agencies and 2) the extent to which agencies are integrated and coordinated through a central authority. Centrality was examined by studying the number of linkages between agencies (i.e., core agency centrality) and the level of influence of core agencies (i.e., concentration of influence). Questionnaires mailed to key personnel and follow-up interviews were used to assess the various aspects of network integration.

Effectiveness was assessed using data obtained from a small (59–80 subjects) random sample of adult clients in each community who had severe mental illness, their family members, and their case managers. Individual-level outcome domains included quality of life, functioning, symptomatology, and satisfaction. The study authors conducted a factor analysis with these data, resulting in a four-factor structure: quality of life/satisfaction (consumer reported), psychiatric/medical status (consumer reported), family-reported effectiveness, and case manager–reported effectiveness. The consumer and family member responses were then combined to produce one score of network effectiveness, and case manager ratings were used as another.

The authors of this study did not find a relationship between interconnectedness or core agency centrality and consumer-reported network effectiveness but did find that concentration of influence was correlated with consumer-reported network effectiveness. Systems with agencies that had concentrated influence were rated as most effective on the basis of consumer and family member data. No relationship was found between any measure of integration and case manager reports of network effectiveness.

The two studies mentioned (Provan and Milward 1995; Reed and Babigian 1994) are informative but are limited by their design and measurement. The bulk of our knowledge about systems integration within the adult mental health system comes from two well-financed cross-site studies, both of which used quasiexperimental designs with comparison groups. In 1985 the Robert Wood Johnson Foundation (RWJF) established the Program on Chronic Mental Illness to address the needs of persons who are chronically mentally ill by developing a mental health authority in each community (i.e., city or county) with centralized administrative, fiscal, and clinical authority for mental health service delivery. RWJF provided $29 million during a 5-year period to nine cities in the United States to develop and implement a centralized mental health authority. It was expected that these agencies would be responsible for planning, funding, and coordinating a wide range of services for people with mental illness as well as overseeing the delivery of services. The expectations were that centralized mental health authorities could expand resources and services, that this expansion would result in continuity of care, and that continuity of care would result in enhanced quality of life and psychosocial functioning at the individual level. There was no specific emphasis on services delivered other than case management to improve service coordination.

The demonstration sites established local mental health authorities, but the performance of the community support system, as determined by the analysis of interagency relations (i.e., density, centralization, and fragmentation), was not viewed as having been sufficiently enhanced (Morrissey et al. 1994). Admitting that their approach had some limitations, the authors noted that the lack of an enhanced community support system may undermine the production of more positive individual-level outcomes.

Lehman et al. (1994) obtained data from two cohorts of respondents at four of the nine RWJF sites. Cohort 1 involved participants who entered the service system in the early stages of the demonstration, whereas those in cohort 2 entered the service system between 3 and 20 months later. The value in comparing cohorts 1 and 2 is based on a program maturation hypothesis. Specifically, it is assumed that the demonstration would take time to achieve maximal success and that those entering the treatment system at later points in time would receive better continuity of care and achieve greater individual-level benefits compared with those entering the system earlier. Client reports were used to assess service process variables (e.g., case management services and continuity of care) and change in individual-level outcomes (e.g., quality of life, symptoms, level of functioning).

More respondents in cohort 2 had case managers at 2 months postbaseline compared with those in cohort 1, but this finding disappeared at 12 months postbaseline. Continuity of care, as indicated by fewer reported changes in case managers, was also found to be greater for cohort 2. No significant differences were found between cohorts on needs met or for the perceived helpfulness of services received. Similar findings were obtained for client outcomes. Symptom scores at 12 months postbaseline were the only area in which a significant main effect was found. In this case, those in cohort 2 were found to have higher symptom scores. Analysis of the process and outcome variables was complicated by numerous interactions between cohort and demonstration site. Specifically, there was great variability across all service sites included in this study. In more recent work, it has been suggested that variability in the quality and availability of case management services might partially account for the lack of outcome differences (Ridgely et al. 1996).

Shern et al. (1994) conducted an evaluation of the RWJF demonstration in Colorado. Five waves of data (baseline plus one yearly assessment) were obtained from almost 800 respondents meeting criteria for serious and persistent mental illness. Respondents obtained services from either the demonstration site (Denver) or a comparable site in Colorado. Self-report data were obtained in three service process areas: continuity of care measures (contacts with service providers and service breaks), met and unmet needs (assess need and receipt of care), and satisfaction with services. Clinical effectiveness was assessed by examining client-reported quality of life, symptoms, and self-esteem.

A discussion of the results from this study is complicated by the fact that the authors' hypotheses included the expectation of site-by-year interactions because of a financial crisis halfway through the demonstration period. As a result, the authors of this study expected significant site differences in the initial years in favor of the demonstration site, followed by no site differences. The systems integration effort was found to have an initial impact on continuity of care as indicated by increased contact with service providers and decreased terminations. However, as expected, financial problems in later years led to the elimination of case manager staff positions and resulted in no differences between the sites. Findings concerning unmet needs were equally complex and generally conformed to the findings for continuity of care. Specifically, early gains in addressing unmet needs were lost as a result of increasingly limited resources in the final years of the demonstration. Respondent satisfaction with services was found to increase over the first 3 years at the demonstration site but decreased following the financial crisis, again in keeping with the authors' hypotheses. These data suggest that important process changes are associated with the systems integration intervention, at least in the initial years of the demonstration.

However, the initiative did not have the expected impact on clinical effectiveness, a finding that is consistent with the Lehman et al. (1994) study. Modest gains were found in only a few areas. The only quality of life indicator that met the expected site-by-year interaction was safety. Demonstration site clients reported feeling safer in the first 3 years, but these differences were not present in later years. Patients at the control sites had more psychotic symptoms in the later years than those at the demonstration site.

The final adult study to be reviewed here is the Access to Community Care and Effective Services and Supports study (ACCESS). The goals of the ACCESS study were to assess the impact of service systems integration on access to services and outcomes for people with serious mental illness who are homeless and to assess whether outcomes are mediated through accessibility and continuity of services (Rosenheck et al. 1998). Nine states obtained funding to implement systems integration efforts at a demonstration site (selected randomly from two comparable sites in the state) and evaluate the outcomes for consumers in this site with those at a comparison site. The demonstration sites were expected to use a variety of policy and organizational strategies to enhance integration (Randolph et al. 1997). Both the demonstration and comparison sites obtained funds to enhance their outreach and case management capabilities.

Early findings indicated that clients in both the demonstration and comparison sites had significant increases in service use in many areas of obvious importance for this population (psychiatric care, substance abuse care, medical care, housing services, income support, and job assistance). Most of the increase was seen within 3 months of obtaining services. One exemplar of this change was that only 5% of clients receiving services had independent housing (i.e., apartment or house) at baseline, yet 44% had independent housing 1 year into the program (Rosenheck et al. 1998). The authors found that systems integration had a direct effect on independent living at 12 months as well as an indirect effect mediated through the increased use of housing services at 3 months. However, systems integration did not appear to affect other types of service use, contradicting an expectation that systems integration would have an additive impact in nonhousing resource use. These findings were replicated in a follow-up study involving two cohorts of ACCESS participants (Rosenheck et al. in press). The replication study also examined client-level clinical outcomes associated with systems integration. The only significant finding was that there were higher levels of depression among those at the more integrated sites.

SYSTEMS INTEGRATION IN CHILD MENTAL HEALTH SERVICES RESEARCH

It seems self-evident that children and adolescents with behavioral health disorders would benefit from integrated service systems because the context of their experiences and problems involves their families, their schools and, often, other categorical child service agencies. Problem resolution in these situations requires accessibility to and coordination of multiple services both within and across service programs. The next section of this chapter concerns recent research on integrated services to children and adolescents.

A series of publications and reports (Knitzer 1982; Saxe et al. 1988; Stroul and Friedman 1986) revealed that mental health service systems for youth were incomplete, fragmented, and uncoordinated; did not meet the needs of children; and were ineffective. In response, Stroul and Friedman (1986) promoted the need for a system of services based on the federal Child and Adolescent Service System Program (CASSP) philosophy of an array of service systems rooted in values and principles, for example, the importance of involving families of youth with mental disorders or the merit of serving children in the least restrictive settings. They added that services must encompass all child-serving systems, especially education and child welfare, and must be coordinated and integrated. Numerous states initiated projects designed to expand the array of services and shift care to less restrictive services (Rosenblatt et al. 1992). Federal agencies as well as private foundations launched multiple projects designed to develop programs that met the service needs of children, added to local arrays of services, developed new revenue sources, and fostered systems and service coordination and integration (Cole and Poe 1993; Lourie et al. 1998; Meyers and Davis 1997). In addition, diminishing resources have put systems of care under pressure to demonstrate accountability and cost-effectiveness (Nixon 1997). A sample of research and demonstration projects is described below to illustrate related development and research issues.

The Alaska Youth Initiative (VanDenBerg 1993) was based on the CASSP concept of a system of care but used state-level leadership to create local-level, interdisciplinary community service teams to provide unconditional, individualized, or wraparound interventions. The objectives of the Alaska Youth Initiative were to limit out-of-home placements and transition back to Alaska youth who had been placed out of state. After 2 years almost all youth who were in residential treatment programs out of state were returned and served in less restrictive programs in Alaska. The study employed simple program evaluation, rather than experimental design, and did not gather child-specific clinical outcomes.

Vermont's New Directions (Santarcangelo et al. 1998) developed and implemented multiple community programs to enhance the array of services and reduce out-of-state placement. The program included specialized education, respite care, crisis stabilization, therapeutic case management, and interagency collaboration and integration. One year after implementation, there were desired shifts in service use. These included a reduced use of residential programs (from 40% to 10% of youth in residential and from 23% to 8% in foster care); increased independent living arrangement (2% to 17%) and residence with family (17% to 23%); and increased use of innovative community-based programs, such as therapeutic case management (16% to 40%). A providers' survey elicited information on improved collaboration, for example, an increase from 27% to 83% of respondents reporting collaboration with other agencies. Consumer satisfaction was in the good to excellent range (e.g., average of 4.34 out of 5 for satisfaction with treatment), and recipients of therapeutic case management had a higher average (4.37) than recipients of other services. Client-level clinical data revealed meaningful and statistically significant reduction in negative behavior, physical aggression, property damage, suicide attempt, sexual abuse, fire setting, and so on. The frequency of monthly incidents by a group of 27 youths declined from 177 to 52 and from an average of 6.6 to an average of 1.9.

A national project, the Alternative to Residential Treatment Study (ARTS), was implemented about in the late 1980s. The study was designed to systematically describe five "mature," integrated community-based programs across the country that served seriously emotionally disturbed youth and their families. The programs were the Alaska Youth Initiative, New Directions, Kaleidoscope in Chicago, Pressley Ridge Youth Development Extension in Pennsylvania, and the Ventura, California project. Recognizing the complex nature of consumer outcomes, the ARTS collected data from youths ($n = 163$, almost equally distributed over the five systems) and their caregivers, local professionals, and case records, using multiple methods and standardized instruments. Analysis consisted mostly of changes over 12 months and produced mixed but encouraging results. There were statistically significant improvements in academic performance in both reading and mathematics, reduction of behavioral problems, and increased functioning but no impact on substance use, social competence, and family functioning. There was some indication of a shift of service provision to less restrictive settings, but many youth remained in state custody. There was also a delay in providing needed services.

The California Assembly mandated a reduction in the use of and expenditures for public residential services for youth and funded replications of the Ventura project in three counties. All participating counties engaged in structured planning, developed in Ventura, to reduce the use of out-of-home placements through creation and maintenance of coordinated and effective community-based services. Multiple time series analysis of aggregated county-level number of placements and related costs during a 10-year period were used to compare the counties with each other and against similar state data. Costs were adjusted for inflation, and all data were adjusted for population size. The rate of placement was lowered in the demonstrations and, although the cost per placement has steadily increased, these counties decreased their total expenditures. The project did not address child-specific, clinical, school, and quality of life outcomes. Furthermore, the Ventura model is a planning model and does not specify particular programs that counties must implement to achieve the desired effects. The lack of child-specific outcomes and the different county systems precluded findings about the nature, quality, and effectiveness of the alternative services and service systems.

In 1988 the RWJF funded a multisite national demonstration project, the Mental Health Services Program for Youth (MHSPY), designed to test the feasibility of creating coordinated and integrated services across child-serving agencies. The integrated systems were expected to reduce out-of-home placements and make more efficient use of available resources (Cross and Saxe 1997; England and Cole 1992). Eight sites were funded to 1) restructure the organization and financing of services to achieve coordination and integration, decategorize funding streams, maximize federal financing, and increase revenues; and 2) serve 200 children with the most severe emotional disorders. A three-pronged evaluation of the MHSPY consisted of 1) case studies of the organization and financing of services, 2) a site-specific client information system to support the integrated services, and 3) clinical assessment conferences to ascertain the impact of interagency systems integration on the quality of care. The sites implemented new services, although these developments varied from one project site to another. Most changes in financing involved Medicaid waivers that allow financing of services not previously covered by state plans (e.g., case management) and enabled states to shift service financing from fee-for-service to managed care.

The Kentucky MHSPY project, Bluegrass IMPACT, stimulated legislation that expanded the project and created the statewide Kentucky IMPACT (Illback et al. 1998). Evaluation aimed at 1) assessment of systems changes in the array of services, nature of collaboration, shifts to services in least restrictive settings, and cost impacts; 2) impacts on participating youth—behavioral changes, achievement, family, and school adjustment; 3) family satisfaction; and 4) determinants of desired outcomes. Automated information and specially collected data via standardized instruments provided the data for the evaluation. The results revealed 1) substantial improvements in behavioral problems, 2) lesser, but mostly significant, gains in social competence, 3) high family satisfaction, 4) dramatic reduction in psychiatric hospitalization but increased use of residential treatment, 5) increased stability of placements, and 6) 36% reduction in costs to the system.

The Fort Bragg Evaluation Project (Bickman et al. 1995) established a continuum of services modeled on the CASSP systems of care (Stroul and Friedman 1986). The study employed rigorous evaluation, a comparison group, and consumer-level outcomes. It examined the implementation of the model and its impact in terms of six dimensions: access, service type, service mix, volume, timing, and continuity of services received by youth. Comparing services, costs, and clinical outcomes at Fort Bragg and two other systems without a formally organized service continuum, the researchers expected improved mental health, lower cost per case, quicker recovery, and higher client satisfaction in the demonstration program. The results, however, were mixed. The implemented continuum of service was true to the model. It produced better access, and a greater proportion of youth received services in the Fort Bragg system (8% compared with 2.7% and 4.5% in the other two systems). There was a reduction in inpatient services, although the newly developed intermediate services seemed to draw children from both inpatient and outpatient services. Services were more timely, as Fort Bragg children received services within 17 days of their assessment compared with 38 days for the comparison sites. There were better linkage and follow-up services at the demonstration; 93% of Fort Bragg children received community services following discharge from a residential treatment center compared with 47% at the comparison sites and tended to remain longer in service. Satisfaction ratings were also higher at the Fort Bragg demonstration site than at the comparison sites. There were no differences, however, between the demonstration and comparison sites on the various clinical outcome measures.

The Fort Bragg Evaluation Project has stimulated a more rigorous replication in the Stark County Evaluation Project (Bickman et al. 1997, 1999). The project is based on the CASSP model and involves multiple initiatives: implementation of a complete array of integrated services, interagency agreements, case management, and improved financial mechanisms. Research questions address clinical outcomes of the systems intervention, child and family determinants of outcomes, use patterns over time, and relationships between service utilization and outcomes. The project has three unique and desirable features: 1) study participants have been randomly assigned to experimental and control conditions in the same treatment community; 2) it is a longitudinal study that encompasses four follow-up interviews; and 3) the primary data collection was accomplished by means of interactive computerized interviews. An extensive battery of instruments used in the interviews has yielded a detailed description of the participants and is beginning to produce a great deal of important information. All children in the study had a serious emotional disorder, and more than 80% of their families received public assistance.

Results from the Stark County Evaluation Project indicate that children in the demonstration condition had greater access to services, received more timely services (i.e., within 30 days of intake in the study), and were much more likely to receive case management and home visits. Nonetheless, these children did not differ from those in the control condition in any of the individual-level clinical outcome domains (e.g., symptoms, functioning, caregiver strain).

Discussion

The results for all these studies are summarized in Table 14–1. The breakdown of dependent variables into four conceptual domains provides us with an interesting vantage point from which to make a number of observations. The various systems integration efforts appear to have a generally positive impact on system, service involvement, and service process variables in both the adult and child studies. This finding is important because it demonstrates that change can be brought about in relatively short periods of time in critical areas such as the development of an array of services, network integration, service use patterns, and continuity of care.

TABLE 14–1. Cross-study outcomes of systems integration

Study	Outcome areas			
	System Continuum of care Coordination	Service involvement Access to care Costs Hospital use Treatment length Service mix Housing Incarceration	Service process Satisfaction Therapeutic relationship Working alliance Continuity of care	Individual-level clinical Symptoms Functioning Empowerment Recovery Quality of life
Rochester Capitation Experiment (Reed and Babigian 1994)	+	+		
Four mental health systems (Provan and Milward 1995)			+/–	
Robert Wood Johnson Foundation (Morrissey et al. 1994)	+/–			
Robert Wood Johnson Foundation (Lehman et al. 1994)			+/–	0
Robert Wood Johnson Foundation (Shern et al. 1994) (precrisis results)			+	0
ACCESS (Rosenheck et al. 1998, in press)		+/0		0/–
Alaska Youth Initiative (VanDenBerg 1993)		+		
Vermont's New Directions (Santarcangelo et al. 1998)		+	+	+

TABLE 14–1. Cross-study outcomes of systems integration *(continued)*

Study	System	Service involvement	Service process	Individual-level clinical
	Continuum of care / Coordination	Access to care, Costs, Hospital use, Treatment length, Service mix, Housing, Incarceration	Satisfaction, Therapeutic relationship, Working alliance, Continuity of care	Symptoms, Functioning, Empowerment, Recovery, Quality of life
Alternatives to Residential Treatment Study		+/–		+/0
Ventura Project		+		
Mental Health Services Program for Youth (Illback et al. 1998)		+/?	+	+
Fort Bragg Evaluation Project (Bickman et al. 1995)	+	+/?	+	0
Stark County Evaluation Project (Bickman et al. 1997)	+	+/?		0

Note. Empty cell indicates that the outcome area was not studied. (+) indicates a positive finding for systems integration. (–) indicates a negative finding for systems integration. (0) indicates there was no difference between a control or comparison group and systems integration group. Notice that we use (+/?) in the service involvement boxes in reviewing the children's studies. The (+) refers to the decrease of inpatient hospitalizations and out-of-home placements. The (?) refers to an increase in the use of services and costs for those children in the systems integration demonstrations. Some might view this as positive because of the criticism that mental health services are underfunded. Others might view this added cost as a negative.

The studies involving children focus heavily on altering service involvement, especially changes in inpatient hospitalization and out-of-home placement. This might not be surprising given that the impetus for systems integration efforts in the children's area was partially driven by overdependence on inpatient treatment and out-of-home placements.

An equally important finding is that there is no current evidence that systems integration efforts have any impact on individual-level clinical outcomes in those studies using comparison or control group designs. The three studies reported here that do show an effect (Duchnowski et al. 1998; Illback et al. 1998; Santarcangelo et al. 1998), all in the children's area, are severely limited by the use of designs that are susceptible to numerous threats to internal validity. The Fort Bragg Evaluation Project (Bickman et al. 1995) and Stark County Evaluation Project (Bickman et al. 1999) used much stronger designs and found no effect for systems integration. Although the current sample of systems integration studies is admittedly small, the studies using rigorous designs provide consistent results concerning impact on individual-level clinical outcomes.

Two related arguments for not finding more positive individual-level outcomes are that there is an implementation lag between service systems change and a learning curve in how clinicians use the new system to maximize benefit for the consumer. It takes time to change systems that have been entrenched in previous operating patterns, and it takes time to make improvements in how efficiently services are delivered through coordination and continuity of care. Recall that Morrissey et al. (1994) did not find that interagency relations were sufficiently enhanced at the RWJF sites. However, as noted earlier, all studies found improvement in the service system, service involvement, and service processes. This suggests that important changes can take place within a few years, but are these the critical changes that need to be brought about? Also, it may take years for service providers to maximize the use of the new system created for them. The data suggest that clinicians change their prescription of service use (e.g., create new programs, use inpatient services less), but how long does it take them to determine which of the new services are appropriate for which clients? Current systems integration research efforts might have evaluated systems before they fully "matured."

However, recall that Shern et al. (1994) followed up with people for 5 years and found no differential improvement over time. Lehman et al. (1994) used a lagged-cohort design (2 years postimplementation versus 4 years postimplementation) and found no differences between groups. Finally, Bickman et al. (1996) did not find differential effects by date of entry into the evaluation. These results raise the question of how long it might take systems to mature to have an impact on individual-level outcomes.

Belief in the strength of systems integration to produce change at the individual client level is so strong that it may produce circular reasoning. Namely, some might assert that the reason no individual-level benefits have been found is that systems integration has not been satisfactorily implemented. The problem with this logic is that null results are dismissed as evidence of poor implementation, even though the studies reviewed here generally find evidence that change has occurred at the system and services levels. We think it is fruitful to consider the reasonable alternative explanation—systems integration is probably not necessary and certainly not sufficient to produce positive individual-level outcomes.

Systems Integration and Individual-Level Outcomes: Weakness in Service Effectiveness

There seems to be growing concern that systems integration interventions are not having their expected impact on clinical effectiveness because the services delivered are not maximally effective and are not improved by increased integration (Goldman et al. 1994; Ridgely et al. 1996; Salzer and Bickman 1997). Mental health professionals used to confidently point to psychotherapy and psychopharmacology laboratory-based research (efficacy studies) as evidence that what they do is effective. However, recent distinctions have been made between laboratory-based findings and treatment delivered in normal private practice or clinic settings (effectiveness studies) (Hoagwood et al. 1995). The effectiveness of mental health services is being increasingly challenged and current meta-analyses have yet to demonstrate that mental health services delivered routinely in the field are effective (e.g., Weisz et al. 1992). However, it should be remembered that relatively few studies, especially hard-to-implement randomized studies, were conducted in natural settings.

If basic mental health services (i.e., inpatient, partial hospitalization, psychotherapy) are not individually effective, could greater systems integration enhance their effectiveness so that improved clinical outcomes are seen? This is unlikely, because the systems integration efforts do not target clinical practices beyond changes in service mix, such as prescribing less restrictive services, and providing consumer access to a greater array of services. In fact, one study of case manager activities in the first 3 years of the RWJF project found very little change in activities during this time period (Ridgely et al. 1996). The use of "best practices" or practice guidelines is not part of systems integration. It seems reasonable to suggest that the most direct way to enhance clinical outcomes is through the development and use of empirically validated services.

Promoting More Rigorous and Alternative Systems Integration Research Practices

Recent large-scale studies provide examples of exemplary systems integration research. The hallmarks of these studies (RWJF, ACCESS, Fort Bragg Evaluation Project, and Stark County Evaluation Project) include their use of sophisticated quasiexperimental designs (in the case of the Stark County Evaluation Project, an experimental design) that enhance the interpretation of results and are critically important in addressing threats to internal validity. These studies also involve large samples to enhance the power of detecting small effects. Finally, they use state-of-the-art tools in assessing change in all measurement domains.

Burns et al. (1998) reviewed the disappointing individual-level clinical outcomes in the child area and recommended convening a panel of experts to draw a national research agenda and suggest approaches to better research. Maloy (1997) and Poole (1997) promoted *emic* (indigenous) case studies rather than *etic* (universal) assessment as the most productive methods for understanding major innovations in complex systems that are very different from each other. Clearly, integrated service systems are very complex. Akin to services for adults, mental health services for children emerged out of at least four different systems: 1) public-funded, agency-based mental health services; 2) private, provider-based services; 3) mental health services provided by the primary care system; and 4) mental health services provided by categorical child-serving agencies such as child welfare. Now, and especially in managed care environments, these discrete systems are being blended in an interacting, open system that consists of multiple levels. First is the child and his or her family and context. Then there is a specific intervention on behalf of the child and family. Each intervention involves the consumer, at least one clinician, and a treatment or service, the efficacy of which depends on both the clinician and the method. Often the intervention is nested within a program element, such as inpatient, residential, outpatient, and community support, which in turn is nested within a larger behavioral health program that interacts with other service systems. Any ineffective link in this chain precludes findings of relationships between systems integration and clinical outcomes. An attempt to research the effectiveness of such a complex system, while treating its layers and dimensions as a "black box," is not likely to be productive.

Summary: Centralized Authority and Single Funding Stream—The Untried Systems Integration Model

Finally, it is important to understand that although systems integration efforts have become more sophisticated, there are important problems with all of the systems integration interventions reviewed in this chapter. None of them really has a single centralized program and clinical management structure that is consolidated with a single funding stream. Particularly in the public sector, funding for services for adults and children is fragmented, not well coordinated, and provided by a wide array of funding streams (Hadley 1996). This lack of consolidated or unified funding may have severely limited the effects of systems integration efforts. At the conceptual level, systems integration efforts assume that integration will result in substantial changes in the organization of services, the continuity of care, and the type and quantity of services delivered to clients.

Although changes in organization, continuity, and type and quantity of services have been documented, it appears that most systems integration efforts have resulted in better organized services (largely of existing types) being delivered to the same clients. In general, none of the studies reviewed in this chapter have a truly integrated clinical and financial system. In most cases, the existing financial incentives were unchanged so that integration was created by goodwill and commitment to the goals of the project, but there was little capacity to actually affect the specific types of services delivered to the specific client. Even in most public managed environments where there is more control, the specifications of what services should be delivered to which clients are often chaotic and without clinical guidelines. In environments in which providers or managed care entities are at financial risk for all services, the effectiveness of services and their client "outcome" becomes a more important issue that may yet permit systems integration efforts to have an impact on client outcomes.

REFERENCES

Agranoff R: Human services integration: past and present challenges in public administration. Public Administration Review 51:533–542, 1991

Bickman L, Guthrie PR, Foster EM, et al: Evaluating Managed Mental Health Services: the Fort Bragg Experiment. New York, Plenum, 1995

Bickman L, Lambert EW, Summerfelt WT, et al: Rejoinder to questions about the Fort Bragg evaluation. Journal of Child and Family Studies 5:197–206, 1996

Bickman L, Summerfelt WT, Noser K: Comparative outcomes of emotionally disturbed children and adolescents in a system of services and usual care. Psychiatr Serv 48:1543–1548, 1997

Bickman L, Noser K, Summerfelt WT: Long term effects of a system of care on children and adolescents. J Behav Health Serv Res 26:185–202, 1999

Bittner E: Police discretion in emergency apprehension of mentally ill persons. Soc Probl 14:278–292, 1967

Burns BJ, Hoagwood K, Mailtsby LT: Improving outcomes for children and adolescents with serious emotional and behavioral disorders: current and future directions, in Outcomes for Children and Youth with Behavioral and Emotional Disorders and Their Families: Programs and Evaluation Best Practices. Edited by Epstein MH, Kutash K, Duchnowski AJ. Austin, TX, pro.ed, 1998, pp 685–707

Cole R, Poe S: Partnership for Care: Systems of Care for Children with Serious Emotional Disturbances and Their Families. Washington, DC, Washington Business Group on Health, Robert Wood Johnson Foundation Mental Health Services for Youth, 1993

Cross TP, Saxe L: Many hands make mental health systems of care a reality: lessons from the mental health services program for youth, in Evaluating Mental Health Services: How Do Programs for Children "Work" in the Real World? Edited by Nixon CT, Northrup DA. Thousand Oaks, CA, Sage Publications, 1997, pp 45–72

Donabedian A: Explorations in Quality Assessment and Monitoring: The Definition of Quality and Approaches to Its Assessment. Ann Arbor, MI, Health Administration, 1980

Duchnowski AJ, Hall KS, Kutash K, et al: The alternative to residential treatment study, in Outcomes for Children and Youth with Emotional and Behavioral Disorders and Their Families: Programs and Evaluation Best Practices. Edited by Epstein MH, Kutash K, Duchnowski AJ. Austin, TX, pro.ed, 1998, pp 55–80

England MJ, Cole RF: Building system of care for youth with serious mental illness. Hospital and Community Psychiatry 43:630–633, 1992

Goldman HH, Morrissey JP, Ridgely MS: Evaluating the Robert Wood Johnson Foundation program on chronic mental illness. Milbank Q 72:37–47, 1994

Green TM: Police as frontline mental health workers: the decision to arrest or refer to mental health agencies. Int J Law Psychiatry 20:469–486, 1997

Hadley TR: Financing changes and their impact on the organization of the public mental health system. Adm Policy Ment Health 23:393–405, 1996

Hoagwood K, Hibbs E, Brent D, et al: Introduction to the special section: efficacy and effectiveness studies of child and adolescent psychotherapy. J Consult Clin Psychol 63:683–687, 1995

Illback RJ, Nelson CM, Sanders D: Community-based services in Kentucky: description and 5 year evaluation of Kentucky IMPACT, in Outcomes for Children and Youth with Behavioral and Emotional Disorders and Their Families: Programs and Evaluation Best Practices. Edited by Epstein MH, Kutash K, Duchnowski AJ. Austin, TX, pro.ed, 1998, pp 141–172

Knitzer J: Unclaimed Children. Washington, DC, Children's Defense Fund, 1982

Konrad EL: A multidimensional framework for conceptualizing human services integration initiatives. New Directions for Evaluation 69:5–19, 1996

Lambert W, Salzer MS, Bickman L: Clinical outcome, consumer satisfaction, and ad hoc ratings of improvement. J Consult Clin Psychol 66:270–279, 1998

Lehman AF, Postrado LT, Roth D, et al: Continuity of care and client outcomes in the Robert Wood Johnson Foundation program on chronic mental illness. Milbank Q 72:105–122, 1994

Lourie IS, Stroul BA, Friedman RM: Community-based systems of care: from advocacy to outcomes, in Outcomes for Children and Youth with Behavioral and Emotional Disorders and Their Families: Programs and Evaluation Best Practices. Epstein MH, Kutash K, Duchnowski AJ. Austin, TX, pro.ed, 1998, pp 20–30

Maloy KA: The Tennessee children's plan: how do we get there? in Evaluating Mental Health Services: How Do Programs For Children "Work" in the Real World? Edited by Nixon CT, Northrup DA. Thousand Oaks, CA, Sage Publications, 1997, pp 117–145

Meyers JC, Davis KE: State and foundation partnerships to promote mental health systems reform for children and families, in Evaluating Mental Health Services: How Do Programs for Children "Work" in the Real World? Edited by Nixon CT, Northrup DA. Thousand Oaks, CA, Sage Publications, 1997, pp 95–116

Morrissey JP, Calloway M, Bartko WT, et al: Local mental health authorities and service system change: evidence from the Robert Wood Johnson Foundation program on chronic mental illness. Milbank Q 72:49–80, 1994

Nixon CT: How does evaluation of mental health services for children work in the real world? in Evaluating Mental Health Services: How Do Programs for Children "Work" in the Real World? Edited by Nixon CT, Northrup DA. Thousand Oaks, CA, Sage Publications, 1997, pp 1–15

Poole DL: The project: community-driven partnership in health, mental health, and education to prevent early school failure. Health and Social Work 22:282–289, 1997

Provan KG, Milward HB: A preliminary theory of interorganizational network effectiveness: a comparative study of four community mental health systems. Adm Sci Q 40:1–33, 1995

Randolph F, Blasinsky M, Leginski W, et al: Creating integrated service systems for homeless persons with mental illness: the ACCESS program. Psychiatr Serv 48:369–373, 1997

Reed SK, Babigian HM: Postmortem of the Rochester capitation experiment. Hospital and Community Psychiatry 45:761–764, 1994

Ridgely MS, Morrissey JP, Paulson RI, et al: Characteristics and activities of case managers in the RWJ Foundation program on chronic mental illness. Psychiatr Serv 47:737–743, 1996

Rosenblatt A, Attkisson CC, Fernandez AJ: Integrating systems of care in California for youth with severe emotional disturbance, II: initial group home expenditure and utilization findings from the California AB377 Evaluation Project. Journal of Child and Family Studies 1:263–286, 1992

Rosenheck R, Morrissey J, Lam J, et al: Service system integration, access to services, and housing outcomes in a program for homeless persons with severe mental illness. Am J Public Health 88:1610–1615, 1998

Rosenheck R, Morrissey J, Lam J, et al: Service system integration and housing outcomes for homeless people with mental illness: a tale of 18 cities, in Housing and Residential Care for Persons with Serious Mental Illness. Edited by Osher F, Newman S. London, England, Gordon and Breach, in press

Rossi PH: Program outcomes: conceptual and measurement issues, in Outcomes Measurement in the Human Services: Cross-Cutting Issues and Methods. Edited by Mullen EJ, Magnabosco JL. Washington, DC, National Association of Social Workers, 1997, pp 20–34

Rubin A: Is case management effective for people with serious mental illness? a research review. Health Soc Work 17:138–150, 1992

Salzer MS, Bickman L: Delivering effective children's services in the community: reconsidering the benefits of system interventions. Applied and Preventive Psychology 6:1–13, 1997

Salzer MS, Nixon CT, Schut LJ, et al: Validating quality indicators: quality as relationship between structure, process and outcome. Eval Rev 21:292–309, 1997

Santarcangelo S, Bruns EJ, Yoe JT: New direction: evaluating Vermont's statewide model of individualized care, in Outcomes for Children and Youth with Behavioral and Emotional Disorders and Their Families: Programs and Evaluation Best Practices. Edited by Epstein MH, Kutash K, Duchnowski AJ. Austin, TX, pro.ed, 1998, pp. 117–140

Saxe L, Cross T, Silverman N: Children's mental health: the gap between what we know and what we do. Am Psychol 43:800–807, 1988

Shern DL, Wilson NZ, Coen AS, et al: Client outcomes, II: longitudinal client data from the Colorado treatment outcome study. Milbank Q 72:123–148, 1994

Stroul BA, Friedman R: A System of Care for Children and Youth with Severe Emotional Disturbances. Washington, DC, Georgetown University Child Development Center, CASSP Technical Assistance Center, 1986

VanDenBerg JE: Integration of individualized mental health services into the system of care for children and adolescents. Adm Policy Ment Health 20:247–257, 1993

Weisz JR, Weiss B, Donenberg GR: The lab versus the clinic: effects of child and adolescent psychotherapy. Am Psychol 47:1578–1585, 1992

Wells KB, Brook RH: The quality of mental health services: past, present, and future, in The Future of Mental Health Services Research. Edited by Taube CA, Mechanic D, Hohmann AA. Washington, DC, U.S. Government Printing Office, 1989, pp 203–224

15

Assessing Quality of Care

Allen S. Daniels, Ed.D., L.I.S.W.
Karl W. Stukenberg, Ph.D.

The measurement of clinical outcomes has been the subject of significant focus in the evolution of managed care. At the facility level, the quality of care has been monitored through the standards of the Joint Commission on the Accreditation of Healthcare Organizations (JCAHO) and the Commission on Accreditation of Rehabilitation Facilities (CARF). The National Committee for Quality Assurance (NCQA) has established standards for measuring quality and improvement. An examination of the scope and influences of these accreditation bodies provides a framework for analyzing some of the principal forces driving the need to monitor and evaluate quality of care and outcomes in behavioral health care systems.

In response to the influence of accreditation groups, a number of organizations have developed performance indicators to monitor and track service and operational quality. A review of existing performance standards gives us a framework for examining the tools that measure clinical processes and outcomes across delivery systems. This review of quality and accountability requirements provides a vantage point from which to examine their impact on delivery systems and providers of care. An important factor in evaluating the measurement of quality is the cost of the evaluation and the impact of that expense on the delivery of care and the allocation of clinical resources. To meet these quality and accountability requirements, provider systems have developed their own performance standards to measure quality and to benchmark their results against similar organizations.

Vast arrays of clinical outcomes measures are currently being used throughout the spectrum of behavioral health care delivery systems. These include measures that are available in the public domain and those that are proprietary. Some of the tools are designed to measure both physical and emotional symptom levels and changes, whereas others are constructed to examine specific behavioral health diagnoses and conditions. An analysis of the components that make up the spectrum of behavioral health care quality improvement systems and outcomes analysis provides a guide for the design and implementation of such programs. This examination includes a review of the episode of care as a unit analysis and a consideration of how this approach can foster evaluation of outcomes and quality improvement.

There is a fundamental relationship between accreditation standards, performance measures, and the evaluation of clinical outcomes. Each of these components is linked in a sophisticated quality improvement program (see Figure 15–1). The relationship between these components will necessarily define the scope and focus of the program. In some cases, these components may involve collaboration between clinicians, treatment services, payors, and other stakeholders.

An important component in the evaluation of a quality improvement program, outcomes measurement system, and accreditation program must include consideration of the ethics and values inherent in the process. As the health care industry sharpens the focus on quality and accountability standards, there is an essential mandate to consider the rights of consumers of care and the contributions to the science that guides this care. A review of the values and ethics that underlie quality improvement programs and the potential for fraud and abuse serves as a foundation to examine the future evolution of this important aspect of behavioral health care.

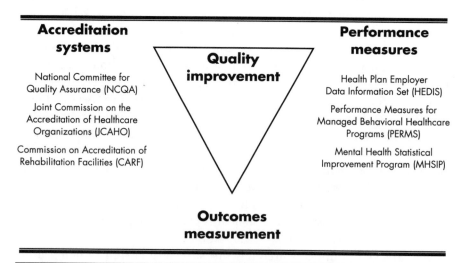

FIGURE 15–1. Relationship between outcomes measurement, accreditation systems, and performance measures in quality improvement.

ACCREDITATION AND ACCOUNTABILITY IN BEHAVIORAL HEALTH CARE

The push for greater accountability and for accreditation has grown substantially in recent years. Employers and purchasers of health care have mandated that insurers and providers establish standards and accountability for the quality of the programs they provide. Historically, the organization that has been the strongest in this area has been the JCAHO. This organization has been the standard for accreditation and accountability for hospitals and facility-based care systems. In behavioral health care the CARF has become involved in the review and certification of facility-based care programs that may be more separate or independent from hospital programs. Health plans have also become subject to accreditation and accountability standards set forth by the NCQA.

Each of the established accreditation systems has a unique focus. The spectrum includes facility and provider systems and health plans. These accreditation systems have a number of important influences on behavioral health care. For the JCAHO, there has been a push to establish a standard outcomes measurement system within facility-based care (Joint Commission on Accreditation of Healthcare Organizations 1998). This will then facilitate the potential for comparison across systems and a common outcome benchmark standard for facility-based care.

The NCQA has also established various sets of standards that affect behavioral health care. These include standards for managed care organizations; the Health Plan Employer Data and Information Set (HEDIS), a standard data reporting set; and a spectrum of accreditation opportunities for physician organizations, credentialing verification organizations, and other related managed care components. In addition, the NCQA has established standards for managed behavioral health care organizations (MBHOs) (National Committee for Quality Assurance 1999). The impact of the NCQA has been to increase the accountability of payors and their constituent providers and to monitor and measure the process and outcome of care. This has led to a greater focus on the quality of care throughout the continuum of care and the coordination of the measurement of outcomes across delivery systems and various levels of care. The impact of the NCQA on quality and accountability has led MBHOs to implement a set of ongoing required studies. These include prevention activities and outcomes studies involving both children and adults. As a result, MBHOs are increasingly involving provider systems in their studies and projects. Of all the medical specialties, behavioral health care has perhaps the greatest level of accountability standards and accreditation opportunities.

PERFORMANCE STANDARDS

Along with accreditation standards, behavioral health care has also developed a broad array of performance measures. These have been developed by constituent organizations as a means to measure and track the performance of providers and systems across sites and programs. These standards have been developed for use in public mental health systems, facility and provider organizations, and managed care organizations. Some of the principal measurement systems include the HEDIS, Mental Health Statistical Improvement Program (MHSIP), and Performance Measures for Managed Behavioral Healthcare Programs (PERMS).

The HEDIS is a comprehensive measurement system for the evaluation of health plan performance. It was designed to give employer groups and purchasers of care a standard system with which to evaluate and compare health plans. The system is designed to provide a comprehensive review across medical care, and it focuses primarily on general health measures. There are some components related to behavioral health care, and recent improvements have focused on this area. The principal goal is to use claims data to measure the performance of particular health plans. For behavioral health care, the indicators have focused on items such as the ambulatory follow-up of patients posthospitalization and the rates of rehospitalization.

The MHSIP system has been developed to track the performance of behavioral health care systems in the public sector. This measurement tool is heavily weighted toward consumer involvement, satisfaction, and outcome in behavioral health care. It examines performance in the domains of access, clinical appropriateness, outcomes and satisfaction, prevention, and cost. It has been an effective measure of the performance of systems and providers in publicly funded mental health care.

The American Managed Behavioral Healthcare Association (AMBHA) developed the PERMS (American Managed Behavioral Healthcare Association 1998). These performance indicators have been established to examine care within MBHOs. The domains include access to care, quality of care, consumer satisfaction, and leadership testing set. One of the goals is to provide a standard system for measuring the performance of organizations and to establish a method for comparing their operations. Each of the measures selected must be meaningful, measured, and manageable.

A common goal of any performance indicator is to provide a set of benchmarks for the comparison of organizations and to foster their continuous improvement. The HEDIS, MHSIP, and PERMS indicators have been developed by their constituent organizations to foster this approach. One of the risks of this type of system is that the indicators tracked may fail to accurately measure the targeted activity. The Institute for Behavioral Healthcare

National Leadership Council has conducted a study (Kramer and Daniels 1997) that examines the cost effectiveness and utility of many performance indicators.

The National Leadership Performance Indicator Project was designed to examine the utility of various indicators in different industry sectors. These include managed care organizations, behavioral group practices, integrated delivery systems, and community mental health centers. Utility was measured along the following axes: time required for tracking, costliness of tracking, perceived value of internal quality improvement, perceived value of external reporting, and cost effectiveness of the indicators. The results varied for each of the industry segments, but overall the findings supported measures of satisfaction, utilization, and outcome.

The impact of measuring performance standards may lead to the goal of meeting external accountability, and the established standards will become minimal expectations. Programs may then be designed to meet these minimum standards, rather than meet targets for continuous improvement. The central goal of any quality improvement program must be to evaluate the outcome of care and the improved well-being of those being served. It is hoped that competitive market focus will push both providers and managers of care to improved levels of organization and enhanced clinical outcomes. The way to achieve that aim is detailed below.

MANAGED CARE AND OUTCOMES MEASUREMENT

To build on outcomes evaluation programs, it is important to examine their evolution and structure. The managed care revolution has led to shifts in the measurement of clinical outcomes (Berman et al. 1998), which can be characterized as a movement from discrete outcome studies through program evaluation to an outcomes management approach that is continuously collecting, managing, and interpreting clinical data (Dickey et al. 1998). As the industry moves toward service integration and more consistently uses outcomes management, it is important that our thinking about the evaluation of the provision of care not remain mired in older, site-specific models of data collection. Instead, measuring an episode of care that cuts across the integrated behavioral continuum; includes outpatient, inpatient, partial hospital, or community residence programs; and evaluates the effectiveness of the response to the patient and to this particular episode of the illness allows for more effective management of the entire treatment process (Daniels 1995).

Measuring quality of care requires determining what outcome domains are of interest. Four are generally assessed: service, cost, clinical, and satisfaction. Service outcome assessment includes timeliness of appointments, number of times the patient is seen, and how the treatment plan is developed. Cost outcomes assessment involves measurement of the expenditure involved in the provision of service and its variance. Clinical outcome is a crucial measurement (Ciarlo et al. 1986) and is the most frequently measured outcome domain (Lambert and Bergin 1994). Measurement can range from measuring changes in presenting symptoms to changes in social or occupational functioning, family functioning, or quality of life. Patient satisfaction measures are the newest and most controversial means of measuring outcomes (Lambert et al. 1998). They can be measures of overall satisfaction with the treatment process and/or measures of satisfaction with process factors that may be important to the patients' perceptions of the quality of care they have received.

Managed care entities have historically focused largely on evaluating patient satisfaction with the provision of care. A recent survey suggested that managed care companies use and rely on patient satisfaction as the most important determinant of the quality of clinical care (Bilbrey and Bilbrey 1995). This may be because it is relatively easy and inexpensive to assess treatment outcome at one time only—posttreatment (Lambert et al. 1998). Unfortunately, the easy solution to a problem is not always the best. Correlations between satisfaction with treatment and clinical outcomes fluctuate, but are generally poor (Lambert 1998). Truly managing the outcome of a mental health intervention involves elements from all four outcome clusters and overreliance on just one is likely to be fraught with problems (Lambert et al. 1998).

Managed care's reliance on satisfaction as a measure evolved in an environment in which the assessment of quality was site specific. Providers in mental health service sites wanted to market their practice to third-party payors and to demonstrate that payors would receive value when they used the site. Satisfaction measures focus on measuring qualities that are not specific to a particular diagnostic group. Thus, for an outpatient practice that is largely treating individuals with adjustment disorders, depressed affect, and anxiety disorders, measurement of patient satisfaction and even self-report measures of changes in common symptoms may be useful measures of the quality of the service provided. In particular, when third-party payors are choosing a mental health provider, it is important for their employees to be satisfied with the service they receive. Because most of the patients will need only outpatient treatment, this large group and its satisfaction are important for minimizing the number of complaints that employees will bring to their human resources departments.

As managed care increases market penetration and funding models focus on prepayment of service costs, it will be increasingly important to manage clinical, service, and cost outcomes. A consistent criticism of more elaborate outcomes measures has been the expense involved (Seligman 1995). As more complex disorders are being treated, the cost of treating them consumes a larger portion of the managed care dollar, and investing in the evaluation of treatment effectiveness is justified. Denying access to mental health treatment is neither an ethical nor an economical option. There is the risk that many of those denied mental health treatment will seek more expensive medical care. The management of health costs needs to be integrated across the health and mental health care spectrums.

Outcomes Measurement Program Design

Kramer (reprinted in Daniels et al. 1997; see Figure 15–2) developed a framework for the design of outcomes management programs. The decision tree supports the development and design of clinical outcome programs. This resource guides the organization in the determination of key components and methodologies for the program.

Outcomes Evaluation and the Episode of Care as a Unit of Analysis

The second author's (K.S.) wife's pregnancy led to a pleasant copayment surprise at the first appointment with her "birthing team." The office manager stated that the copayment for that visit would be the sole copayment for the pregnancy. The pregnancy and birth are seen by this practice as being one episode of care and, rather than billing office visits, hospital stays, and various other procedures individually, the consumer is charged based on the entire episode of treatment for one entity—a pregnancy. Although billing for mental health treatment in this manner might seem problematic for several reasons, those evaluating the quality of care in an integrated behavioral health continuum have much to learn from this model. Specifically, quality of care should be client focused and based on the episode of care rather than on the location in which service is provided.

We believe that using the episode of care as a unit in the evaluation of the quality of care provided would involve a number of shifts in measuring response to provided care. First, all clients who presented for treatment to a mental health entity would be screened for inclusion in a "study." Those patients who qualified would receive a thorough evaluation of their clinical states at entry, would be followed through the course of the episode of care, and would be evaluated at set periods of time after the initial evaluation. Second, the measurement of the quality of care would be more specific to the difficulties of the group in question than an evaluation of a global entity like patient satisfaction. Finally, the evaluation would cut across multiple sites, and the client's response to the system as a whole rather than to a particular element or site in that system would be the focus of concern.

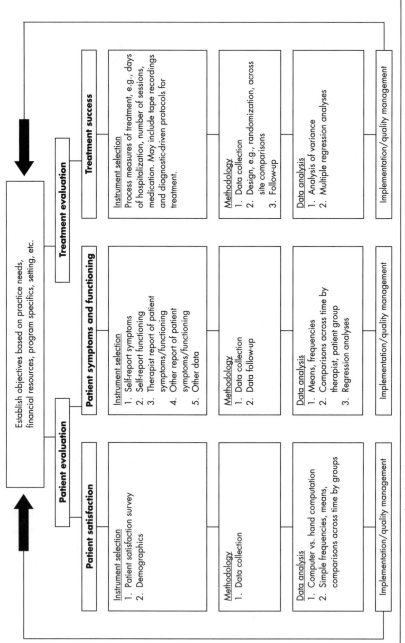

FIGURE 15–2. Decision tree for developing outcomes management program.

Source. Reprinted from Daniels et al. 1997. Used with permission.

EPISODE OF CARE AS A MEASURE OF QUALITY OF CARE

The first characteristic of the episode of care assessment model is that a particular subset of the client population must be selected for evaluation. Measuring clinical outcomes and cost outcomes can be done more precisely by working within a diagnostic group (Beutler and Berrin 1998), as opposed to satisfaction that can, theoretically, be assessed across diagnoses. Comparing the clinical or cost outcome of the treatment of an episode of depression with the treatment of an episode of schizophrenia or of borderline personality disorder is, clearly, like comparing apples and oranges. Instead of comparing across diagnoses, a specific diagnostic category needs to be more thoroughly evaluated.

Designating the diagnostic group or groups of interest should be based on several factors. First, the group should be symptomatically severe enough that a continuum of behavioral health care will be used. Furthermore, the investment of time and energy in tracking the consumers should be offset by the expected expense of treating them. Bipolar disorder, the schizophrenias, severe personality disorders, and severe major depression are all candidates for episode of care quality evaluation. Severity of disturbance may be an important element to assess independently, but it is unlikely to be a good single determinant of inclusion, because the resulting heterogeneity of the sample would cause confusion about the clinical outcome evaluation.

Choosing the diagnostic group of interest should be determined. If there are practitioners within the behavioral health continuum who have a specialty, either in assessment or treatment, it makes sense to track and use the resources of those with special interests and expertise. Choosing instruments to assess clinical outcomes should be based on the specific diagnostic group that is being followed. In the example, we are assuming an interest and expertise in tracking and treating depression. Two self-report measures of depression, the Beck Depression Inventory (Beck and Beck 1972) and the Zung Self-Rating Depression Scale (Zung 1965), have been demonstrated to be effective at screening depression in outpatient populations (Stukenberg et al. 1990). These are inexpensive to administer and score. For those patients who score above a relatively high cutoff, interviewer-rated measures, including the Hamilton Rating Scale for Depression (Hamilton 1960), would then be administered.

Once a group of participants has been identified and initial measures have been administered to evaluate their inclusion in the tracking group, regular contact with them across the course of their care is established. Those who are willing to participate will be contacted on a regular basis, to be determined by the expected course of their diagnosis. At the time of contact, service, cost, and clinical outcomes as well as satisfaction can be measured. In the example of tracking a group that has depression, an interval of 6 months is a typical time period to evaluate progress. At 6-month intervals, service and cost outcomes can be determined in part by a review of the records since the last contact. Clinical outcomes can be evaluated based on readministration of the Beck, Zung, and/or Hamilton instruments. Satisfaction measures can also be administered, in part to allow comparisons across diagnostic groups.

Collection of data is facilitated by the patient's participation in a managed care system that manages care across a continuum of care. The collection and management of these data will involve dedicating administrative and clinical resources to the project. Use of instruments that are nonproprietary would allow for comparison with other care providers. It would also facilitate evaluation on a par with other outcomes research, thus furthering the science of understanding psychological treatment. Finally, it allows for the evaluation of service, cost, and clinical outcomes, and satisfaction measures could easily be added at the termination of treatment or at preset intervals during the episode of care.

The importance of evaluating the outcome of clinical care across the continuum is evident in the quality improvement process. A well-designed program can promote both efficiency and effectiveness of care. With an increased focus on the management of care, outcomes are a vital component. In addition, the manner in which these programs are designed will have an effect on their utility.

ETHICS OF QUALITY IMPROVEMENT

There is a broad spectrum of issues that must be considered in any review of quality improvement programs. Issues range from confidentiality and respect for patient rights to the impact on scientific knowledge and process. The goal of the quality improvement process is to evaluate the impact of the interventions and the outcome of clinical programs while striving to achieve continuous improvement. Meanwhile, a significant focus of accreditation and external review agencies has been to establish standards for the operation and measurement of performance in health care organizations. A risk is that quality improvement programs will become compliance monitoring systems and lose sight of the ultimate goal of improved health care for patients.

Any quality improvement program must have a set of intrinsic goals, principles, and values. These must become the moral guiding principles for the programs. The proliferation of quality improvement requirements by accreditation agencies and external accountability systems poses a threat to the integrity of these programs unless they are well grounded in the structure and integrity of the organization.

There are substantial and inherent risks for the abuse of the quality improvement process, to both providers and patients, as organizations compete in an increasingly cost-conscious environment. As these organizations strive to meet the requirements of external reviews, there is a potential threat to the process of results being created to meet accountability standards and to stretch the limits of the findings.

Most accreditation programs require the measurement of patient symptom and functional change. Within the process of quality improvement or accreditation standards there is little guidance on what factors protect patient rights of participation and confidentiality. Outcomes evaluation programs are not mandated to have the informed consent of patients, and there are no clear guidelines for the use of the studies' findings. Furthermore, there is no external monitoring of the data collection and analysis of these outcomes studies. Therefore, a potential exists for the abuse of the scientific process and the compromise of the fundamental rights of patients.

Within the context of science, there are clearly established standards for the design and implementation of investigations. There is a process and an outcome that guides the course of any investigation. The public presentation of findings provides the opportunity for public scrutiny and replication of methods and results. These aspects are absent from the established process of quality improvement studies. In addition, the proprietary nature of the business competing in the health care industry leads to an enormous potential for scientific fraud and the abuse of the quality improvement process. The risk that findings will be fabricated or that legitimate findings will be held in proprietary secrecy is a substantial threat to the integrity of health care.

Several recommendations can be made to address the ethical concerns raised about outcomes evaluation and quality improvement programs,. First, any evaluation of patient clinical data that can be linked to an individual patient must include an informed consent process. The standards for this must be as rigorous as for any other segment of scientific inquiry. Second, any clinical programs or instructions that are made based on these findings must be subject to public report and scrutiny. The failure to do so runs the risk of propagating false knowledge. Finally, quality improvement research must develop a means of detecting, reporting, and dealing with scientific fraud. The failure to accomplish these tasks can pose a significant threat to all scientific investigation.

REFERENCES

American Managed Behavioral Healthcare Association: Performance Measures for Managed Behavioral Healthcare Programs (PERMS). Washington, DC, American Managed Behavioral Healthcare Association, 1998

Beck AT, Beck RW: Screening depressed patients in family practice: a rapid technique. Postgraduate Medicine 52:81–85, 1972

Berman WH, Rosen CS, Hurt SW, et al: Toto we're not in Kansas anymore: measuring and using outcomes in behavioral health care. Clin Psychol Sci Pract 5:115–132, 1998

Beutler LE, Berrin MR: Integrative Assessment of Adult Personality. New York, Guilford, 1998

Bilbrey J, Bilbrey P: Judging, trusting, and utilizing outcomes data: a survey of behavioral health care papers. Behav Healthc Tomorrow 4:62–65, 1995

Ciarlo JA, Brown TR, Edwards DW, et al: Assessing mental health treatment outcome measurement techniques. Rockville, MD, National Institute of Mental Health, 1986

Daniels A: University-based single specialty group: university managed care, in The Complete Capitation Handbook: How to Design and Implement At-Risk Contracts for Behavioral Healthcare. Edited by Zieman GL. San Francisco, CA, Jossey-Bass, 1995

Daniels A, Kramer T, Zieman G: The Comprehensive Quality Tool Kit. Tiburon, CA, CentraLink, 1997

Dickey B, Hermann RC, Eisen SV: Assessing the quality of psychiatric care: research methods and application in clinical practice. Harv Rev Psychiatry 6:88–96, 1998

Hamilton Rating Scale for Depression

Joint Commission on Accreditation of Healthcare Organizations: Using Performance Measurement to Improve Outcomes in Behavioral Health Care. Washington, DC, Joint Commission on Accreditation of Healthcare Organizations, 1998

Kramer TL, Daniels A: NLC performance indicators: second study. Behav Healthc Tomorrow 6:59–61,1997

Lambert MJ, Bergin AE: The effectiveness of psychotherapy, in Handbook of Psychotherapy and Behavior Change. Edited by Garfield SL, Bergin AE. New York, Wiley, 1994, pp 1432–1489

Lambert W, Salzer MS, Bickman L: Clinical outcome, consumer satisfaction, and ad hoc ratings of improvement in children's mental health. J Consult Clin Psychol 66:270–279, 1998

National Committee for Quality Assurance: Managed Behavioral Healthcare Organizations (MBHO) Standards for Accreditation. Washington, DC, National Committee for Quality Assurance, 1999

Seligman ME: The effectiveness of psychotherapy: the consumer reports study. Am Psychol 50:202–208, 1995

Stukenberg KW, Dura JR, Kiecolt-Glaser JK: Depression screening scale validation in an elderly, community-dwelling population. psychological assessment: J Consult Clin Psychol 2:134–138, 1990

Zung WK: A self-rating depression scale. Arch Gen Psychiatry 41:949–958, 1965

16

A Consumer View of an Episode of Care and How Self-Help Helps

Edward L. Knight, Ph.D.

Ike Powell

Joanne Forbes, R.N., M.S.

Partnership between consumers and providers is fundamental to the concept of an integrated delivery system. To realize that partnership, it is necessary for providers to understand how consumers view an episode of care and how they become involved and responsible for their own recovery at all levels of care along the continuum.

TREATMENT AND ITS EFFECTS

To most consumers an episode of illness is fundamentally a trauma, and most care is feared as an addition to that trauma. Treatment is in no way looked forward to or anticipated with joy.

All along the continuum, the functions of care and the beliefs, attitudes, and manner of professionals affect consumers. Especially at the most intensive levels of care, consumers experience a sense of containment. Most consumers live with a root fear that it will happen again, that they will be contained. No amount of psychological double talk about the patient's real need for safety will change the reality of being locked up.

Deskilling

To quote Turkelson et al. (1993), "hospitalization is automatically deskilling." It involves a decrease in self-efficacy. It shakes people's confidence in their abilities and in themselves, especially their ability to make decisions or in any way rely on their own minds. The loss of rationality in an episode has that effect automatically, and the effect is increased by containment. What is "validated" by containment is the person's own inability to be trusted. In other words, containment is invalidating.

Decreased Self-Esteem

One of the major struggles for people with mental illness who are undergoing an episode of care and containment is the struggle with self-esteem (DeMasi et al. 1996). The invalidation and loss of skills they experience causes self-esteem to plummet.

A positive self-image results when people feel they can act in their own best interests and can influence their lives by their own actions. Often this positive feeling is devastated by the symptoms of a mental illness, side effects of medication, social stigma, and demeaning manner in which many professionals relate to people receiving services from the mental health system.

Loss of Hope

When the focus of the treatment is primarily on stabilizing the symptoms and providing adequate custodial care, it is quickly communicated to patients that this focus is based on the belief that they cannot think for themselves and need to be taken care of by someone else perpetually. This "We know what's best for you. You just need to trust us and be obedient" approach communicates to patients that they cannot trust themselves. It is the first step toward deskilling and "learned dependence," which are often labeled as negative symptoms and are detrimental to the recovery process.

The most influential aspect of the service provider–service recipient relationship is the image that the provider has of the recipient's potential for recovery. A person committed to a hospital is often in a vulnerable condition and is looking for help—for release of some of the confusion and pain. When a professional, who is the authority and the source of help, communicates that recovery is probably not possible and the whole approach to treatment supports that belief, the patient often gives in and gives up.

The question, then, is how can the deskilling and invalidation, loss of self-esteem, and loss of hope during an episode of care be decreased? Unfortunately, they cannot be eliminated within the context of treatment, but they can be diminished.

Consumer Involvement

The solution is to shift treatment to a more self-help– and recovery-oriented experience. When a system shifts its treatment philosophy from stabilization and custodial care to self-help and recovery, the entire environment of the system begins to change. This shift is based on three beliefs: 1) that people who receive a diagnosis of mental illness can and do recover; 2) that these people can play an active role in their own recovery by learning to cope with or manage symptoms, recognize triggers, reduce stress, and participate in determining the services that they feel they need; and 3) that they can benefit by sharing with and learning from other consumers who have been through or are going through similar experiences.

The system environment shifts to a partnership approach in which the power is not concentrated in the hands of professionals and the attitude of "staff knows best" is avoided. Because patients with mental illness are able to think—to reflect and learn from their experiences—they are listened to because of their wisdom rather than talked down to because of their supposed ignorance. This approach produces an environment based more on respect, dignity, and hope than are traditional systems.

Several principles govern the shift to self-help and recovery. First, the consumer's involvement in the recovery process must be immediate and as inclusive as possible from the onset of the care episode to ensure that the effects of treatment are minimized.

Second, self-help and recovery services are provided only on request, are strictly voluntary, and are offered in the spirit of partnership and goodwill. This guiding factor is important in supporting paradigm change because it accomplishes two things critical to any successful, lasting shift: 1) it stimulates curiosity, a subtle competition (always present in a system accustomed to scant resources), and motivation to find out more; and 2) it mirrors and models one of the tenets of the consumerism movement—respect for what a group or an individual *wants*, not what someone thinks they *should* have (even if it is something as self-evident as the benefits of self-help).

Third, the partnership between providers and consumers must extend beyond the doctor–patient relationship into other aspects of the treatment/care delivery experience. The patients see other consumers playing vital roles in all aspects of the service delivery system. This has a positive impact on the experience of an episode of care.

TECHNIQUES AND MODELS OF CONSUMER INVOLVEMENT ACROSS THE CONTINUUM

Self-Help

One way to minimize invalidation and help consumers build good feelings about themselves and improve their self-efficacy is to involve them in self-help groups. Even the most restrictive settings can accommodate groups run by consumers. One self-help group, for example, is reaching into jails, prisons, and forensic settings because of the efforts of Howie Vogel, a consumer with a dual diagnosis and the founder of Double Trouble in Recovery (DTR). DTR is a 12-step program adapted from Alcoholics Anonymous, with steps adjusted for dual diagnoses of substance abuse and mental illness. Consumers with this dual diagnosis completely and very successfully run DTR programs.

Howie Vogel's DTR program started originally in New York but is now spreading nationally. In New York City he started a group in a forensic program for people with dual diagnoses and a history of violence. A psychiatrist on staff has said that the DTR group is making a large positive impact. In fact, Vogel has been asked to establish a group for these same people in the outpatient system into which they will be discharged. This will give continuity from the inpatient to the outpatient setting, continuing the self-efficacy–creating activities and helping to counter the deskilling effects of containment. The New York state prison system has also approached Vogel about establishing DTR for people with dual diagnoses in the state prisons. In addition, he and the consumers he has trained have established DTR in the Atlanta city jail system. Given the growth of this program, the National Development and Research Institutes is studying it on a 5-year grant from National Institute on Drug Abuse.

Customer Representatives

South Beach Psychiatric Center, a state hospital in New York, has found multiple ways to minimize deskilling. For example, following training, recipients of mental health services are employed as "customer representatives" at South Beach Psychiatric Center's Staten Island facility. The position fulfills two purposes.

First, serving as a customer representative gives recipients of services a set of useful skills, an image of themselves as supporters of other people's recovery, and recognition as people who are on the cutting edge of the shift in mental health services from a focus on stabilization and custodial care to self-help and recovery. It enhances their ability to function as local role models and statewide leaders in the consumer movement.

Second, a customer representative contributes to the care experience of others. Soon after admission, patients are visited by a representative who welcomes them and lets them know that he or she has been where they are now and has been able to deal with the hospital experience and move back into the community. This decreases invalidation caused by the loss of rationality and being locked up and gives the patient the hope of a successful return to community life. Bandura (1977) pointed out that vicarious experience—having another person with a disability as severe or more severe than your own show that something can be done—is a powerful way to build self-efficacy.

Customer representatives fulfill a variety of other roles that reinforce self-efficacy. The representative becomes a peer for patients to talk with, and he or she visits each ward regularly to hold self-help mutual support meetings with patients and carry on a dialogue with patients and staff.

Consumer Dialogues

Consumer dialogues, created by the Mental Health Empowerment Project, Inc., are 60- to 90-minute participatory facilitation processes that enable a group of 10–30 people to have in-depth dialogue about a variety of topics, such as How do you sustain hope in your life? What has been helpful in your recovery? What about the experience of being given a diagnosis of mental illness has been disempowering and/or empowering? What has been the role of spirituality in your recovery? What is friendship, and how have friends been important to you? What is the role of stress in your life? The dialogues affirm the fact that people can learn from their experiences and can help one another when they have had common experiences. This has a tremendous impact on consumer self-efficacy. Participants in the dialogue can be all consumers or a mixture of consumers and nonconsumer professional staff. Consumers facilitate these dialogues in the community, in the outpatient clinics, and on the hospital wards.

The dialogues most frequently requested by staff and consumers are the Dialogues on Hope. It gives consumers the opportunity to share ideas and feelings about a concept that is basic to recovery. It is especially important in-hospital on the "back wards," where both the staff and the patients seem to have given up all hope. The first time this dialogue was conducted in that setting at South Beach Psychiatric Center, staff described it as "the most important thing that has happened on this ward in 20 years." It was a powerful experience as well for the three recipients of mental health services who conducted that dialogue.

A short case example helps to illustrate the power of the dialogue.

Dialogues on Hope

A patient who was on 24-hour suicide watch attended one of the Dialogues on Hope. This person was silent during the entire experience. The next morning he angrily shared with the staff that the experience had robbed him of his "no-hope" stance to life and that he was having difficulty justifying to himself the desire to take his life. He is now living in the community in a Fairweather Lodge and returning to the hospital as a volunteer to facilitate the dialogues.

The Consumer Network

The Consumer Network, a place and a philosophy of recovery for mental illness, provides direct services aimed at diminishing the deskilling effects of longer-term inpatient hospitalization. Through its services, The Consumer Network reaches directly into this population with a message of hope, empowerment, and recovery. Run by consumers for consumers, the network's offerings include regular Hope Dialogues, Recovery Dialogues, Self-Help 101, tutoring, patient's rights, and advocacy.

The Consumer Network's "The Faces of Recovery" series promotes the theme that recovery is doable, that recovery is self-determined and self-initiated. The series is also designed to debunk the myths beginning to bubble up from nonbelievers: that a consumer in recovery is a rare commodity, that high-functioning consumers have obviously been given a misdiagnosis, and that there is a predefined notion of recovery for which all consumers should strive.

Consumer-Run Supported Housing

Restrictive models of housing, group homes, and intensive supportive apartments are also amenable to self-efficacy approaches based on mutual support. The least restrictive mental health housing, supported housing, on the model established by Paul Carling is actually run by consumer agencies in New York. Carling's model is one of generic housing supported by rent stipends and freely chosen wraparound services. Peers supply support services for the consumer residences.

These supported housing agencies were either started by or given assistance from the Mental Health Empowerment Project They are made up of and run entirely by consumers from the public system. Their boards, staff, and management are consumers who were given diagnoses of schizophrenia, bipolar disorder, or serious depression. They are powerful consumer examples of self-efficacy.

Housing Options in Gowanda achieved the most spectacular success. This agency took 30 long-term patients from Buffalo Psychiatric Center and successfully placed 29 of them in supported housing, where they have lived for 6 years. These were patients who had been hospitalized for 10 years or longer.

Bridger Project Programs

When patients are ready for discharge, the consumer-run Bridger Project helps them make the transition from hospital to community by providing a peer mentor. The Bridger Project connects the patient with peer support, advocacy, and mutual support groups in the community so that the patient continues to be connected to peer supports throughout the care episode. This provides continuity to models of self-efficacy and maximizes the chances of recovery.

Harvey Rosenthal created the Bridger Project program model in cooperation with the Mental Health Empowerment Project. The New York State Association of Psychosocial Rehabilitation, Rosenthal's organization, runs six Bridger Project programs in New York State. In the South Beach Psychiatric Center catchment area, there is The Brooklyn Peer Advocacy Project, a consumer-run organization that provides many support services to recipients living in the community. Colorado Health Networks, a ValueOptions partnership, is starting Bridger Project programs in Colorado Springs, and ValueOptions partners in New Mexico are starting similar mentor programs there. A large managed care company, ValueOptions is willing to promote such projects because they extend community tenure.

Mutual Support Groups

In many states, most prominently New York, Pennsylvania, Ohio, California, Georgia, Colorado, and New Mexico, mutual support groups are available for consumers who live in their own or parents' housing and go to outpatient clinics. New York has more than 600 such groups, as does Pennsylvania. The groups are for consumers with the least connection with treatment settings; consumers find that the mutual support helps them in times of loneliness and frustration. Mutual support groups help them stay out of hospitals and in the least restrictive environment.

Open Charting

Open charting is a simple practice that involves consumers in their own recovery. In open charting, consumers are permitted to read progress notes and make entries of their own. The mystery of what is being written in charts is removed, demystifying the disease process. Open charting decreases the potential for paranoid feelings created by something done behind the consumers' backs, something in which they cannot, by definition, be involved. It opens up the setting to participation rather than closing it as hidden charting does.

What does it take to change a paradigm of care? South Beach Psychiatric Center provides a case example:

South Beach Psychiatric Center

In the late 1980s a large urban state-operated mental health system began a journey that would end in the creation of a very different service delivery system for people receiving a diagnosis of mental illness. This particular mental health system originated and developed in the 1960s and early 1970s, incorporating the spirit and philosophy of both the community mental health movement and the civil rights movement.

Services developed in neighborhoods and were easily accessible and blended in with the usual businesses and storefronts found on any urban street. Community residents who were "sent away" 20, 30, or more years before to state hospitals far from their homes were repatriated and helped to reintegrate into neighborhoods where family and friends resided. Community education was an integral part of lessening stigma as well as encouraging neighborhood residents to access treatment for mental illness at an early stage. Alliances were developed with local family organizations that were quickly forming to give voice and representation to this largely forgotten and underrepresented group. The initial plan was to avoid hospitalizing anyone but instead, through an ambitious plan of sophisticated medication use and individual/group/family treatment plus community supports, to ensure that outpatient treatment was the primary modality for everyone. This paradigm failed over time.

Eventually the first inpatient beds opened. Treatment teams comprising professionals from multiple disciplines were charged with the care and discharge of all patients. A patient's treatment became the responsibility of the whole team, not just the sacrosanct territory of one or two professional disciplines.

Despite these efforts, despite a culture that supported community tenure, despite a length of stay that averaged only 9–11 days, and despite the best efforts of highly trained and caring staff, many patients still became dependent on the system. Young men and women alike were caught in the revolving door of a system designed to keep them out. (At that point, this mental health system had even eliminated the more artificial barriers to community tenure by integrating the outpatient and inpatient systems under one administrative manager and by having joint inpatient and outpatient rounds.) To some it would seem that patients elected to stay in the hospital, resisted all attempts at discharge, and seemed to settle in.

Innovative treatment approaches were introduced: token economies were instituted and McFarlane multifamily psychoeducational approaches were promulgated. Discharges continued unabated, yet the sense of frustration, failure, and confusion kept growing. The one thing that never changed was the collective "never give up" spirit that was part of the brick, mortar, and culture of South Beach Psychiatric Center.

Consumer mutual support to encourage self-efficacy had not been a part of this model. In spite of the best intentions, the model had remained professional through and through. Like an answer to a prayer, a path presented itself in the late 1980s.

The Caring Community Alliance for the Mentally Ill affiliates regularly sponsored conferences in conjunction with South Beach Psychiatric Center. Each conference was designed to bring in cutting-edge information for families, professionals, and the surrounding communities. At one such conference, Joe Rogers, a very well-known consumer leader, was invited to speak on consumerism. That speech would become the catalyst for the widespread changes that would be implemented at South Beach Psychiatric Center during the next decade. That day, Joe Rogers, by sharing his experience, strength, and hope, demonstrated that not only could people with serious mental illness get better, they could lead the way and create opportunities for those with similar devastating illnesses to have a life of quality and substance.

What followed that conference was a journey that led this enormous, urban, multifaceted, state-operated mental health system to embrace self-help, empowerment, advocacy, and recovery and to integrate those components into its mental health delivery system.

The consumer movement that Joe Rogers spoke about had been gaining converts and momentum for many years. Supporting this movement were the first author (E.K.) and other consumer/survivors who were creating options and role models that would pave the way. On a visit to the National Self-Help Clearinghouse in Philadelphia, Rogers patiently explained how to institute self-help—how to create a consumer movement at South Beach Psychiatric Center. At the time, we best summarized his advice with a mantra: "Listen to what consumers are saying. Really listen. Shut up and get out of the way. Create as many opportunities for consumers to say what they want as possible. Find someone who knows how to get a self-help group going and let them do it."

And that is what was done. A local consumer recommended by Rogers was asked to begin a self-help group. Out of those efforts, Friends United to Understand Recipient Empowerment (FUTURE) was born. Professional staff members were involved in providing technical assistance, securing a meeting place and time, spreading the word, and calming the fears of other professionals. In retrospect, this alliance of staff served to pass the baton—to allow consumers and professionals a transition time in which the power of the professional was transferred to the leaders of the self-help group.

There were other events that would serve to challenge the existing paradigm for administration and middle managers. The first author (E.K.) held a series of Empowerment Dialogues with the groups. Sharing humanness and problem solving helped shatter the "us/them," "we know/you don't," and "helpful/helpless" splits that were accepted in psychiatry at that time.

About this time, South Beach Psychiatric Center began to use another concept to promote change—pools of difference. A *pool of difference* represents an area in which change could begin, where consumers could become change agents in a manner that stimulated interest and curiosity, not in a way that would trigger overt resistance, resentment, and sabotage. Ingredients that would sustain these efforts were quiet persistence and commitment to persevere.

The blossoming of more local self-help groups created another opportunity to establish pools of difference. For many years the chief executive officer of South Beach Psychiatric Center had meetings with the leadership of local family organizations. The years of experience with these meetings highlighted the ongoing tension between what families wanted and what patients wanted. Conflicts over medication compliance, housing options, and the need for inpatient hospitalization were particularly difficult. Including leaders of the self-help groups in these meetings gave voice to these issues. Partnership on issues affecting multiple stakeholders became another pool of difference.

Another opportunity to create a difference presented itself as a new job training option was created. Customer representatives were hired on state

Office of Mental Health Patient Rehabilitation lines to represent the consumers (customers) of South Beach Psychiatric Center. Deployed at the request of the multiple outpatient sites, these people focused on fostering self-help, empowerment, and advocacy services at each site. Mental Health Empowerment Project trained interested people in dialogue and group facilitation techniques. These individuals then facilitated Recovery Dialogues at each service site. The results of the dialogues provided a template for others to follow. More important, the dialogues provided yet another chance for consumers to find their voices, to express directly what helped them, and to discover common themes and bonds.

Along with the addition of customer representatives came a change in the organizational structure of the hospital. The Department of Community Relations was renamed the Department of Customer Services to highlight and underscore the paradigm shift taking place. A consumer was hired as customer service coordinator to organize and support all the efforts of the customer reps. The entire department was focused on multiplying the pools of difference. To support the effort, customer reps and others attended local, statewide, and national conferences regularly. The networking and information sharing added to the creative process and knowledge base.

Leadership training was also offered to all interested consumers. The training covered a range of topics—self-help, mental health systems, advocacy, entitlements, and housing options. The diversity of topics was designed to attract consumers, empower customer representatives, and create curiosity among staff and professionals. The training has been an important pool of difference, and consumers access training often reserved only for staff.

The Ambassador Project is another initiative that used the pool of difference concept. A staff member who had been exposed to consumerism indirectly contacted customer service to ask whether a consumer could visit one of the inpatient units. The staff person said that someone was needed to come in and instill hope—an ambassador of hope. The notion of the Ambassador Project was born. Ambassadors are consumers who volunteer to lead self-help groups on inpatient services. The project crystallized the guiding principle that services are provided only on request. So, to that end, ambassadors were recruited, trained, and deployed only on request. It was not entirely surprising to observe that a year later an ambassador group was being held on each of the inpatient units.

Since South Beach Psychiatric Center introduced consumerism, all of these efforts have provided multiple opportunities for consumers to find their voices and a chance to "reskill"—to use atrophied skills, express opinions, and experiences. "Helpees" have become helpers, modeling the process of regaining parts of life that had been lost or given up on.

Since South Beach Psychiatric Center gave up its acute care function several years ago, the inpatient population has come to represent consumers who from one perspective "have been given up on" or "have given up on themselves." In response, South Beach Psychiatric Center began using The Consumer Network. The daily availability of The Consumer Network staff members has allowed all levels of staff to consult them on myriad issues. Their skillful, diplomatic handling of requests supports the paradigm shift. The partnership between The Consumer Network and other advocacy and self-help agencies provides a concrete resource for consumers and staff to use. Consumers are linked to these resources before and after discharge.

In addition to the creation of pools of difference, multiple opportunities are created to expose consumers and staff to the principles behind self-help and recovery. To that end, we have used town meetings, focus groups, dialogues, and the Interactive TV Recovery show, which is broadcast biweekly to the inpatient units.

In addition to these opportunities for consumers to speak about issues directly, there have been growing chances for them to represent their constituencies on planning and policy-making entities. Consumers are voting members of local advisory boards, which are attached to each service and designed to promote vital, dynamic communication loops between the services, the people, and the communities they represent. Consumers are members of various committees and have direct input into policy issues. They have been active in screening applicants to a new residential option based on the Fairweather Lodge model. A Bridger Project program supports members and graduates of the Ocean View Lodge training program in their efforts at community reintegration.

CONCLUSION

Changing from stabilization and custodial care to self-help and recovery is not easy. An overriding factor is that for most consumers used to relying on external prompts, judgments, and definitions of self, learning to celebrate and build on their own expertise is a novel experience. Waiting for others, such as experts and family members, to tell them who they are and what they want has become a way of life. They are so deskilled that it seems almost impossible to turn things around.

This massive deskilling was recently demonstrated during a series of focus groups with consumers who had been receiving outpatient services for a number of years. These were consumers with significant histories of hospitalizations who had now attained community tenure. When questioned about what it took to accomplish that, answers were not readily available. Only after a consumer-driven intervention did the volume and depth of information come forth. Before the consumer intervention, trite clichés of the professional world about mental illness were all that was available to most consumers: Take your medications, avoid stress, and so on. After the consumer intervention, consumers had in-depth knowledge about how to find new meaning in their lives and how to hold on to that meaning.

When the self-help and recovery paradigm is fully embraced, change can occur. All along the continuum of services, consumers have access to powerful opportunities to change how they perceive themselves and the system offering them services. Likewise, staff are exposed regularly to events and activities that underscore that they are partners in care and not benevolent dictators.

REFERENCES

Bandura A: Self-efficacy: toward a unifying theory of behavioral change. Psychol Rev 84:191–215, 1977

DeMasi M, Videka-Sherman L, Knight EL, et al: Specifying the dimensions of recovery. Paper presented at the 6th annual National Conference on State Mental Health Agency Services Research and Program Evaluation, Arlington, VA, February, 1996

Turkelson K: A Dialogue Between Psychiatrists and Recipients (videotape). New York, New York State Office on Mental Health, 1993

17

Behavioral Health Care Systems Relating to Other Systems

Andres J. Pumariega, M.D.

Interagency systems of mental health and human services gained increasing attention and significance during the 1990s. The field of community-based systems of care involves the study and implementation of innovative approaches to improve access to and use, financing, and clinical and cost effectiveness of mental health and social services within the communities and natural environments of clients and families. These approaches, which are guided by principles that ensure that the strengths and individuality of clients and their families are valued, bring together diverse agencies/services to maximize their impact and reduce duplication. The ultimate goal of these systems of care is to fully integrate clients and families served into the fabric of their community and culture.

A number of important trends have led to the growing importance of this field. First, increasing use of and need for mental health services in the United States have spurred their rapid growth. Although mental illness and emotional disturbance were once thought to be relatively rare, recent studies suggest overall prevalence rates of 25% among adults and 15%–19% among children and adolescents, with 3%–10% for serious mental illness and emotional disturbance (Robins and Regier 1991; Tuma 1989). Morbidities associated with mental illness and emotional disturbance are increasing at alarming rates. These include suicide, homicide, substance abuse, homelessness, child abuse and domestic violence, teenage pregnancy, school dropout and underemployment, welfare dependence, crime, and associated institutionalization and incarceration. All human service agencies serving children, adults, and families (schools, social welfare agencies, child protective agencies, juvenile justice, adult corrections, public health) have experienced the increasing impact of psychosocial morbidity. Typically, these agencies address different pieces of the service system puzzle, with little to no coordination with other agencies that most often serve the same population (Knitzer 1982).

In interagency systems of care for mental health, the most extensive work to date, both conceptually and in implementation, has focused on children with serious emotional disturbances (SED) and their families. In this chapter I use that work as a template for discussing interagency systems of care, while also referring to work in that area with adults with serious mental illness and their families.

HISTORICAL BACKGROUND

Mental health services for adults were originally focused in large state-operated institutions, based on the work of pioneers such as Dorothea Dix. The orientation of that work was toward providing sanctuary, or asylum, to those dealing with mental illness and sheltering them from the demands of the outside world. However, from their earliest origins, mental health services for children have emphasized a community orientation. These services began in the United States in response to the perceived need for counseling juvenile offenders rather than incarcerating them with adult offenders. In the 1890s and 1900s, the United States, much as today, was undergoing rapid cultural changes as a result of immigration as well as economic changes resulting from industrialization and urbanization. These social pressures led to marked increases in a number of new social problems, such as child abuse and neglect, child industrial labor, decreased school attendance and behavior problems, and crime committed by juveniles. The first state compulsory education laws had been enacted in the 1860s, and the first child abuse laws were fashioned in the 1880s after the animal cruelty laws. These were followed by the first child welfare, juvenile justice, and public health services in the nation in the next two to three decades.

The first mental health clinic for children was founded at the University of Pennsylvania in 1896 with a focus on school problems. The juvenile court clinics in Chicago and Boston were founded in the early 1900s, giving rise to the first interdisciplinary child mental health services in the nation, staffed by physicians, social workers, and psychologists. The success of these clinics led the Commonwealth Foundation to commission a study that in 1922 recommended and funded the development of child guidance clinics throughout the United States. These clinics were to be staffed with interdisciplinary teams of professionals who could serve the child and the family. At first these clinics were primarily staffed by social workers but in time attracted pediatricians, psychologists, psychoanalysts, and psychiatrists; they later served as the bases for the first child psychiatry programs in the nation. These clinics were quite different and removed from the specialty-driven medical system that was evolving in tertiary medical centers, and they did not encourage the practice of hospital-bound care. They provided low-cost services oriented to the needs of the child and the family, with treatment modalities evolving to include individual psychodynamic psychotherapy, family therapy, crisis intervention, and even day treatment programs. Many of these clinics have survived to this day. They served as models for the community mental health centers that were developed in the 1960s under federal legislation and that sought to decrease the large populations of institutionalized adults in state mental hospitals (Berlin 1991).

Advances in psychopharmacotherapy facilitated the deinstitutionalization of adults to the community under the care of the new mental health centers. However, the medicalization in psychiatry starting in the 1970s served to paradoxically move psychiatric services toward a more hospital-based, tertiary care model. This left the child guidance clinics and the community mental health centers without significant psychiatric participation. Community-based services were neglected, leaving these clinics generally understaffed, underfunded, and with narrow choices of interventions (medication, counseling, or multiple hospitalizations). The United States also experienced a rapid increase in the population of poor and minority children and adults with higher levels of need for mental health services. Many of these children were placed in the custody of child welfare agencies or placed in out-of-home residential care and juvenile detention facilities, whereas children with insurance coverage were placed in the new medicalized psychiatric facilities, thus overtaxing the resource capacity of many agencies and funders. The lack of integrated services under this approach led to a marked increase in homelessness among adults who were seriously mentally ill as well as families in the late 1970s and 1980s. The increase of children with SED also overtaxed the resources of public school districts, which faced funding cuts as a result of political pressures to cut property taxes (England and Cole 1992; Shore 1989).

The modern era of community-based systems of care for children was ushered in by the publication of Jane Knitzer's (1982) groundbreaking book *Unclaimed Children*, which exposed the aforementioned consequences of neglecting to provide community-based mental health services for children and their families. Her advocacy and that of others led to the development of the Child and Adolescent Service System Program (CASSP), which helped all 50 states develop an infrastructure for publicly funded community-based services (Lourie and Katz-Leavy 1986). The CASSP initiative was modeled on the conceptual work of Stroul and Friedman (1986), who coined the term *community-based system of care for children with SED*. CASSP advocated interagency coordination among child-serving agencies in the provision of services for children with SED and related family support services. It proposed that such services be delivered as close to the child's home and community as possible, avoiding the use of more restrictive levels of care that often separated children from natural family and community supports. Families were to be involved as partners in the effective treatment of the child. Stroul and Friedman's work spurred the development of various innovative community-based treatment modalities as well as a number of model demonstration programs in different parts of the United States. These programs embody the use of community-based treatments and interventions within the context of an organized interagency system of care and include more than 50 model demonstration community-based systems of care sites funded by the federal Center for Mental Health Services, eight model demonstration sites funded by the Robert Wood Johnson Foundation, and four community-based and -governed service demonstration sites funded by the Casey Foundation (England and Cole 1992).

In the area of services for adults, community-based systems of care principles have been implemented through a number of new initiatives, including demonstration projects under the Community Support Programs of the Center for Mental Health Services. Programs for consumer empowerment, which resulted from the mental health consumer movement, have employed consumers providing advocacy and case management services for other consumers under the principle that a consumer's experience with the system of care can be invaluable for the recovery of other consumers (Mowbray et al. 1996). Programs serving people who are mentally ill and homeless have integrated mental health and social services into community shelter environments and programs for subsidized housing, combining the resources of those agencies and progressively addressing many of the needs of this population. The advent of the Assertive Community Treatment programs (Stein and Test 1980) has also advanced the concept of intensive community-based treatment for adults with serious mental illness, averting costly and disruptive recidivism into hospitalization or incarceration.

PRINCIPLES OF COMMUNITY-BASED SYSTEMS OF CARE

The CASSP initiative for children's mental health services set forth the initial principles inherent in the concept of community-based systems of care. The key aspects of these systems include access to a comprehensive array of services; treatment individualized to the child's needs; treatment in the least restrictive environment possible (with full use of the resources of the family and the community); full participation of families as partners in the planning and delivery of services; interagency coordination; use of case management for services coordination; prohibition of ejection or rejection from services because of lack of "treatability" or "cooperation" with interventions; early identification and intervention; smooth transition of youth into the adult service system; effective advocacy efforts; and nondiscriminating, culturally sensitive services (Stroul and Freidman 1986).

The principle of cultural competence is an integral aspect of the philosophy of community-based systems of care. The literature on the mental health of culturally diverse children strongly indicates the presence of diagnostic biases toward children of color, disproportionate referral to more restrictive levels of care, and lower access to community-based mental health services (Cohen et al. 1990; Cuffe et al. 1995; Kilgus et al. 1995; Pumariega et al. 1998; Shyne and Schroeder 1978). The principles of community-based systems of care seek to address these problems by requiring that practitioner guidelines be instituted for the attitudes, skill, and knowledge base necessary to serve minority and culturally diverse children and families in their communities and that policies and procedures be put in place to remove barriers to service access. Community-based systems of care approaches were found to be consonant with the cultural values of ethnic minority populations, which emphasize strong extended family involvement in the life and upbringing of children, and the use of natural community resources first, to deal with the emotional and physical problems of family members (Cross et al. 1989; Pumariega and Cross 1997). These values have been shown to protect against some of the morbidities associated with emotional disturbance, such as substance abuse and suicidality (Pumariega et al. 1992).

Another important principle inherent in community-based systems is that of targeting services to children who are termed *seriously emotionally disturbed*. This designation includes the presence of an Axis I diagnosis under DSM-IV (American Psychiatric Association 1994), but it places equal emphasis on the child's level of function in his or her life domains (e.g., school, home, socially with peers). This principle addresses the difficulty that many children and their families have had in accessing necessary services when their diagnosis was not "severe enough" despite serious disruption in function, particularly when the child received a diagnosis of disruptive disorder. Studies indicate that the level of care children receive is only partially accounted for by their clinical diagnosis, with much of it accounted for by their level of function and psychosocial stressors (Silver et al. 1992).

CHARACTERISTICS OF INTERAGENCY SYSTEMS OF CARE

Interagency systems of care embody a series of paradoxes that reflect their, at times, conflicting missions and visions (Friesen and Briggs 1995). The main paradoxes are outlined below:

- *Individualized versus systemic.* The primary goal of interagency systems of care is to provide services that are individualized to the needs of the children and families being served. However, for the overall system to serve the broader population of children with SED and/or serious mental illness (SMI) as well as those at risk, a more systemic approach to service delivery is adopted than is traditionally seen in the individual agencies, incorporating aspects of public health population models.

- *Autonomous versus accountable.* A subjective approach that is responsive to the needs of the family and the community is promoted, but a more objective approach is taken when assessing the quality and outcomes of services delivered. This is akin to the philosophy of total quality management, which has been adopted by American and global industry. In total quality management, teams of employees address issues and problems in the system using a combination of objective analytical tools and subjective consumer input for guidance.

- *Flexible versus systematic.* Although greater flexibility to meet consumer needs is promoted, the use of systematic approaches to data collection, policies and procedures, and measurement is also emphasized.

- *Professional/clinical versus nonprofessional/nonclinical.* The professionalism inherent in social service agencies is promoted through increased training and credentialing requirements. However, the use of extenders, paraprofessionals, and consumer providers moves away from having service delivery become the sole province of trained professionals. The expertise of family members and consumers in navigating a sometimes complex system and their ability to determine more accurately the true focus of need and interventions are highly valued.

Interagency collaboration within systems of care is facilitated by a number of organizational and structural characteristics. Formal interagency agreements have been increasingly implemented to improve coordination of services, either to overlapping populations of consumers or to high-risk populations. A number of other structural mechanisms short of formal agreements have been used to facilitate interagency collaboration. Collocation of staff or services allows multiple agencies to provide services to overlapping consumers at common sites. Agencies can provide services at each other's sites or at neutral community-based sites such as schools, churches, or community centers where consumers feel a greater sense of comfort and less stigma. Interagency plans constructed by interagency teams as well as consumers and families formally outline the accountability for different services by different agencies and the coordination of these services. The plans are usually associated with the designation of lead agency status, with the lead agency being responsible for the case management of the plans. Blended funding agreements have also been used to facilitate the purchase of flexible services from the budgets of multiple participating agencies for common consumers/clients. This blended funding allows for the purchase of wraparound services that fall outside but complement the categorical services delivered by different agencies, for example, the purchase of tutoring services, a shadow for a child, or home repair service for a family (Fox and Wicks 1995; Friesen and Briggs 1995).

Escalating need and limited funding have increased pressures on public mental health and social service agencies to demonstrate improved clinical and cost effectiveness. State and federal governments have adopted new philosophies of downsizing, streamlining, and privatization of governmental services. There has also been a progressive devolution of responsibility, and services are being funded by more local levels of government.

Agencies are increasingly turning to managed care to finance and organize mental health and social services. However, managed care approaches are relatively new in mental health and human services, and those that exist were developed for adult and private-sector populations. These approaches have relied on a priori benefit restrictions based on actuarial approaches that select out poorer populations who are high users of services, and augment large pools of relatively healthy, minimally impaired populations from higher socioeconomic backgrounds who are lower users of services. When applied to child mental health services, the usual benefits restriction approach in traditional behavioral managed care results in depriving poor, underserved, and more impaired children of timely and effective intervention/prevention. This results in fragmentation of care and shifting of the burden of services and cost to other child-serving agencies and systems. These effects raise the potential for significantly increased morbidity. Managed care models for children's mental health need to emphasize community-based treatment and prevention of such morbidity through enhancing family and community resources and reducing psychosocial stressors for the child as well as providing clinical services (Brokowski 1995; Pumariega et al. 1997).

CHALLENGES OF COLLABORATION WITH OTHER AGENCIES

Although human service agencies interfacing with the mental health of children and families have common challenges and pressures, some challenges are unique to the scope of responsibility of particular agencies. Specific challenges are outlined below.

Welfare/Social Services

The population of children in state custody is well known to be at high risk for serious emotional and behavioral disturbances (Pumariega et al. 1995).

The child welfare system has traditionally been a high consumer of mental health services, both directly for its wards and for the treatment of parents/family members in the service of reunification. Rising rates of SED/SMI in this population have had a significant impact on the recovery of traumatized children from serious abuse and neglect, the ability to reunify families after abuse, and the ability of families on the welfare rolls to care for children with SED/SMI. Given the cutbacks in public child mental health services associated with downsizing and managed behavioral health, increasing numbers of families have returned to the practice of giving up children to state custody because they are unable to care for them. This aggravates the already critical shortage of out-of-home residential placements available for children in state custody, particularly therapeutic and nontherapeutic foster homes.

The high prevalence of serious mental illness and substance abuse among the adult homeless population presents a major challenge for social service agencies, which often require the assistance of volunteer and religious entities to provide support services (Culhane et al. 1998). A recent issue is the increasingly important role that adequate levels of mental health services play in the ability of families on welfare to return to work under a number of welfare reform initiatives in many states (Bazelon Center for Mental Health Law 1996). This has placed a greater premium on improved family functioning so that former welfare recipients can participate in the workforce (Bazelon Center for Mental Health Law 1996). It is clear that welfare reform has a much greater impact on adults with serious mental illness, a fact that has implications for the success of subsequent waves of these programs as they encounter a harder core population of persons with mental illness (Cohen 1997; Salomon et al. 1996).

Various initiatives have been developed to address the integrated mental health and social service needs of this large at-risk population. Some states have moved into managed welfare services under capitated or case rate mechanisms, with providers credentialed to provide the whole array of social, residential, and mental health services, with built-in incentives to step down to least restrictive levels of care and reunification. The collocation of mental health services within the offices of governmental welfare agencies, volunteer welfare programs, and shelter programs is now becoming widely accepted and facilitates integrated service delivery greatly. Another promising modality for integrated service delivery is that of family preservation services with strong case management components. These approaches attempt to prevent out-of-home placement, or to transition children with SED back to families with multiple needs, with promising initial results (Rivera and Kutash 1994).

Employment Services

Another important development is a greater collaboration between vocational rehabilitation and adult mental health agencies. The therapeutic value of work has been well known for some time, and capacity for self-sufficiency has been associated with better self-esteem and community tenure. This collaboration ranges from the collocation in community mental health programs of vocational specialists who focus on the development of job skills and opportunities for adults with mental illness to the creation of supported employment programs for these populations. Early results from these programs indicate positive outcomes in employment as well as improved social skills (Blankertz and Robinson 1996; Bond et al. 1997).

Education

The educational system faces the impact of increased educational demands for average students because of the growing technological and informational demands on our society. In addition, the increasing needs of children with learning disorders and SED are placing added burdens on schools. This situation occurs in the context of underfunding of school districts because of downward pressures on property taxes and other means of funding education. The lack of funding is especially felt in the area of special education services. Many school districts actively avoid the mandates of federal laws such as the Individualized Disability Education Act (IDEA) and Section 504 (which outlines services for children who are mentally ill/emotionally disturbed), often underidentifying children with covered disabilities and meeting their needs informally through the services of regular classroom teachers to prevent added service commitments.

A recent salutary development in the area of interagency systems of care is the renewed interest in school-based services. They go beyond traditional school mental health consultation and involve the collocation of health and mental health professionals within schools to provide a wide array of direct and indirect preventive health and mental health services. School-based mental health services serve as an ideal core service for a children's system of care, providing an excellent accessible portal of entry that is nonstigmatizing, and a naturalistic setting to observe behavior and integrate interventions into a child's environment. Often these services are paid for through blended Medicaid fee-for-service and managed care funding augmenting limited school funding. A number of these models have been implemented in Baltimore, Maryland; rural South Carolina; Charlotte, North Carolina; and other locations, with documented success in reducing adverse morbidity and increasing access to needed services (Casat et al. 1999; Flaherty et al. 1996; Motes et al.

1996). Innovative approaches to legislation involving IDEA-mandated services have been promoted in California through a law that mandates interagency collaboration in the development and implementation of individualized educational plans when they involve areas outside formal education services (Schacht and Hansen 1999).

Juvenile Justice

A number of studies have documented high rates of serious emotional disturbance among youth in the juvenile justice system (Atkins et al. 1999; Otto et al. 1992). Typically these youth are diverted into this agency because of their propensity to display aggressive or disruptive behaviors and subsequent to successive disciplinary interventions in the schools and out-of-home placements. However, typically they have underused mental health services when compared with cohorts that remain in the mental health system (Pumariega et al. 1999). There is also greater racial disparity in the population of youth that are served by juvenile justice. This may be due to the poverty and adversity that they face as well as the lack of culturally competent services in mental health and other agencies/systems.

Despite the similarities in their populations, the juvenile justice and mental health systems have significant differences in their service orientations and philosophies. The juvenile justice system has itself faced a recent split in its orientation between those who still promote the rehabilitation of its consumers and those who promote a more purely punitive and containment/public safety approach. This often clashes with the treatment mentality and orientation of the mental health system, although the latter suffers because of the lack of focus on behavioral containment and long-term follow-up.

Areas of natural collaboration between these systems are in preventing entry into juvenile justice, particularly into detention/incarceration, and the treatment of youth with SED in the juvenile justice system. Multisystemic therapy, a therapeutic approach combining home-based and wraparound interventions within a systemic context, has been tested with youth at risk of detention and incarceration and resulted in significant reductions in out-of-home placement, externalizing criminal behaviors, rates of arrest and incarceration, and treatment costs (Borduin 1999; Henggeler et al. 1993). There is an increasing focus on the mental health treatment of incarcerated youth and its impact on recidivism (Melton and Pagliocca 1992).

Adult Corrections

An increasing trend of incarcerating adults who have a serious mental illness in local jail facilities as well as state and federal penitentiaries has been clearly documented since the deinstitutionalization of patients from state mental hospitals was initiated. This new institutionalization has raised concerns about the factors that lead to the incarceration of people who are mentally ill as well as the adequacy of psychiatric and mental health services available in jails and prisons. The increasing public outcry for community safety and security, deinstitutionalization from state mental hospitals, and criminalization of substance abuse seem to have been significant factors contributing to the trend (Metzner et al. 1990).

There has been increasing openness by law enforcement and corrections officials toward integrating mental health services in correctional services. This has included the development of new standards for mental health services in correctional facilities, diversion programs for offenders who are mentally ill, and aftercare programs for inmates with mental illness and substance abuse (Condelli et al. 1994; Metzner et al. 1990, 1994; Steadman et al. 1995). Some services researchers have even proposed using incarceration rates as a means to measure the performance of community mental health programs, given their critical importance in diverting individuals who are mentally ill from jails and prisons (Pandiani et al. 1998).

Public Health/Primary Care

Children and adults served in primary care settings, particularly in public settings, are known to have a higher risk for mental illness and emotional disorders (Costello 1986). Primary care integration of mental health services has long held the promise of providing greater access because of its lower stigmatization and regular contact with covered individuals. The benefits of integration include the potential to provide earlier, more preventive services and even screen for risk for mental illness/emotional disturbance as a part of routine maintenance health care, potentially leading to reductions in the cost of higher-end services and improved mental health of the population (Shandle and Christianson 1988). There is even a special version of the DSM developed for the recognition of subthreshold mental disorders by primary care practitioners (Jellinek 1997). On the other hand, the collaboration between community mental health agencies and public health departments has been minimal over time, especially as the latter have a diminishing role in the service system (Polivka et al. 1997).

In some publicly funded health plans, mental health services are being integrated into general health services, with primary care practitioners having a greater role as direct mental health providers and psychiatrists and other mental health professionals serving in consulting or supporting roles. This has been especially attractive in rural communities, which have suffered from chronic shortages of mental health services and professionals (Bird et al.

1998). There are limitations in this model because of the lack of training for primary care practitioners in detecting, diagnosing, and treating mental disorders. Additionally, the limited contact time that primary care physicians and practitioners have with clients limits their abilities to effectively screen and diagnose mental health problems (Glied 1998). There is also hesitation by Medicaid-funded programs to proceed into carve-in models of integrated health/mental health delivery for fear of increasing the use of mental health services and exceeding the cost reductions gained by earlier intervention (Pires et al. 1995). Decision support protocols can ensure consistent diagnostic and treatment services and timely consultation (van der Feltz-Cornelis et al. 1997).

CARE PROCESS IN INTERAGENCY SYSTEMS OF CARE

A community-based treatment approach to services begins with access to services facilitated through multiple portals of entry, including direct referral or referral through multiple agencies (such as the school, juvenile justice, social services, or public health). A triage system should direct clients and families to services and providers appropriate to their special needs. A full interdisciplinary team, including a psychiatrist, should be involved in the development of triage procedures and protocols. Comprehensive mental health assessments should be made by licensed credentialed providers in consultation with a psychiatrist (or child/adolescent psychiatrist as indicated). Such assessments should include clinical/diagnostic, functional, developmental, family, and cultural/community evaluations of the needs *and* strengths of the client and family. Standardized measures should be reliable, valid, clinically useful, culturally competent for the population being served, and useful for programmatic evaluation (Silver et al. 1992).

Clients and families who require time-limited, less intensive services should have an initial care plan developed by a licensed mental health professional in consultation with a psychiatrist. The initial care plan for children or adults requiring more extensive treatment should be developed by an interdisciplinary team, including all relevant mental health and social service professionals. The care plan should identify problem areas and strengths that are relevant to the client's and family's functioning, as well as community-based interventions to address these needs. The client and his or her family should be equal participants in the development and implementation of the plan of care. Plans of care should be individualized to the needs of the client and family, including attention to cultural issues, and should follow the client continuously throughout all levels of care, being amended as needed. The plan of care should promote continuous coordination and integration of all applicable services and agencies that have responsibility for providing services to the client and family, such as primary health care, juvenile justice, schools, and social services (Stroul and Friedman 1986).

Treatment and other services should be specific to the unique needs of clients and their families and use approaches that maintain clients in, or reintegrate them into, their families and community. Service protocols should be developed to ensure that clients' developmental, physical, mental, and emotional needs are addressed. The system should have as many diverse therapeutic interventions as possible, particularly those that have demonstrated effectiveness. These include traditional and intensive outpatient services, nonresidential community-based interventions (including family preservation, wraparound services, day treatment, assertive community treatment programs, and school-based services), community-based residential services (such as therapeutic foster homes and group homes), and brief acute inpatient services (Pumariega et al. 1997).

Case management services are essential in community-based treatment, including assessment of problem areas, measurement of functioning level, determination of needs, linkage with necessary resources, care coordination, advocacy, and monitoring of services provided as well as their outcomes. The client and family should be assigned a case manager who has the necessary skills to ensure seamless coordination of care across all levels, different providers, and the full time course of the illness/disturbance. The frequency and intensity of case management services should be proportional to the intensity of services and level of care. The client and family should be full participants in the case management process, sharing responsibilities with case managers for using and coordinating services. Case management protocols should facilitate the coordination of multiagency, multisystem interventions; the integration of services from various responsible providers and agencies; and the coordination of services with primary care physicians and health providers (Stroul 1995).

RESEARCH IN INTERAGENCY SYSTEMS OF CARE

Child mental health services research has focused on the evaluation of both interagency community-based interventions and demonstration interagency systems. This has included the evaluation of community-based residential approaches; nonresidential intensive community-based approaches; and clinical, functional, and cost outcomes of interagency systems of care (Kupermine and Cohen 1995; Pumariega and Glover 1997; Rivera and Kutash 1994).

A number of innovative community-based techniques for children that provide intensive and individualized services are undergoing initial evaluation studies, including different types of day treatment programs, school-based interventions, wilderness programs, mobile crisis outreach teams, therapeutic in-home emergency services, time-limited hospitalization with coordinated community services, intensive case management, and family support services. Studies involving these modalities have demonstrated significantly better outcomes than with traditional outpatient or residential services. Outcomes include reduced levels of externalizing and internalizing symptoms, improved family functioning, and reduced use of more restrictive services (Burns et al. 1996; Evans et al. 1996; Ichnose et al. 1994; Kupermine and Cohen 1995).

The wraparound model of care embodies this approach toward multimodal community-based interventions. The model emphasizes aggressive outreach; use of least restrictive treatment options; and individualized, flexible, and unconditional child- and family-centered services for children imminently at risk for or already in out-of-home placements. A number of studies of wraparound programs have reported positive outcomes, such as reduction of externalizing behavioral problems and out-of-home placement, improved child and family level of function, and consumer/family satisfaction (Eber et al. 1996; Hyde et al. 1996; Rivera and Kutash 1994).

Studies of community-based service systems for children that use innovative interventions along with interagency coordination and family empowerment are being undertaken. Initial outcome data on overall service system function in community-based systems of care in Vermont; New York; and Ventura County, California, have demonstrated reduced hospitalization rates and days, decreased out-of-home placement and less restrictive placements, significantly lower incidence of negative behaviors severe enough to put children at risk of out-of-home placement, and lower rates of overall problem behaviors (Bruns et al. 1995; Evans et al. 1996; Jordan and Hernandez 1990).

The Fort Bragg Demonstration Project has been the largest systems of care demonstration project attempted so far. The project developed a comprehensive continuum of care for the children of military dependents at Fort Bragg, North Carolina, including ready access to outpatient and intermediate levels of care but relatively restricted use of residential and inpatient services. The initial results suggest that the program did achieve significantly lower restrictiveness of care, higher consumer satisfaction, greatly increased access to services, and greater funding spent in less restrictive services than usual Comprehensive Health and Mental Health Programs for the Uniformed Services (CHAMPUS) at other sites. However, clinical and functional outcomes were not significantly different overall, with split differences in various diagnostic subgroups. Costs were not significantly different and were even somewhat higher in the demonstration site (Bickman et al. 1996).

Research on community-based interagency approaches for adults has also had promising results. Research has included the outcomes of supported employment programs (Bond et al. 1997), assertive community treatment programs (Burns and Santos 1995), step-down programs for inmates with psychiatric disorders (Condelli et al. 1997), and screening programs for mental illness in primary care settings (Reifler et al. 1996). To date, such projects have focused on the interface between mental health and another agency or entity in the system of care, with no comprehensive system of care demonstration projects to date.

FUTURE DIRECTIONS OF INTERAGENCY SYSTEMS OF CARE

The emerging community-based systems of care model is being tested at several pilot demonstration sites, including community-based programs funded by the Center for Mental Health Services in different communities with strong child mental health services infrastructures and community-based and -governed program sites funded by the Casey Foundation. Future studies of child and adult mental health epidemiology and service use and outcomes should provide data to help us understand the extent of need for mental health services on a national scale. Such studies should also provide information on the effectiveness of our current service systems and of our evaluation and research methods. Despite research activity under way, there are still significant deficits in some areas of our knowledge base of interagency systems of care. Areas in which further research is needed include acceptability of services and consumer satisfaction with services, effectiveness of culturally competent services, factors that contribute to effective interfaces across agencies, impact of different cost-containment and reimbursement mechanisms, effectiveness of interagency collaboration and coordination (especially under flexible integrated capitation funding mechanisms), and the integration of mental health and primary care services. (Jensen et al. 1996; Rivera and Kutash 1994; Young et al. 1995).

REFERENCES

American Psychiatric Association: Diagnostic and Statistical Manual of Mental Disorders, 4th Edition. Washington, DC, American Psychiatric Association, 1994

Atkins D, Pumariega A, Rogers K, et al: Mental health and incarcerated youth, I: prevalence and nature of psychopathology. Journal of Child and Family Studies 8:193–204, 1999

Bazelon Center for Mental Health Law: An Uncertain Future: How the New Welfare Law Affects Children With Serious Emotional Disturbance and Their Families. Washington, DC, National Technical Assistance Center for Children's Mental Health, 1996

Berlin I: Development of the subspecialty of child and adolescent psychiatry, in Textbook of Child and Adolescent Psychiatry. Edited by Weiner J. Washington, DC, American Psychiatric Press, 1991, pp 8–15

Bickman L, Heflinger C, Lambert E, et al: The Fort Bragg managed care experiment: short-term impact on psychopathology. Journal of Child and Family Studies 5:137–160, 1996

Bird D, Lambert D, Hartley D, et al: Rural models for integrating primary care and mental health services. Adm Policy Ment Health 25:287–308, 1998

Blankertz L, Robinson S: Adding a vocational focus to mental health rehabilitation. Psychiatr Serv 47:1216–1222, 1996

Bond G, Drake R, Mueser K, et al: An update on supported employment for people with severe mental illness. Psychiatr Serv 48:335–346, 1997

Borduin C: Multisystemic treatment of criminality and violence in adolescents. J Am Acad Child Adolesc Psychiatry 38:242–249, 1999

Brokowski A: Financing case management services within the insured sector, in From Case Management to Service Coordination for Children With Emotional, Behavioral, or Mental Disorders. Edited by Friesen B, Poertner J. Baltimore, MD, Paul H. Brookes, 1995, pp 133–148

Bruns E, Burchard J, Yoe J: Evaluating the Vermont system of care: outcomes associated with community-based wraparound services. Journal of Child and Family Studies 4:321–339, 1995

Burns B, Santos A: Assertive community treatment: an update of randomized research. Psychiatr Serv 46:669–675, 1995

Burns B, Farmer E, Angold A, et al: A randomized trial of case management for youths with serious emotional disturbance. Journal of Child Clinical Psychology 25:476–486, 1996

Casat C, Rigsby M, Sobelewski J, et al: School-based mental health services (SBS): a pragmatic view of a program. Psychology in the Schools 36:403–414, 1999

Cohen C: The impact of welfare reform as perceived by users of mental health services in New York City. Psychiatr Serv 48:1589–1591, 1997

Cohen R, Parmalee D, Irwin L, et al: Characteristics of children and adolescents in a psychiatric hospital and a correctional facility. J Am Acad Child Adolesc Psychiatry 29:909–913, 1990

Condelli W, Dvorskin J, Holanchock H: Intermediate care programs for inmates with psychiatric disorders. Bulletin of the American Association of Psychiatry and the Law 22:63–70, 1994

Condelli W, Bradigan B, Holanchock H: Intermediate care programs to reduce risk and better manage inmates with psychiatric disorders. Behavioral Sciences and the Law 15:459–467, 1997

Costello, E: Primary care pediatrics and child psychopathology: a review of diagnostic, treatment, and referral practices. Pediatrics 78:1044–1051, 1986

Cross T, Bazron B, Dennis K, et al: Toward a Culturally Competent System of Care. Washington, DC, CASSP Technical Assistance Center, Georgetown University Child Development Center, 1989

Cuffe S, Waller J, Cuccaro M, et al: Race and gender differences in the treatment of psychiatric disorders in young adolescents. J Am Acad Child Adolesc Psychiatry 34:1536–1543, 1995

Culhane D, Averyt J, Hadley T: Prevalence of treated behavioral disorders among adult shelter users: a longitudinal study. Am J Orthopsychiatry 68:63–72, 1998

Eber L, Osuch R, Redditt C: School-based applications of the wraparound process: early results on service provision and student outcomes. Journal of Child and Family Studies 5:83–99, 1996

England M, Cole R: Building systems of care for youth with serious mental illness. Hospital and Community Psychiatry 43:630–633, 1992

Evans M, Armstrong M, Kuppinger A: Family-centered intensive case management: a step toward understanding individualized care. Journal of Child and Family Studies 5:55–65, 1996

Flaherty L, Weist M, Warner B: School-based mental health services in the United States: History, current models, and needs. Community Ment Health J 32:341–352, 1996

Fox H, Wicks L: Financing care coordination services under Medicaid, in From Case Management to Coordination for Children With Emotional, Behavioral, or Mental Disorders: Building on Family Strengths. Edited by Friesen B, Poertner J. Baltimore, MD, Paul H. Brookes, 1995, pp 95–131

Friesen B, Briggs H: The organization and structure of service coordination mechanisms, in From Case Management to Service Coordination for Children With Emotional, Behavioral, or Mental Disorders. Edited by Friesen B, Poertner J. Baltimore, MD, Paul H. Brookes, 1995, pp 63–94

Glied S: Too little time? the recognition and treatment of mental health problems in primary care. Health Serv Res 33:891–910, 1998

Henggeler S, Melton G, Smith L, et al: Family preservation using multisystemic therapy: long-term follow-up to a clinical trial with serious juvenile offenders. Journal of Child and Family Studies 2:283–293, 1993

Hyde K, Burchard J, Woodworth K: Wrapping services in an urban setting. Journal of Child and Family Studies 5:67–82, 1996

Ichnose C, Kingdon D, Hernandez M: Developing community alternatives to group home placement for seriously emotionally disturbed special education students in the Ventura County system of care. Journal of Child and Family Studies 3:193–210, 1994

Jellinek M: DSM-PC: Bridging primary care and mental health. J Dev Behav Pediatr 18:173–174, 1997

Jensen P, Hoagwood K, Petti T: Outcomes of mental health care for children and adolescents: II. literature review and application of a comprehensive model. J Am Acad Child Adolesc Psychiatry 35:1055–1063, 1996

Jordan D, Hernandez M: The Ventura Planning Model: a proposal for mental health reform. Journal of Mental Health Administration 17:26–47, 1990

Kilgus M, Pumariega A, Cuffe S: Influence of race on diagnosis in adolescent psychiatric inpatients. J Am Acad Child Adolesc Psychiatry 35:67–72, 1995

Knitzer J: Unclaimed Children: The Failure of Public Responsibility to Children and Adolescents in Need of Mental Health Services. Washington, DC, Children's Defense Fund, 1982

Kupermine G, Cohen R: Building a research base for community services for children and families: what we know and what we need to learn. Journal of Child and Family Studies 4:147–175, 1995

Lourie I, Katz-Leavy J: Severely emotionally disturbed children and adolescents, in The Chronically Mentally Ill. Edited by Menninger W. Washington, DC, American Psychiatric Association, 1986, pp 159–185

Melton G, Pagliocca P: Treatment in the juvenile justice system: directions for policy and practice, in Responding to the Mental Health Needs of Youth in the Juvenile Justice System. Edited by Coccoza J. Seattle, WA, The National Coalition for the Mentally Ill in the Criminal Justice System, 1992, pp 107–139

Metzner J, Frye G, Usery D: Prison mental health services: results of a national survey of standards, resources, administrative structure, and litigation. J Forensic Sci 35:433–438, 1990

Metzner J, Miller R, Kleinsasser D: Mental health screening and evaluation within prisons. Bull Am Acad Psychiatry Law 22:451–457, 1994

Motes P, Melton G, Smith L, et al: Developing Comprehensive School-Based Mental Health Services. Columbia, SC, University of South Carolina, Institute for Families in Society, 1996

Mowbray C, Moxley D, Thrasher S, et al: Consumers as community support providers: issues created by role innovation. Community Ment Health J 32: 47–67, 1996

Otto R, Greenstein J, Johnson M, et al: Prevalence of mental disorders among youth in the juvenile justice system, in Responding to the Mental Health Needs of Youth in the Juvenile Justice System. Edited by Coccoza J. Seattle, WA, The National Coalition for the Mentally Ill in the Criminal Justice System, 1992, pp 7–48

Pandiani J, Banks S, Schacht L: Using incarceration rates to measure mental health program performance. J Behav Health Serv Res 25:300–311, 1998

Pires S, Stroul B, Roebuck L, et al: Health Care Reform Tracking Project: Tracking State Health Care Reforms as They Affect Children and Adolescents With Emotional Disorders and Their Families. Tampa, FL, University of South Florida, Florida Mental Health Institute, Research and Training Center for Children's Mental Health, 1995

Polivka B, Kennedy C, Chaudry R: Collaboration between local public health and community mental health agencies. Research in Nursing and Health 20:153–160, 1997

Pumariega A, Cross T: Cultural competence in child psychiatry, in Basic Handbook of Child and Adolescent Psychiatry, Vol 4. Edited by Noshpitz J, series editor, Alessi N, volume editor. New York, John Wiley and Sons, 1997, pp 473–484

Pumariega A, Glover S: New developments in services delivery research for children, adolescents, and their families, in Advances in Clinical Child Psychology, Vol 20. Edited by Ollendick T, Prinz R. New York, Plenum, 1997, pp 303–343

Pumariega A, Swanson J, Holzer C, et al: Cultural context and substance abuse in Hispanic adolescents. Journal of Child and Family Studies 1:75–92, 1992

Pumariega A, Johnson P, Sheridan D: Emotional disturbance and substance abuse in adolescents in residential group homes. Journal of Mental Health Administration 22:426–431, 1995

Pumariega A, Nace D, England M, et al. Community-based systems approach to children's managed mental health services. Journal of Child and Family Studies 6:149–164, 1997

Pumariega A, Glover S, Holzer C, et al: Utilization of mental health services in a tri-ethnic sample of adolescents. Community Ment Health J 34:145–156, 1998

Pumariega A, Atkins D, Rogers K, et al: Mental health and incarcerated youth. II: service utilization. Journal of Child and Family Studies 8:205–215, 1999

Reifler D, Kessler H, Bernhard E, et al: Impact of screening for mental health concerns on health service utilization and functional status in primary care patients. Arch Intern Med 156:2593–2599, 1996

Rivera VR, Kutash K: Components of a System of Care: What Does the Research Say? Tampa, FL, University of South Florida, Florida Mental Health Institute, Research and Training Center for Children's Mental Health, 1994

Robins L, Regier D (eds): Psychiatric Disorders in America: The Epidemiologic Catchment Area Study. New York, The Free Press, 1991

Salomon A, Bassuk S, Brooks M: Patterns of welfare use among poor and homeless women. Am J Orthopsychiatry 66:510–525, 1996

Schacht T, Hansen G: The evolving climate for school mental health services under the Individual With Disabilities Education Act. Psychology in the Schools 36:415–426, 1999

Shandle M, Christianson J: Mental health care for children and adolescents in health maintenance organizations, in The Financing of Mental Health Services for Children and Adolescents. Washington, DC, National Center for Education in Maternal and Child Health. National Maternal and Child Health Clearinghouse, 1988

Shore J: Community psychiatry, in Comprehensive Textbook of Psychiatry, Vol 2, 5th Edition. Edited by Kaplan H, Sadock B. Baltimore, MD, Williams & Wilkins, 1989, pp 2063–2067

Shyne A, Schroeder A: National Study of Social Services for Children and Their Families. Rockville, MD, Westat, 1978

Silver S, Duchnowski A, Kutash K, et al: A comparison of children with serious emotional disturbance served in residential and school settings. Journal of Child and Family Studies 1:43–59, 1992

Steadman H, Morris S, Dennis D: The diversion of mentally ill persons from jails to community services: a profile of programs. Am J Public Health 85:1630–1635, 1995

Stein L, Test M: Alternative to mental hospital treatment. I. conceptual model, treatment program, and clinical evaluation. Arch Gen Psychiatry 37:392–397, 1980

Stroul B: Case management in a system of care, in From Case Management to Service Coordination for Children With Emotional, Behavioral, or Mental Disorders. Edited by Friesen B, Poertner J. Baltimore, MD, Paul H. Brookes, 1995, pp 3–25

Stroul B, Friedman R: A System of Care for Severely Emotionally Disturbed Children and Youth. Washington, DC, Georgetown University Child Development Center, CASSP Technical Assistance Center, 1986

Tuma J: Mental health services for children: the state of the art. Am Psychol 44:188–199, 1989

van der Feltz-Cornelis C, Lyons J, Huyse F, et al: Health services research on mental health in primary care. Int J Psychiatry Med 27:1–21, 1997

Young S, Nicholson J, Davis M: An overview of issues in research on consumer satisfaction with child and adolescent mental health services. Journal of Child and Family Studies 4:219–238, 1995

Epilogue

The Future of Integrated Behavioral Health Care

Laurel J. Kiser, Ph.D., M.B.A.
Paul M. Lefkovitz, Ph.D.
Lawrence L. Kennedy, M.D.

Health care is undergoing rapid change spurred by a complex set of economic, political, and social forces. In no other branch of medicine are the pressures more intense or the rate of change more rapid than in behavioral health care. The result will no doubt be a drastically altered system of care; the new form is not yet clear. As the factors creating the impetus for change are examined—cost containment initiatives including managed care and risk sharing, consumer rights movement, consolidation, service, and information technology—answers emerge. For although diverse in nature, these pressures converge to create a logical direction to guide the course of change.

As illustrated in Chapter 1, current pressures create multiple opportunities for building interdependencies and for blurring distinctions and boundaries between previously separate entities and ideas. Take, for example, the assumption of risk. As providers assume risk, prospects for new collaborative relationships develop between providers and payors, different types of providers, providers and consumers, and providers and the general population. With each opportunity taken, behavioral health care moves a step closer to achieving integration.

The promise for integrated behavioral health care is great; reaching its potential is the challenge. Throughout the system of care—from the organizational level through direct service delivery—integrating care creates major implications for quality, effectiveness, and efficiency. With many different, and often competing, models for developing the basic infrastructures necessary to support integrated systems and for building wide-ranging service arrays, this volume offers a comprehensive conceptual foundation for service delivery integration.

This model for service delivery integration takes advantage of the many prospects for change by redefining static dimensions of organizational existence into dynamic forces that reinforce coordination of efforts while reducing boundaries and barriers. A number of integrative mechanisms are explored that facilitate such transformation, including organizational alignment, centralized patient access, coordination of care, systemwide milieu, continuum-based staffing, the continuous medical record, and a host of others. An infinite number of integrative mechanisms are likely to exist and can be brought to light by a vision for system-oriented thinking within the context of the continuum of care.

A major focus of this model for service delivery integration is on the clinical processes and mechanisms fundamental to caring for patients within a seamless continuum of care. Beyond a review of the levels of care, we detail the decisions, processes, and practices necessary to match patient care needs smoothly and efficiently with available services.

One of the particularly exciting aspects about this model of integrated health care systems is that it emphasizes creativity in meeting patient needs just as in the 1960s when clinicians were encouraged to develop new ways of treating patients and many new modalities developed. It is within this framework that we put forth a comprehensive definition for access to integrated care that supports responsibility for treatment at the population level. It is within this framework that we analyze and discuss the changes inherent in therapeutic and milieu processes as a patient moves from one level of care to another. It is within this framework that we explore avenues for improving therapeutic alliance by truly investing consumers with responsibility and inclusion in all aspects of the treatment delivery process. It is within this framework that we look at how integrated behavioral health delivery systems relate to a variety of other systems and provide a vision for how behavioral health care can sensitively address the needs of each individual within the broader medical and sociocultural context.

We present our model with a clear understanding that major barriers remain that will hamper progress toward realization of the goals. Thus, we look to the future with guarded optimism.

THE IMMEDIATE FUTURE

To the extent that financial forces significantly influence service delivery integration, signs of uncertainty may be present. The managed care industry has not passed along risk to providers to the degree that was envisioned in the early 1990s. Managed care has been challenged by legal, regulatory, and marketplace forces that have moderated its impact on the industry. Also, new forays into large-scale managed health care such as managed Medicaid and managed Medicare have met with mixed success at best. The vision of behavioral health providers having a financial incentive to embrace integrated service delivery does not appear to be in the immediate picture in most settings. As the industry moves through its current cycle of change and adaptation, however, new models for financial risk sharing are likely to evolve.

Similarly, there are signs of growing caution surrounding the vertical integration of behavioral health entities. Many efforts to develop integrated delivery systems have failed, typically because of barriers around organizational alignment. The "panic" of the early 1990s that prompted providers to enter into partnerships to ensure survival has relaxed in more recent years. That may lead to less numerous but more judicious and, therefore, more successful alliances. Overall, observers will increasingly question the wisdom of assuming "bigger is better" without the careful consideration of a host of other factors.

Technology may well be a more influential benefactor of service delivery integration in the immediate future. Electronic documentation and medical record processes offer great promise for enhancing service delivery integration. During the next few years, products should become more attractive to providers through refinements in ease of use as well as cost. Many systems of care will seriously consider and adopt electronic documentation, much to the benefit of integrated care.

Service delivery integration may also receive support from ongoing efforts to define best practices, clinical benchmarks, critical pathways, and shared protocols. A growing body of literature is likely to become increasingly available to support uniform and coordinated care. Professional organizations may continue to provide leadership in promoting standardized care throughout the continuum.

There may also be added emphasis on clinical integration as a result of the more strident posture assumed by the Joint Commission on Accreditation of Healthcare Organizations (JCAHO) with respect to accreditation following its 1999 challenge from the Office of the Inspector General. Rigorous interpretation of standards and random unannounced surveys will likely have a significant industry impact. Greater attention to the JCAHO standards contained throughout this volume will further the interests of service delivery integration.

The immediate future, therefore, presents a number of avenues for continued strides in behavioral health integration. However, progress will continue, gradually and steadily, until financial incentives are properly aligned within the industry. At that point, the evolution is likely to be transformed into a revolution of service delivery integration.

Pushing the Envelope

Evolution to fully integrated continuums for service delivery requires a long-term focus for providers to assume responsibility and accountability (fiscal and clinical) for the emotional wellness of a specific population. Necessarily, provider organizations will not be able to achieve integration without substantial changes from other industry stakeholders—payors, employers, other purchasers of behavioral health care services, educators, and so on.

To be realistic, many of the forces behind health care reform and development of new delivery systems have been and will continue to be financial. It is indeed possible to create reimbursement mechanisms that align financial incentives with the provision of services matched closely to patient needs. As illustrated in the chapters on reimbursement (Chapters 12 and 13), if providers receive a fixed amount to treat the patient (capitation), they can decide on the best use of their time for this purpose. Furthermore, if they are responsible (clinically and fiscally) for this same patient over time, they will provide services (disease management and health promotion) designed to achieve and maintain health and wellness longer term.

Successful models for risk sharing will emerge, bringing better integration between financing and service delivery and minimizing or eliminating incentives for under- or overtreatment. These models will probably be tied to improved measurement of clinical outcomes that provide accurate (valid and reliable) indicators of change. In turn, improvements in our ability to measure outcomes can be tied to organizational evaluation, staff credentialing, and consumer choice.

In addition to the shifts necessary from others, behavioral health care educators and provider organizations will need to continue work on several fronts. The future in integrated behavioral health care will probably be difficult (require adaptation) for most professional groups because it will mean change in traditional practice patterns. Therefore, new and differently trained clinicians may have to promote the organizational and clinical changes necessary to achieve integration. This will require modifications to education and training programs, adding an enhanced focus on systems thinking, biopsychosocial models, prevention, and wellness. Training programs will also have to provide clinical rotations in treatment settings beyond those traditionally mandated—inpatient and outpatient.

Professional changes will likely include expanded participation in multidisciplinary teams. Improvement in multidisciplinary team functioning through development of models outlining role distinctions, common language, incentives for cooperation, decreased competition, and improved communication will aid this work.

Providers will adopt a longer-term perspective on treatment, moving beyond treatment in a specific level of care to treatment of an episode of care and eventually interventions designed to address the course of an illness. Such efforts will be enhanced by development of episodic treatment plans and course-of-illness treatment plans and planning processes.

Finally, society will mandate (and providers will respond to) an increased focus on wellness. Under the current system, dollars spent on treatment exceed dollars spent on prevention/wellness. To change this, mental health prevention efforts would begin early in life and would extend into primary care and educational systems. Such efforts would include information on attachment, parenting practices, emotional development, and protective factors given to new or expectant parents and emphasized at the same level as are breast-feeding or immunizations. Most important, mental health wellness efforts would become de rigueur components of every level of care along the behavioral health care continuum.

The future of integrated behavioral health care awaits us.

Index

Page numbers printed in **boldface** type refer to tables or figures.